PROBLEMS IN GENERAL SURGERY

REVIEWING SURGICAL TOPICS

Series Editors: Thomas King, M.D. and Keith Reemtsma, M.D.
Columbia University College of Physicians and Surgeons
New York, New York

THE METABOLIC MANAGEMENT OF THE CRITICALLY ILL
Douglas W. Wilmore, M.D.

PROBLEMS IN GENERAL SURGERY
Jack Pickleman, M.D.

PROBLEMS IN GENERAL SURGERY

JACK PICKLEMAN, M.D.
Loyola University Stritch School of Medicine
Maywood, Illinois

SPRINGER SCIENCE+BUSINESS MEDIA, LLC

Library of Congress Cataloging in Publication Data

Pickleman, Jack.
Problems in general surgery.

(Reviewing surgical topics)
Includes bibliographical references and index.
1. Surgery. I. Title. II. Series. [DNLM: 1. Surgery, Operative—Problems. WO 18 P597p]
RD31.P53 617 81-22702
ISBN 978-1-4757-1757-0 ISBN 978-1-4757-1755-6 (eBook) AACR2
DOI 10.1007/978-1-4757-1755-6

Originally published by Plenum Publishing Corporation, New York in 1982
Softcover reprint of the hardcover 1st edition 1982

To Brenda B. Pickleman

FOREWORD

All around us, in this age of consumerism, are expressions of public expectations regarding the quality of medical care. Among the responses of the medical profession to this growing public demand has been a crescendo of interest in continuing education. Continuing education is not a new concern for the physician. Most major professional organizations were founded to increase the exchange of information among members.

But something new is in the wind. Both inside and outside the profession, the question is becoming more and more insistent: What does attendance at meetings or exposure to other types of prepared materials have to do with the quality of care that is provided? Recertification, reexamination, and peer review of outcomes of practice—subjects only recently unmentionable—have become common issues before specialty boards, legislatures, hospital boards, insurance carriers, and even medical societies. As of October of 1979, all 22 of the member boards of the American Board of Medical Specialties had made commitments to the principle of periodic recertification of their members. Most boards have explicitly acknowledged that the cognitive skills measured in the objective examination do not assure clinical competence. An assumption behind information-assessing recertification efforts is that, though mastery of the current knowledge upon which clinical decisions should be made does not guarantee competent practice, the lack of it probably impairs competent practice.

The immense cost of postgraduate courses and national conventions and conferences is, of course, passed on to the patient; a cost-conscious public someday may ask for evidence that the costs of these meetings are defensible business expenses with some measurable value. When the cost of these continuing education programs—travel and hotel expenses, fees, program production costs, and time lost from productive practice each year—are added to the other high costs of doing business for the practicing physician, the public may demand evidence that such activities improve the physician's care of his patients. Considering the money and effort invested in these programs, it seems surprising that so little evidence of their value can be found.

But is it surprising? Consider what is known about human learning. A body of research has been accumulating over the past four or five decades, much of which seems to lead to certain evidence about the characteristics of efficient learning experiences in adults. An analysis of this evidence would lead the dispassionate observer to conclude that, as typically conducted, continuing education programs ought to be inefficient learning experiences giving rise to very little change in the behavior of the passive audiences.

Efficient learning takes place in response to specific, perceived need, not in anticipation of need. It requires active involvement of the learner. The learner must have an opportunity to practice what he would learn; similarly, he will learn the skills he practices. Without early application of new knowledge to real problems in the natural setting, very little will be retained.

Can we easily reconcile the profession's long-felt need to upgrade itself and society's newly enunciated need for quality assurance with the best existing evidence on the learning process? The learning for which we should strive should not be an episodic escape from daily professional activity but an integral part of it. It should be oriented to realistic clinical problems and be carried out in the setting in which such problems need to be solved, using the tools and resources that are part of the clinician's usual environment.

This series is an approach to continuing education of surgeons with methods designed in accord with good learning experiences. It is problem-oriented, as is life. It can be carried out at the learner's own pace, it provides immediate feedback of the correct or preferred responses, an informative resume of the rationale for the answer, and some references for the learner to increase his understanding of the subject matter should he desire or need to do so.

We acknowledge that these efforts do not measure clinical competence. The assumptions behind the project are that awareness of current information upon which good clinical decisions should be made is worth cultivating and that this facility, unlike technical skills, is reasonably easy to assess and can be acquired by a motivated surgeon. These assumptions seem reasonable

In this series the authors structure their volumes around the significant generalizations that they believe epitomize the most important concepts in a given surgical area. For each of these generalizations, a series of questions is constructed or a representative clinical problem developed that requires mastery of the fundamental concepts for solution. A critical analysis of the problems is presented, which provides the background information required for solution, including discussion of the misunderstandings that might have led to selection of distractor responses.

This series, then, provides the surgeon with a method of learning by solving problems. The success of this approach depends not simply on the acquisition and analysis of information, but rather on the application of this new information to the care of patients.

Thomas C. King, M.D.
Keith Reemtsma, M.D.

New York, New York

PREFACE

This book represents an attempt to discuss current surgical knowledge in a problem-solving format. It is not intended to be a complete text of general surgery, but rather to deal with areas of controversy and clinical importance to the practicing surgeon. It is not anticipated that each reader will desire to work through all of the problems, merely those with which he feels less secure. It is hoped that the problem-solving format and the immediate feedback it provides will educate, entertain, and stimulate the participant to read further from the quoted references.

The work represents the thinking and practice of one general surgeon and, as such, not all will agree with the reasoning and the judgments that are put forth. This is healthy, for the practice of surgery grows by analysis and discussion of our differences, and this too can be a learning experience.

Finally, I want to express my gratitude to my secretaries, Ms. Linda Schultz and Ms. Sally Blangin, who prepared many drafts of the manuscript and who above all spurred me on when the project seemed to be flagging.

Jack Pickleman, M.D.

Maywood, Illinois

A note on units. Throughout the book, blood pressure is measured in millimeters of mercury, pulse rate is measured in beats/minute, and respiration rate is measured in breaths/minute.

CONTENTS

1. Esophagus

1.1 Reflux Esophagitis and Stricture 2
1.2. Incarcerated Traumatic Diaphragmatic Hernia 6
1.3. Paraesophageal Hernia 10
1.4. Achalasia 14
1.5. Carcinoma 16
1.6. Zenker's Diverticulum 18
References 20

2. Peptic Ulcer Disease

2.1. Complications of Duodenal Ulcer 24
2.2. Duodenal Ulcer: Choice of Operation 26
2.3. Parietal Cell Vagotomy 28
2.4. Perforated Duodenal Ulcer 30
2.5. Complications of Duodenal Ulcer Surgery 33
2.6. Alkaline Reflux Gastritis 35
2.7. Elevated Serum Gastrin 38
2.8. Stress Ulceration 40
2.9. Stress Ulceration: Gastritis 42
2.10. Stress Ulceration: Multiple Gastric Ulcers 44
References 46

3. Portal Hypertension

3.1. Treatment of Variceal Hemorrhage 52
3.2. Balloon Tamponade for Variceal Hemorrhage 54
3.3. Vasopressin for Variceal Hemorrhage 56
3.4. Distal Splenorenal (Warren) Shunt 58
3.5. Portal Vein Thrombosis 60
3.6. Budd–Chiari Syndrome 62

3.7. Varices Secondary to Splenic Vein Thrombosis 64
3.8. Treatment of Intractable Ascites 66
References 68

4. Pancreatico-Biliary Problems

4.1. Treatment of Acute Cholecystitis 72
4.2. Treatment of Acute Cholecystitis 74
4.3. Acute Ascending Cholangitis 77
4.4. Treatment of Asymptomatic Gallstones 78
4.5. Chenodeoxycholic Acid Treatment of Gallstones 80
4.6. Treatment of Recurrent Common Duct Stone 82
4.7. Treatment of Retained Common Duct Stone 84
4.8. Acalculous Cholecystopathy 86
4.9. Gallstone Pancreatitis 92
4.10. Acute Pancreatitis (Prognostic Factors) 94
4.11. Pancreatic Pseudocyst 95
4.12. Pancreatic Abscess 97
4.13. Pancreatic Ascites 98
4.14. Chronic Pancreatitis 100
References 103

5. Bowel Obstruction

5.1. Large Bowel Obstruction 108
5.2. Superior Mesenteric Artery Embolus 112
5.3. Superior Mesenteric Vein Thrombosis 115
5.4. Sigmoid Volvulus 116
5.5. Cecal Volvulus 120
5.6. Small Bowel Obstruction 124
5.7. Postoperative Small Bowel Obstruction 126
5.8. Gallstone Ileus 130
5.9. Partial Mechanical Small Bowel Obstruction 133
5.10. Recurrent Small Bowel Obstruction 135
5.11. Intussusception 137
References 139

6. Inflammatory Bowel Disease

6.1. Perforated Sigmoid Diverticulitis 142
6.2. Colovesical Fistula 143

6.3. Diverticulitis with Abscess Formation 145
6.4. Appendiceal Abscess 147
6.5. Appendiceal Phlegmon 150
6.6. Complications of Crohn's Disease 152
6.7. Treatment of Crohn's Disease 154
6.8. Ulcerative Proctitis 156
6.9. Toxic Megacolon 157
6.10. Granulomatous Colitis 160
6.11. Amebic Colitis 163
6.12. Ischemic Colitis 165
6.13. Radiation-Induced Rectovaginal Fistula 168
References 170

7. Gastrointestinal Cancer

7.1. Esophageal Carcinoma 174
7.2. Adenocarcinoma of the Gastroesophageal Junction 176
7.3. Gallbladder Carcinoma 178
7.4. Carcinoma of the Hepatic Duct Bifurcation 180
7.5. Pancreatic Carcinoma 183
7.6. Small Bowel Carcinoid 186
7.7. Malignant Colon Polyp 188
7.8. Rectal Villous Adenoma 190
7.9. Colon Carcinoma 191
7.10. Role of Carcinoembryonic Antigen 192
7.11 Treatment of Liver Metastases 193
7.12. Carcinoma of the Anus 195
References 197

8. Endocrine Surgery

8.1. Cushing's Disease 202
8.2. Cushing's Syndrome 204
8.3. Aldosteronoma 206
8.4. Pheochromocytoma 207
8.5. Adrenal Crisis 210
8.6. Multiple Endocrine Neoplasia I Syndrome 212
8.7. Glucagonoma 214
8.8. Pancreatic Diarrheagenic Tumor 216
8.9. Insulinoma 217
8.10. Nesidioblastosis 219

8.11. Primary Hyperparathyroidism 220
8.12. Graves Disease 222
8.13. Thyroid Nodule 224
8.14. Radiation-Induced Thyroid Cancer 226
8.15. Anaplastic Thyroid Cancer 228
8.16. MEN-II (Sipple's Syndrome) 230
8.17. Renovascular Hypertension 232
References 234

9. Breast

9.1. Treatment of Breast Cyst 240
9.2. Breast Carcinoma: Role of Adjuvant Chemotherapy 241
9.3. Breast Carcinoma: Treatment of Metastatic Disease 242
9.4. Noninvasive Intraductal Carcinoma 244
9.5. Inflammatory Carcinoma 246
9.6. Lobular Carcinoma 249
9.7. Paget's Disease 250
9.8. Male Breast Carcinoma 252
9.9. Cystosarcoma Phyllodes 254
References 255

10. Postoperative Complications

10.1. Wound Infection: Etiology 258
10.2. Wound Infection: Prophylactic Antibiotics 259
10.3. Wound Dehiscence 260
10.4. Subphrenic Abscess 261
10.5. Anastomotic Dehiscence with Fistula 264
10.6. Ileus 266
10.7. Atelectasis 267
10.8. Adult Respiratory Distress Syndrome 270
10.9. Adult Respiratory Distress Syndrome and PEEP 272
10.10. Renal Failure 274
10.11. Hepatic Failure 275
10.12. Septic Shock 276
References 278

11. Thromboembolic Disease

11.1. Pulmonary Embolus: Diagnosis 282
11.2. Pulmonary Embolus: Treatment 284

11.3. Suspected Pulmonary Embolus: Treatment 287
11.4. Vena Caval Interruption 290
11.5. Pulmonary Embolus and Shock: Treatment 292
11.6. Fibrinolytic Drugs 293
11.7. Prevention of Deep Venous Thrombosis 294
11.8. Phlegmasia Cerulea Dolens 296
References 298

12. Trauma

12.1. Blunt Abdominal Trauma 302
12.2. Stab wound of the Abdomen 304
12.3. Esophageal Perforation 305
12.4. Duodenal Hematoma 308
12.5. Gunshot Wound of the Colon 312
12.6. Splenic Rupture 314
12.7. Liver Trauma 317
12.8. Pancreas Trauma 320
12.9. Renal Trauma 322
12.10. Pelvic Fractures and Hemorrhage 324
12.11. Blunt Trauma of the Thorax 327
12.12. Gunshot Wound Arterial Injury 330
12.13. Anterior Compartment Syndrome 332
12.14. Tetanus 334
References 336

Index 341

1
ESOPHAGUS

1.1. A 46-year-old woman has had persistent heartburn and a feeling of acid regurgitation for 6 years, only partially controlled by antacids. She gives a 3-month history of progressive dysphagia and a feeling of food sticking in her throat substernally. An upper GI tract X ray series is performed and is shown as Figures 1-1 and 1-2. Esophagoscopy reveals a stricture in the distal esophagus; biopsy discloses only inflammatory tissue. Treatment should consist of:

A. Bougie dilatation.
B. Antireflux procedure.
C. Weight loss and cimetidine.
D. Dilatation and antireflux procedure.
E. Esophageal resection with colon interposition.

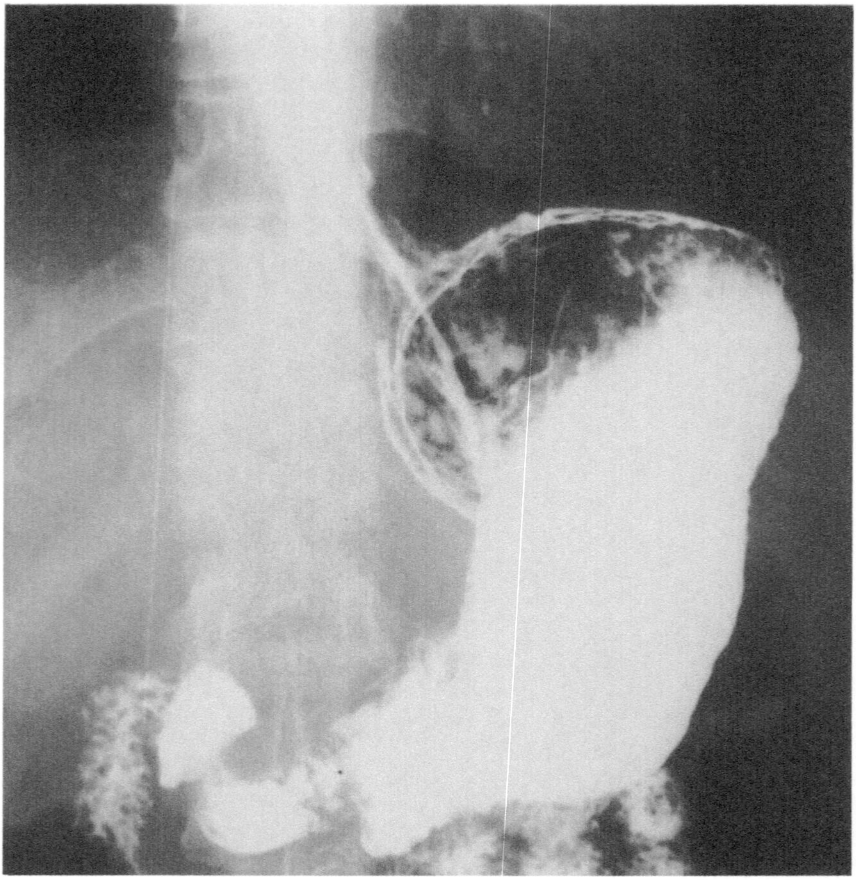

Figure 1-1

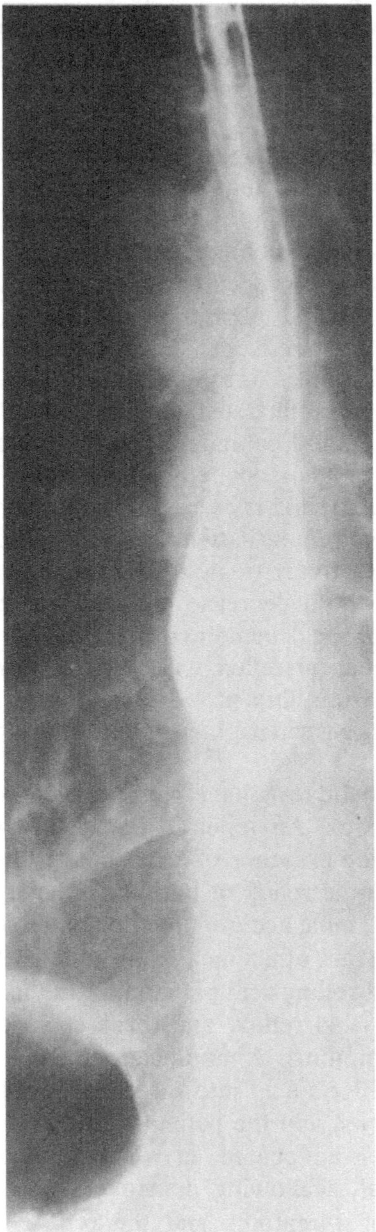

Figure 1-2

This patient has a small hiatus hernia with long-standing reflux that has progressed to an esophageal stricture. The biopsy discloses only inflammatory tissue, and although this does not absolutely rule out the possibility of a coexistent malignancy, it renders this possibility far less likely. This circumstance represents an end stage of esophageal reflux and surely could have been prevented by earlier operative treatment of this patient.

Uncontrolled reflux esophagitis can lead to other complications besides stricture. Mucosa in the injured area may be replaced by columnar epithelium (Barrett's esophagus), and there is some indication that this represents a premalignant lesion. Bleeding from an area of esophagitis is not uncommon, either in an occult fashion or presenting as a massive upper GI tract hemorrhage. Aspiration into the lungs can also occur, although probably not as frequently as thought in the past. Using very rigid criteria for the diagnosis of aspiration, one series demonstrated that only 8% of patients with reflux sustained this complication.[1]

At the outset, it should be understood that reflux can occur with or without the presence of an associated hiatus hernia. Therefore, treatment of patients with hiatus hernia is carried out only for those who manifest evidence of esophageal reflux. Patients with an asymptomatic hiatus hernia should not be operatively treated. The cause of reflux has been definitely established to be a decrease in the lower esophageal sphincter pressure. Using esophageal manometric techniques, nearly all patients with significant esophageal reflux will show abnormally low pressures which are raised by antireflux procedures. It has been suggested that decreased endogenous gastrin might account for this decrease in sphincter pressure.[2]

Numerous diagnostic tests have been advocated to confirm the presence of esophageal reflux. An upper GI tract X ray with cineradiography will often determine the presence of an associated hiatus hernia, but will often miss the retrograde reflux of barium. Esophagoscopy with biopsy is considered to be the most accurate method of determining the presence of esophagitis. However, other means are utilized to test for sphincter incompetence. An indwelling acid pH monitor in the distal esophagus will accurately document acid reflux, and these episodes can be correlated with the patient's symptoms. A modification of this test (Bernstein test) instills dilute hydrochloric acid into the distal esophagus along with saline control instillations, and the patient's responses are noted. An acid clearing test has been advocated, in which a given amount of acid is cleared by sequential swallowing maneuvers, and the time taken for the disappearance of symptoms and the return of pH to normal is noted. Many authorities consider this the single best test for sphincter incompetence.[3,4]

The majority of patients with esophageal reflux can be helped with nonoperative therapy alone. Many of these patients are obese, and it has been found that weight loss alone can alleviate many of the reflux sumptoms. Elevating the head of the bed and avoiding tight-fitting garments such as girdles are also beneficial steps. If the patient is a cigarette smoker, cessation of smoking can likewise bring about improvement in symptoms. Numerous medicines have been advocated, and of these, antacids are uniformly beneficial.[5] Bethanechol, an anticholinergic drug, has likewise been utilized to increase lower esophageal sphincter pressure and decrease reflux.[5,6] Metoclopramide also increases lower esophageal sphincter pressure, increases acid clearing from the distal esophagus, and can lead to a decrease in reflux symptoms.[5,7,8]

The operative treatment of hiatus hernia with reflux has enjoyed a resurgence of respect since it has been discovered that the etiologic problem to be solved is the incompetent lower esophageal sphincter and not necessarily the position of the gastroesophageal junction itself. Surely, earlier attempts at hiatus hernia repair were often unsuccessful, with recurrent or persistent symptoms the rule rather than the exception. Currently, three operations are known to be effective: the Nisson, Belsey, and Hill repairs.[9–11] In expert hands, these three operations have demonstrated roughly equal results, with greater than 90% of patients benefitted. Following surgery, measurements of lower esophageal sphincter pressure have been carried out and uniformly demonstrate significant increases that parallel the cessation of reflux symptoms. The Nisson procedure has been the one used most extensively in this country, and therefore has been subjected to the most critical review. One problem following this operation is that as many as 50% of patients cannot vomit afterwards.[12] Another complication following this procedure has been the gas bloat syndrome, which is seen in as many as 50% of patients initially, but decreases to about 10% on long-term follow-up.[9] Also, dehiscence of the Nisson repair and slippage of the repair down around the body of the stomach have been described, as have postoperative gastric dilatation and inadvertant vagotomy.[13,14]

In the patient presented, esophageal dilatation alone would not be expected to bring about any lasting relief, as the underlying reflux would not be benefitted. Likewise, the mere performance of an antireflux procedure alone would leave the patient unable to swallow. The combination of these two has been shown to bring about complete relief in most patients, and more radical procedures such as esophageal resection have been unnecessary.[15–17]

ANSWER: D.

1.2. A 26-year-old man is admitted to the emergency room with left upper quadrant pain and vomiting of acute onset. His only significant past history includes a 3-day hospitalization for observation following an automobile accident 7 years ago. His clinical signs are: temperature, 37.3°C; pulse, 126; blood pressure, 124/80; respirations, 36 and shallow. There appear to be decreased breath sounds at the base of the left lung. A chest X ray is taken, and is shown as Figure 1-3. Treatment should consist of:

A. Pericardiocentesis.
B. Left tube thoracostomy.
C. Left thoracotomy.
D. Left thoracolaparotomy.
E. Laparotomy.

The diagnosis of an incarcerated left diaphragmatic hernia is confirmed by the chest X ray, which discloses a gas-filled viscus, in this case the splenic flexure of the colon, in the left chest. Diaphragmatic defects may be created by either blunt trauma or penetrating stab or gunshot wounds of the torso. Although most hernias are located on the left side, probably because of the relative protection afforded the right hemidiaphragm by the liver, right-sided diaphragmatic hernias can also occur.[18] As would be expected, the stomach and the colon are the most common organs that herniate through diaphragmatic defects.

Symptoms may occur immediately and consist of cardiorespiratory embarrassment, or after many years if the initial injury is overlooked. Many patients with blunt trauma who sustain this injury will not be diagnosed during the initial hospitalization, and symptoms occur years later with the onset of acute incarceration.[19] The radiologic diagnosis can usually be suspected from the chest X ray itself, although confusion with such entities as a diaphragmatic eventration, acute gastric dilatation, or spontaneous pneumothorax can occur.[20] In this situation, the initial step should be the insertion of a nasogastric tube, which should lead to prompt decompression of the stomach if it is herniated. A subsequent chest X ray will demonstrate a disappearance of the defect, and if the patient is not presenting as an acute surgical abdomen, contrast studies of the GI tract can then be carried out. In the patient presented, there was no evidence of strangulation, and because of the apparent haustra seen on the chest X ray a barium enema was carried out, which disclosed the splenic flexure above the diaphragm (Figures 1-4 and 1-5).

To a certain degree, prevention of incarceration can be achieved by an awareness of the possibility of diaphragmatic rupture in any blunt trauma victim along with the careful exploration of the diaphragmatic

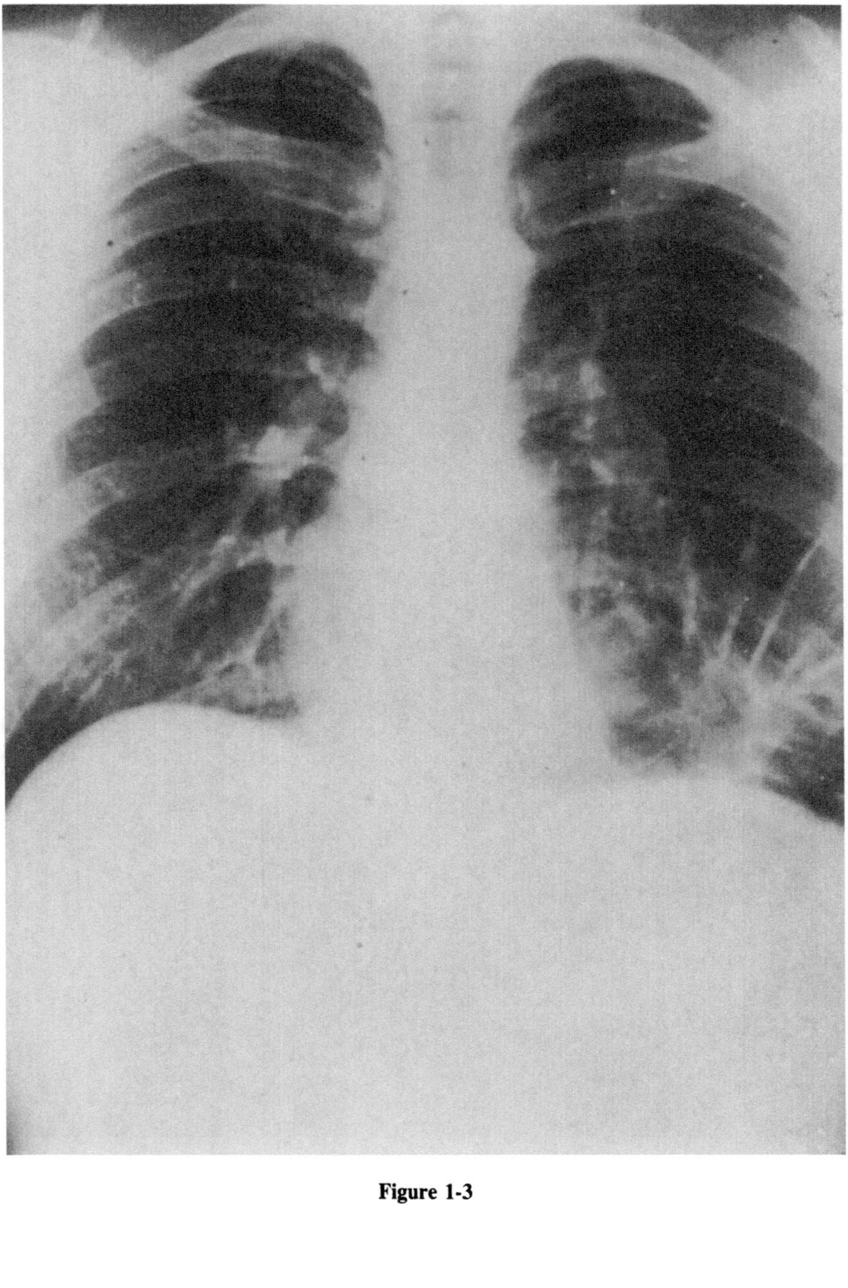

Figure 1-3

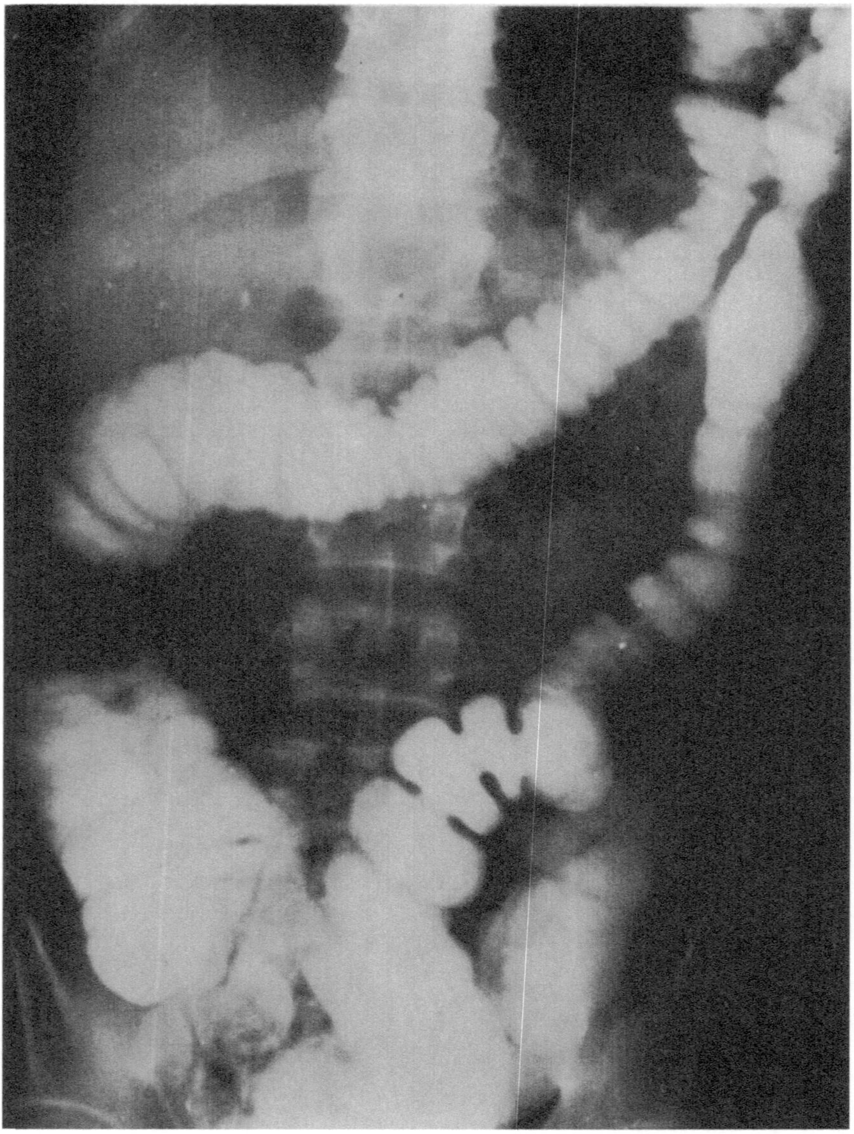

Figure 1-4

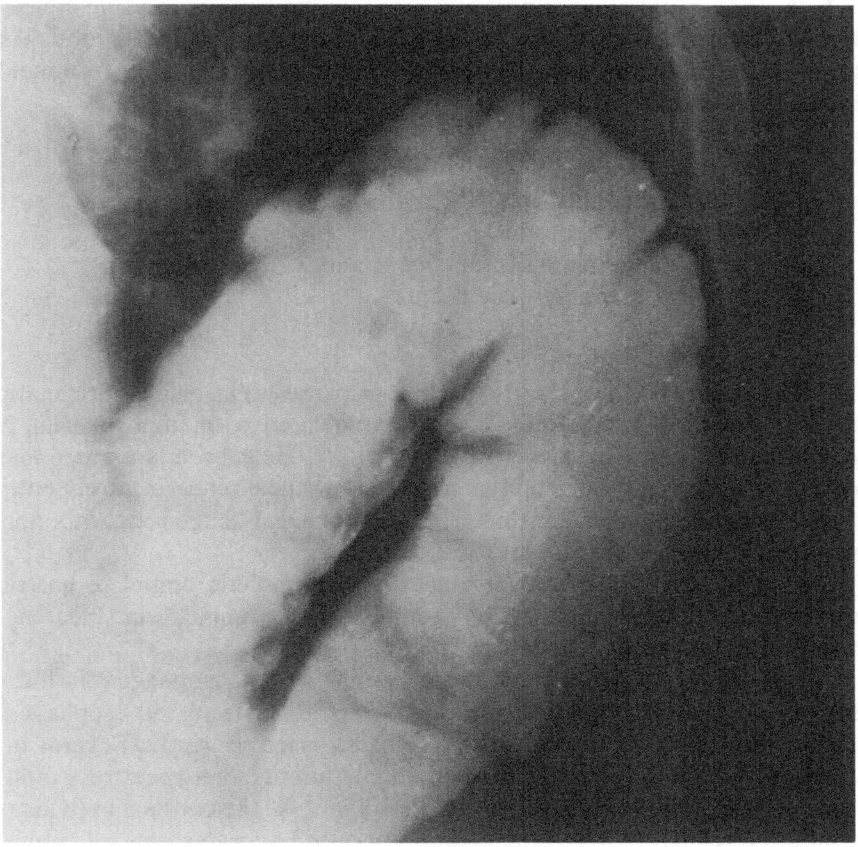

Figure 1-5

surfaces in any patient undergoing celiotomy for blunt or penetrating trauma. In the acute situation, a celiotomy is preferred rather than a thoracotomy, as this enables management of any associated injuries. Reduction of the incarcerated viscera into the abdomen is nearly always possible, as no intrathoracic adhesions have formed. If, however, the patient presents at a time after the acute injury, a thoracotomy is preferred, since there are often dense intrathoracic adhesions present and reduction from below is impossible.[21,22] Repair should be accomplished with nonabsorbable suture material, and recurrence is rare.

ANSWER: C.

1.3. A 75-year-old woman presents with symptoms of increasing epigastric fullness after eating and periodic vomiting of undigested food. An upper GI is obtained and is shown as Figures 1-6 and 1-7. Treatment should consist of:

A. No treatment at the present time.
B. Nisson fundoplication.
C. Parietal cell vagotomy.
D. Cimetidine and small frequent feedings.
E. Repair of diaphragmatic hernia.

The upper GI X ray clearly discloses a paraesophageal diaphragmatic hernia. The most prominent symptom associated with such a hernia is postprandial fullness and occasional vomiting. Heartburn is a much less common symptom, presumably because esophageal reflux is infrequently noted in paraesophageal hernias, as the esophageal hiatus retains its normal fixation below the diaphragm.

Complications of paraesophageal hernias include complete gastric obstruction, incarceration of the stomach, and strangulation, bleeding, and perforation of the stomach.[23]

Despite the designation of these hernias as paraesophageal in location, they generally appear to be more enlargements of the esophageal hiatus with subsequent herniation of the stomach upwards. Several investigators have shown no true diaphragmatic fibers between the esophagus and the paraesophageal hernial defect.[23,24] As the cardia and pylorus tend to be relatively fixed, the greater curvature migrates upward, sometimes associated with rotation of the stomach, leading to gastric volvulus.

Elective operation is indicated in all good-risk patients presenting with a paraesophageal hernia, even if the patient is asymptomatic. In one series, 30% of all patients with paraesophageal hernia presented with incarceration or obstruction and required emergency surgery. If preoperative decompression was not possible, a 50% mortality rate was noted.[25] Another series disclosed a 27% incidence of patients presenting with acute gastric obstruction.[23] A third series followed 21 patients with paraesophageal hernias who were treated nonoperatively because of their mild symptoms. Six of these patients died as a result of the complications of the hernia, and 15 patients underwent elective repair.[26] Most observers have noted the uniformly fatal outcome if strangulation is present.[25]

Recommendations for treatment have been varied, but all stress the necessity of closure of the diaphragmatic defect. Whether a thoracotomy or a celiotomy should be employed has likewise been debated, and the

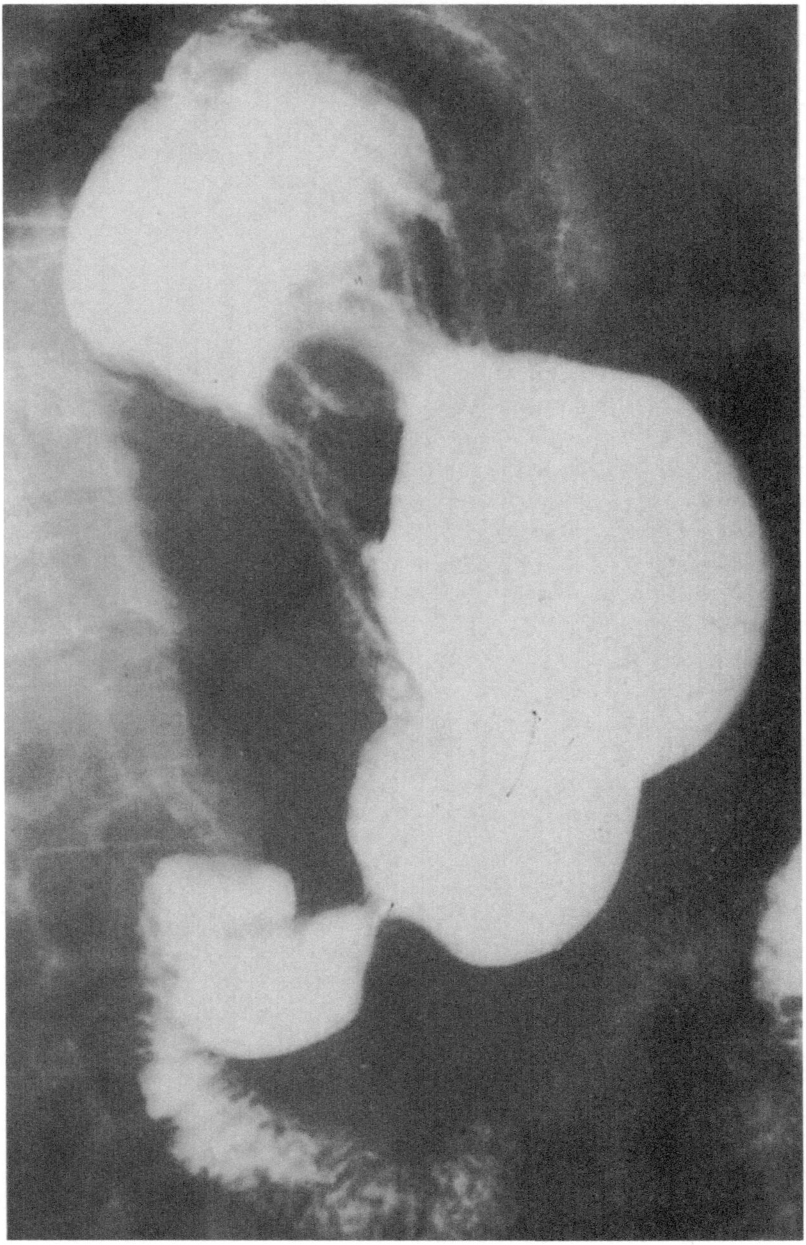

Figure 1-6

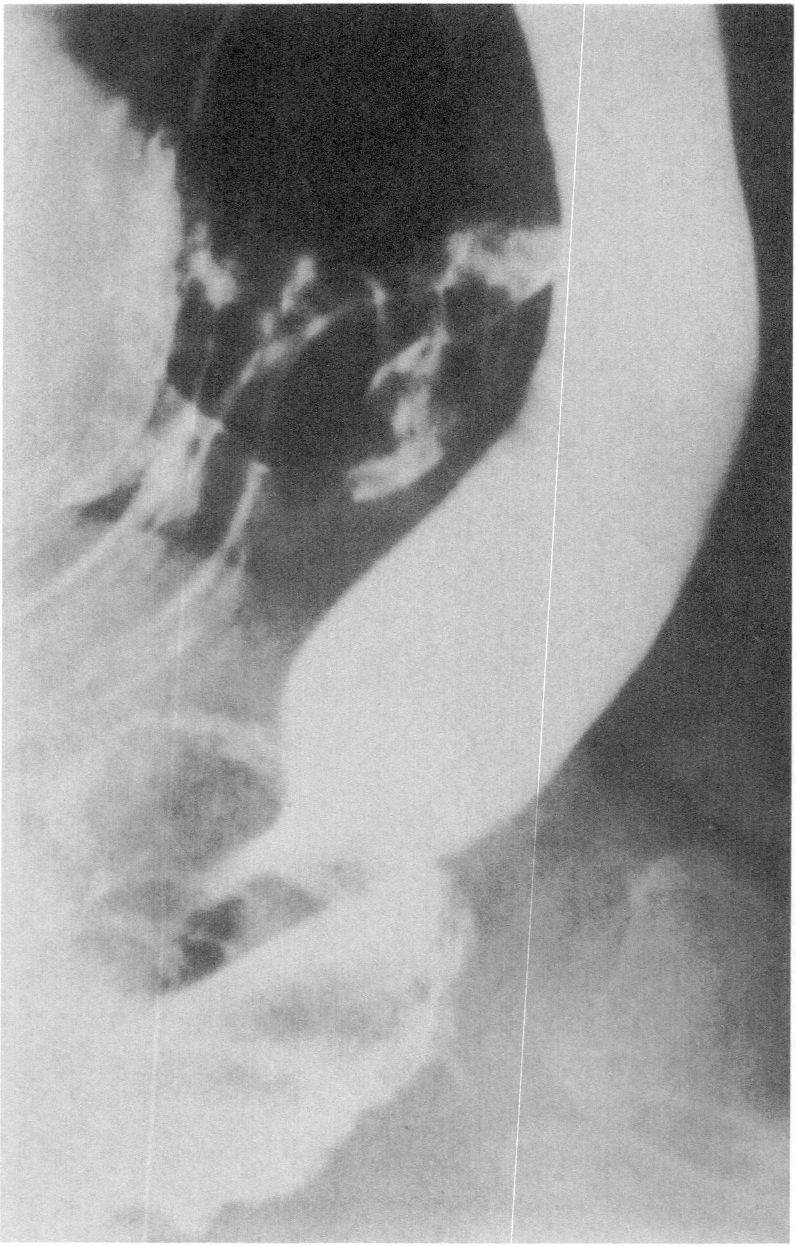

Figure 1-7

need for an antireflux procedure in addition to the hernia repair has been questioned. Some authors have felt that closure of the defect with return of the stomach to the abdomen would lead to reflux esophagitis in the future, whereas others have not noted this occurrence. In addition, some authors have recommended fixing the stomach within the abdomen by either a gastropexy or a tube gastrostomy.[23] At this time, the consensus for treatment would probably be celiotomy for any patient presenting with a paraesophageal hernia with reduction of the stomach into the abdomen, closure of the paraesophageal defect, and no antireflux procedure. All authorities agree that after surgery there is an extremely low recurrence rate of the hernia.[24]

ANSWER: E.

1.4. A 56-year-old man gives a history of progressive dysphagia, nighttime regurgitation, and substernal pain. He occasionally awakens at night coughing violently. He has undergone forceful dilatation of the distal esophagus three times in the past year, with recurrence of symptoms within 2 months on each occasion. A chest X ray is normal. An esophagogram is shown as Figure 1-8. Treatment should consist of:

A. Esophagectomy with colon interposition.
B. Esophagogastrectomy.
C. Heller cardiomyotomy.
D. Fundoplication.
E. Heller cardiomyotomy plus fundoplication.

The X ray discloses achalasia of the esophagus with marked proximal dilatation and stasis present. Achalasia is a disease of disordered motor function of the esophagus and consists of two major abnormalities. Aperistalsis is present throughout the entire length of the esophagus. In addition, there is partial or incomplete relaxation of the lower esophageal sphincter pressure.[27] The complications of this condition include malnutrition and anemia, aspiration of esophageal contents, and squamous cell carcinoma of the esophagus in 5%–10% of cases.[27,28] Medical management of this disorder has had very limited success, and currently two forms of treatment, either forceful pneumatic dilatation or a Heller cardiomyotomy are preferred. In the patient presented, the failure of three prior dilatations indicates that the operation should be performed.

With the advent of the Heller cardiomyotomy, a treatment was available that markedly improved at least 80% of patients. However, about one quarter of these manifested significant esophageal reflux after this procedure. In addition, some patients suffered a recurrent obstruction.[27,29,30] Because of this, most authorities today recommend a Heller cardiomyotomy with the addition of one of the antireflux procedures. No one of the antireflux procedures seems to possess any definite advantage over the others, and excellent results can be expected in about 90% of patients.[31–33]

ANSWER: E.

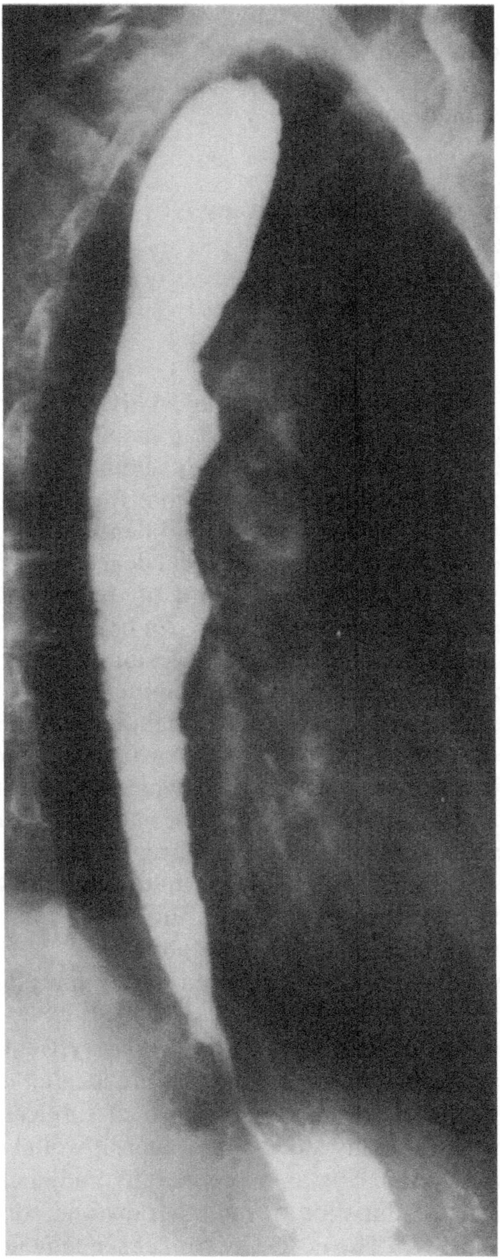

Figure 1-8

1.5. A 72-year-old alcoholic man gives a three-month history of progressive dysphagia and inability to swallow solid food. He has lost 18 lb. A chest X ray is normal. An upper GI tract X ray is shown as Figure 1-9. A liver–spleen scan and carcinoembryonic antigen determination are normal. Treatment should consist of:

A. Radiotherapy.
B. Radiotherapy plus chemotherapy.
C. Esophagectomy.
D. Esophagogastrectomy.
E. Celestin tube intubation.

The history of alcoholism and the clinical history of progressive dysphagia are all indicative of the presence of an esophageal carcinoma. Prior to any definitive treatment, esophagoscopy should be performed, and a biopsy should confirm the nature of the lesion. Because of the uniformly poor results when utilizing any of the treatment modalities, numerous recommendations have been made and a great deal of dispute still persists.

In general, lesions of the lower third of the esophagus and very proximal adenocarcinomas of the stomach can be successfully treated by esophagogastrectomy. For proximal gastric lesions without extension into the esophagus, a left thoracolaparotomy is quite acceptable. For lesions slightly higher in the esophagus, however, right thoracotomy is required. The initial procedure should be a celiotomy, with assessment of the liver and all regional gastric lymph nodes. Following this, the stomach can be mobilized fully and the abdomen closed. Following positioning of the patient for a right thoracotomy, the esophageal portion of the operation can be completed and the stomach pulled up through the widened hiatus for an end-to-side esophagogastrostomy. The merits of concomitant pyloroplasty have been discussed, but it would appear that in most cases, if the vagus nerves have not been severed during the dissection, this is not necessary.[34]

Radiotherapy has been advocated as a primary treatment modality for esophageal carcinomas mainly when they are located in the middle or proximal third of the esophagus, areas in which surgical complications have been greater. After many studies, however, it would appear that the role of radiotherapy should be as a preoperative adjunct, and in some series of patients, a combination of radiotherapy and surgery has given rise to extended survival. The necessity for subsequent surgery has been borne out in studies that have demonstrated residual carcinoma in the resected specimen following radiotherapy.[35] Radiotherapy alone, even

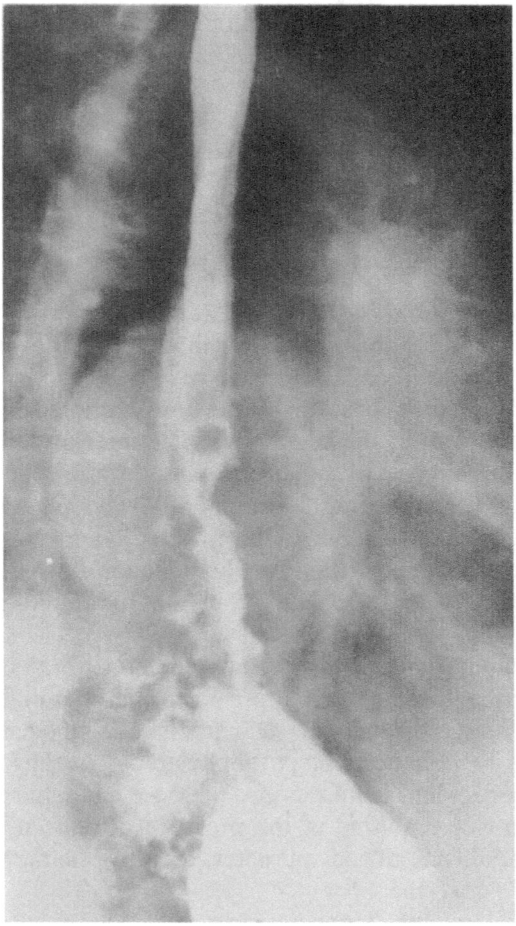

Figure 1-9

utilizing supervoltage equipment, has been associated with such problems as esophageal stricture, tracheoesophageal fistulas, and pulmonary fibrosis.[36] Chemotherapy has been used mainly for recurrent disease. Celestin tube intubation has been utilized with significant success in very poor-risk patients who could not swallow and who were not candidates for any major resectional procedure. Often many months of palliation can be gained utilizing esophageal prostheses.[37]

ANSWER: D.

1.6. A 68-year-old man complains of increasing symptoms of fullness in the throat, dysphagia, and bouts of coughing. An esophagogram is performed and is shown as Figure 1-10. Treatment should consist of:

A. Diverticulectomy.
B. Diverticulectomy plus cricopharyngeal myotomy.
C. Cricopharyngeal myotomy.
D. Bouginage.
E. Esophageal resection.

The esophagogram shows a typical Zenker's diverticulum. This problem probably results from disordered motility of the cricopharyngeus muscle, which is now recognized as a true upper esophageal sphincter. This muscle arises from the lateral borders of the cricoid cartilage, running posteriorly to the wall of the esophagus. The inferior constrictor muscle borders the cricopharyngeus superiorly, and between these two muscles is where the Zenker's pulsion diverticulum always presents. Diverticula of the esophagus may occur in two other areas: In the midesophagus, they may be secondary to a traction phenomenon from inflamed mediastinal nodes; in the lower esophagus, they may be found in an epiphrenic location.

Esophageal manometric studies have demonstrated contractions adjacent to the cricopharyngeus that are abnormal in amplitude, duration, and timing. The significance of such findings is unclear, but it would appear that the basic underlying pathophysiology leading to formation of a Zenker's diverticulum is an incoordination of the pharyngoesophageal peristaltic sequence resulting in the pressure of pharyngeal contraction being exerted against a closed sphincter, thereby leading to a pharyngeal outpouching.[38]

In recent years, treatment appears to be evolving. Originally, diverticulectomy was considered to be the treatment of choice. In one series from the Mayo Clinic, 809 patients were treated with diverticulectomy. Over 90% had excellent relief of symptoms, but there were still a number of symptomatic recurrences with or without a recurrent diverticulum being present.[39] Because of these difficulties, and in view of more recent physiological data concerning the upper esophageal sphincter, cricopharyngeal myotomy has been advocated in addition to diverticulectomy, with excellent results. At this time, it is not clear whether diverticulectomy alone, cricopharyngeal myotomy alone, or the combined operation should be utilized in all patients, but on the basis of the large series of patients accumulated at the Mayo Clinic, the following recommendations have been made: Myotomy without diverticulectomy is reserved for those pa-

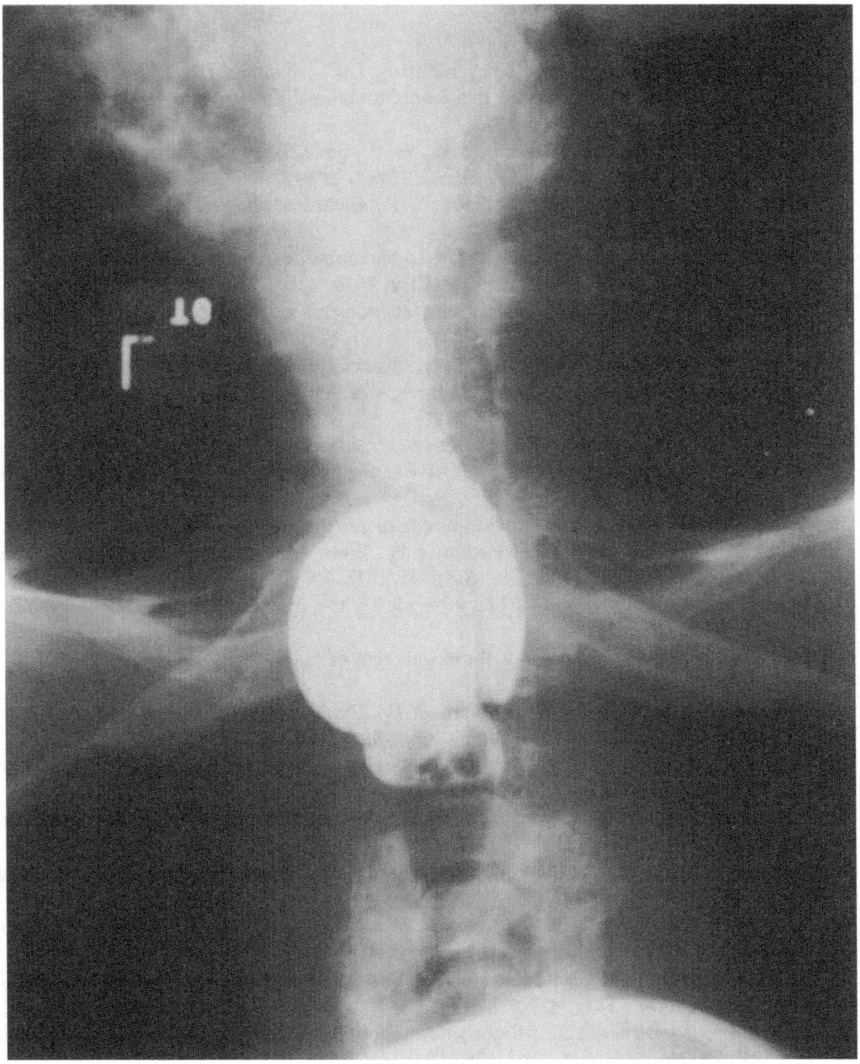

Figure 1-10

tients with small diverticula, whereas excision of the diverticulum and myotomy are employed for patients with diverticula over 5 or 6 cm in diameter. It is not truly known whether diverticulectomy is essential in most patients, as the diverticula often regress following myotomy alone.[38]

ANSWER: B.

References

1. Pellegrini, C.A., DeMeester, T.R., Johnson, L.F., Skinner, D.B.: Gastroesophageal reflux and pulmonary aspiration: Incidence, functional abnormality, and results of surgical therapy. *Surgery* 86:110, 1979.
2. Lipshutz, W.H., Gaskins, R.D., Lukash, W.M., Sode, J.: Pathogenesis of lower-esophageal-sphincter incompetence. *N. Engl. J. Med.* 289:182, 1973.
3. Battle, W.S., Nyhus, L.M., Bombeck, C.T.: Gastroesophageal reflux: Diagnosis and treatment. *Ann. Surg.* 177:560, 1973.
4. Behar, J., Biancani, P., Sheahan, D.G.: Evaluation of esophageal tests in the diagnosis of reflux esophagitis. *Gastroenterology* 71:9, 1976.
5. Bennett, J.R.: Medical management of gastro-oesophageal reflux. *Clin. Gastroenterol.* 5:175, 1976.
6. Farrell, R.L., Roling, G.T., Castell, D.O.: Stimulation of the incompetent lower esophageal sphincter: A possible advance in therapy of heartburn. *Digestive Diseases* 18:646, 1973.
7. McCallum, R.W., Ippoliti, A.F., Cooney, C., Sturdevant, R.A.L.: A controlled trial of metoclopramide in symptomatic gastroesophageal reflux. *N. Engl. J. Med.* 296:354, 1977.
8. Stanciu, C., Bennett, J.R.: Metoclopramide in gastroesphageal reflux. *Gut* 14:275, 1973.
9. Bushkin, F.L., Meustein, C.L., Parker, T.H., Woodward, E.R.: Nisson fundoplication for reflux peptic esophagitis. *Ann. Surg.* 185:672, 1977.
10. Belsey, R.: Mark IV repair of hiatal hernia by the transthoracic approach. *World J. Surg.* 1:475, 1977.
11. Hill, L.D.: Progress in the surgical management of hiatal hernia. *World J. Surg.* 1:425, 1977.
12. DeMeester, T.R., Johnson, L.F., Kent, A.H.: Evaluation of current operations for the prevention of gastroesophageal reflux. *Ann. Surg.* 180:511, 1974.
13. Polk, H.C.: Fundoplication for reflux esophagitis: Misadventures with the operation of choice. *Ann. Surg.* 183:645, 1976.
14. Saik, R.P., Greenburg, A.G., Peskin, G.W.: A study of fundoplication disruption and deformity. *Am. J. Surg.* 134:19, 1977.
15. Skinner, D.B.: Complications of surgery for gastroesophageal reflux. *World J. Surg.* 1:485, 1977.
16. Herrington, J.L., Wright, R.S., Edwards, W.H., Sawyers, J.L.: Conservative surgical treatment of reflux esophagitis and esophageal stricture. *Ann. Surg.* 181:552, 1975.
17. Hill, L.D., Gelfand, M., Bauermeister, D.: Simplified management of reflux esophagitis with stricture. *Ann. Surg.* 172:638, 1970.
18. Jarrett, F., Bernhardt, L.C.: Right-sided diaphragmatic injury: Rarity or overlooked diagnosis. *Arch. Surg.* 113:737, 1978.
19. Hegarty, M.M., Bryer, J.V., Angorn, I.B., Baker, L.W.: Delayed presentation of traumatic diaphragmatic hernia. *Ann. Surg.* 188:229, 1978.
20. Grimes, O.F.: Traumatic injuries of the diaphragm: Diaphragmatic hernia. *Am. J. Surg.* 128:175, 1974.
21. Griswold, F.W., Warden, H.E., Gardner, R.J.: Acute diaphragmatic rupture caused by blunt trauma. *Am. J. Surg.* 124:359, 1972.
22. Drews, J.A., Mercer, E.C., Benfield, J.R.: Acute diaphragmatic injury. *Ann. Thorac. Surg.* 16:67, 1973.
23. Wichterman, K., Geha, A.S., Cahow, E., Baue, A.E.: Giant paraesophageal hiatus

hernia with intrathoracic stomach and colon: The case for early repair. *Surgery* 86:497, 1979.
24. Hill, L.D., Tobias, J.A.: Paraesophageal hernia. *Arch. Surg.* 96:735, 1968.
25. Hill, L.D.: Incarcerated paraesophageal hernia: A surgical emergency. *Am. J. Surg.* 126:286, 1973.
26. Skinner, D.B., Belsey, R.H.R.: Surgical management of esophageal reflux and hiatus hernia. *J. Thorac. Cardiovasc. Surg.* 53:33, 1967.
27. Cohen, S.: Motor disorders of the esophagus. *N. Engl. J. Med.* 301:184, 1979.
28. Carter, R., Brewer, L.A.: Achalasia and esophageal carcinoma. *Am. J. Surg.* 130:114, 1975.
29. Rees, J.R., Thorbjarnarson, B.: Achalasia: Results of operation in 84 patients. *Ann. Surg.* 171:195, 1970.
30. Yon, J., Christensen, J.: An uncontrolled comparison of treatments for achalasia. *Ann. Surg.* 182:672, 1975.
31. Hatafuku, T., Maki, T., Thal, A.P.: Fundic patch operation in the treatment of advanced achalasia of the esophagus. *Surg. Gynecol. Obstet.* 134:617, 1972.
32. Menguy, R.: Management of achalasia by transabdominal cardiomyotomy and fundoplication. *Surg. Gynecol. Obstet.* 133:482, 1971.
33. Peyton, M.D., Greenfield, L.J., Elkins, R.C.: Combined myotomy and hiatal herniorrhaphy: A new approach to achalasia. *Am. J. Surg.* 128:786, 1974.
34. Piccone, V.A., LeVeen, H.H., Ahmed, N., Grosberg, S.: Reappraisal of esophagogastrectomy for esophageal malignancy. *Am. J. Surg.* 137:32, 1979.
35. Parker, E.F., Gregorie, H.B.: Carcinoma of the esophagus: Long term results. *J.A.M.A.* 235:1018, 1976.
36. Lowe, W.C.: Survival with carcinoma of the esophagus. *Ann. Intern. Med.* 77:915, 1972.
37. Gallagher, E.G., Zumbro, G.L., Treasure, R.L.: Celestin tube intubation for advanced esophageal carcinoma. *Am. J. Surg.* 136:405, 1978.
38. Ellis, F.H., Schlegel, J.F., Lynch, V.P., Payne, W.S.: Cricopharyngeal myotomy for pharyngo-esophageal diverticulum. *Ann. Surg.* 170:340, 1969.
39. Welsh, G.F., Payne, W.S.: The present status of one stage pharyngoesophageal diverticulectomy. *Surg. Clin. North Am.* 53:953, 1973.

2
PEPTIC ULCER DISEASE

2.1. Which of the following complications of chronic duodenal ulcer represents an absolute indication for operation?

A. Hemorrhage.
B. Obstruction.
C. Intractability.
D. Perforation.
E. None of the above.

While any of the above conditions may result in a situation requiring operation, each may also be treated nonoperatively in selected instances. Surely, hemorrhage of a mild degree that is not recurrent in nature can often be managed successfully over the long term by appropriate medical therapy. Likewise, intractability is a relative indication for surgery. It is possible that with the use of the newly released α-2-histamine blocker, cimetidine, the number of truly intractable duodenal ulcer patients will diminish, but at present this is speculative.

The presence of gastric outlet obstruction associated with duodenal ulcer has been regarded by some as a mandatory indication for operation. However, it is important to realize that this type of obstruction may consist of two distinct entities. One is the acute edematous obstruction associated with a recently activated ulcer. The other is the chronic cicatrix associated with long-standing duodenal ulcer disease. The former situation is often rapidly reversible with nasogastric suction, and perhaps only 25% of these patients go on to require operation for obstruction or other complications within the following 2 years.[1,2] The chronically obstructing duodenal ulcer is often associated with profound electrolyte abnormalities, namely hypokalemia and a hypochloremic alkalosis. This results not only from a small loss of potassium in the nasogastric aspirate, but also from a renal mechanism whereby potassium and hydrogen ions are exchanged, resulting in a loss of potassium with a commensurate retention of hydrogen ion. This latter variety of obstruction is rarely benefited by prolonged trials of nasogastric suction and will generally require surgical relief. These patients are optimally prepared for operation by a 5- to 10-day period of nasogastric suction accompanied by total parenteral nutrition.

In the United States, the usual question regarding the management of perforated duodenal ulcer is which operative procedure is required, either simple plication of the duodenal perforation or a definitive operation for the ulcer diathesis. Little attention has been paid to the nonoperative alternatives for treatment. However, several series of patients with perforated duodenal ulcers have been published in which the results of treatment using only nasogastric suction and intravenous fluids with antibiotics have been associated with an overall mortality of approximately 5%, a figure comparable to those obtained in many series of patients in whom operation has been utilized.[3] In general, it would seem wise to reserve nonoperative management of perforated duodenal ulcer to two groups of patients. One would be those patients who present several days after the onset of perforation symptoms with an obviously sealed off perforation. In the absence of evidence of peritoneal sepsis, conservative management will suffice. The other group would be the extremely poor-risk patients who present with the perforation and are in a state of refractory shock and in whom any operation would be associated with a prohibitive mortality.

ANSWER: E.

2.2. Which of the following operations for chronic duodenal ulcer is associated with the lowest incidence of ulcer recurrence?

A. Vagotomy and pyloroplasty.
B. Vagotomy and gastroenterostomy.
C. Vagotomy and antrectomy.
D. Parietal cell vagotomy.
E. Subtotal gastrectomy.

The mere fact that numerous operations are currently advocated for treatment of the patient with a duodenal ulcer is proof that no one of these operative procedures is clearly superior to all others in all situations. In general, surgeons have sought the operation that gives maximum long-term control of the duodenal ulcer diathesis with a minimum of operative mortality and postoperative dumping symptoms. However, this ideal goal has proved elusive. Vagotomy and pyloroplasty is associated with a lower operative mortality in the hands of many surgeons than is any form of gastrectomy, either antrectomy or subtotal gastrectomy with either Billroth I or II reconstructions. Vagotomy and pyloroplasty can often be accomplished with operative mortalities of 0.5% or less. There is, however, some agreement that the recurrence rates after vagotomy and pyloroplasty are higher than after vagotomy and antrectomy. This is probably related to two factors. One is a higher incidence of gastric stasis after pyloroplasty, and the other is that if an inadequate vagotomy is performed, the patient is more likely to develop a recurrent ulcer after pyloroplasty than after antrectomy.[4] Other groups with extensive experience in performing antrectomy have noted very favorable results. Herrington has reported over 3500 patients in whom this operation was performed with less than a 1% operative mortality and ulcer recurrence rate.[5] Other groups have shown the effectiveness of vagotomy and antrectomy, even if as little as 25% of the distal stomach is removed.[6] Despite this and other data that would support the superiority of vagotomy and antrectomy over vagotomy and drainage procedures,[7,8] others have found that vagotomy and drainage procedures can be performed with a lesser operative mortality and that they are associated with equal ulcer recurrence rates to vagotomy and antrectomy.[9] In addition, at least two large series have been published in which the long-term recurrence rates following vagotomy and pyloroplasty were less than 5%, and the recommendation was made that this operation represents the best choice for treatment of the patient with duodenal ulcer.[10,11]

There is fairly uniform agreement, however, that the least acceptable operation today for the treatment of duodenal ulcer is subtotal gastrectomy without vagotomy.[12] Into this rather unsettled state of affairs has come the latest entry into the field of duodenal ulcer operations, namely parietal cell vagotomy, in which only those vagal fibers innervating the proximal portion of the stomach containing parietal cells are severed, thus leaving the antrum and pylorus normally innervated. Operative mortality as low as that achieved with vagotomy and pyloroplasty has been uniformly noted, and during a relatively short follow-up period, recurrent ulceration has been seen in approximately 5% of cases.[13,14] These series have noted a significantly lower incidence of postoperative dumping symptoms and diarrhea in these patients. Several areas of question remain, however. It is generally agreed that this operation is indicated for only those patients with intractable duodenal ulcer, and is not to be employed for those presenting with gastric outlet obstruction or hemorrhage. Also, there appears to be more difficulty in learning the technical steps of this operation than is the case with the other procedures. Several early series of parietal cell vagotomy were published in which ulcer recurrence rates of 13%–22% were noted.[15–17] The same authors ultimately noted lower ulcer recurrence rates as their operative technique was perfected. The last point to be considered in the discussion of parietal cell vagotomy is that most series of patients in whom this operation has been utilized have not been followed up long enough to know what the ultimate ulcer recurrence rate is going to be. Remembering the lesson derived from the performance of gastroenterostomy alone for the treatment of duodenal ulcer, it was noted that whereas this operation was initially successful for many patients with this disorder, it took up to 25 years for the true, extremely high incidence of ulcer recurrence to manifest itself. In view of this, the true value of parietal cell vagotomy will probably be questioned for many years.

ANSWER: C.

2.3. Which of the following situations is a contraindication to parietal cell vagotomy for intractable duodenal ulcer?

A. Gastric outlet obstruction.
B. The patient is over 40 years of age.
C. The patient is female.
D. The patient has a basal acid output greater than 10 mEq/hr.
E. The patient has a coexistent hiatus hernia without reflux.

Over the past 50 years, numerous operations have enjoyed temporary popularity for the control of the duodenal ulcer diathesis. Gastroenterostomy; subtotal gastrectomy; vagotomy, either truncal or selective, coupled with pyloroplasty or antrectomy; and most recently, parietal cell vagotomy have all had their advocates. Various claims have been made for each of these with regard to diminished operative mortality, ulcer recurrence rates, and postoperative dumping symptoms.

Parietal cell vagotomy is the latest entrant in the field of methods vying for the optimal operative control of duodenal ulcer. In this operation, only the vagal fibers innervating the proximal stomach are sectioned, so that the entire antrum retains its vagal innervation and resultant motility and function. Interest in this operation arose mainly because of dissatisfaction with postoperative diarrhea and dumping symptoms associated with all other gastric operations, not because of high recurrent ulcer rates.

Several early series of parietal cell vagotomies disclosed an unacceptable ulcer recurrence rate, but careful analysis showed this to be due to operative inexperience, and these rates decreased as the operating surgeon gained technical competence with the operation.[15,17]

Other series have shown that the operation can be associated with an extremely low operative mortality and recurrence rates of between 1% and 9%.[18] However, far longer follow-up periods are necessary to be sure that these good results will be sustained. Already, in some studies, a discernible increase in basal and stimulated acid outputs has been noted with the passage of time.

Remembering that it took approximately 25 years for the original operation of gastroenterostomy for duodenal ulcer to fall into disrepute should make one cautious of considering this operation the final chapter in the story of the surgery of duodenal ulcer.

What is agreed by all persons performing this operation is that the patient with gastric outlet obstruction or significant scarring from duodenal ulcer is not a good candidate for the procedure, as the incidence of subsequent obstruction or postprandial fullness is greatly increased in this group. Thus far, no contraindication to the performance of parietal cell vagotomy exists because of the age or sex of the patient, the amount of preoperative acid present, or the presence of a coexistent hiatus hernia.

ANSWER: A.

2.4. A 42-year-old man has been hospitalized on five occasions in the past 8 years for a duodenal ulcer. On his last admission, he underwent a gastric analysis revealing a basal acid output of 11 mEq/hr and a maximal acid output of 20 mEq/hr. He presents to the emergency room with a 2-hr history of severe, diffuse abdominal pain. Examination discloses abdominal rigidity and diffuse peritoneal irritation. Radiographs are obtained, and one is shown as Figure 2-1. Treatment should consist of:

A. Nonoperative management.
B. Vagotomy and pyloroplasty.
C. Vagotomy and antrectomy.
D. Oversewing of the ulcer with an omental patch.
E. Parietal cell vagotomy.

The proper treatment of a perforated duodenal ulcer will depend upon many variables, including the history and age of the patient, his general medical condition, and the time elapsed between perforation and operation. This man obviously has a severe duodenal ulcer diathesis, as manifested by his multiple recurrences over the preceding few years and also the marked hyperacidity noted on the gastric analysis. The acid values obtained are high within the duodenal ulcer range, and the significant response to pentagastrin stimulation probably rules out an associated gastrin-secreting pancreatic islet cell tumor. Both nonoperative management and merely oversewing the ulcer would be inappropriate in such a patient, as he has such a severe ulcer diathesis and would likely require a definitive duodenal ulcer operation at some time in the future. Although initial nonoperative therapy of perforated duodenal ulcer has its advocates,[3,19] few would advocate such a treatment in the patient presented. Many studies have shown that patients who have a chronic duodenal ulcer and present with a perforation will, if the perforation is patched, suffer ulcer recurrence and often need definitive duodenal ulcer surgery in the future. On the other hand, patients who have a short history of ulcer symptoms often have no further problem with their duodenal ulcers following mere plication of the ulcer.[20–23]

Therefore, realizing that this patient requires some form of definitive duodenal ulcer management, the question narrows down to which is the preferable operation. It has been repeatedly shown in series of patients with acute duodenal ulcer perforations that vagotomy and antrectomy, vagotomy and pyloroplasty, and simple plication of the perforated ulcer are all associated with roughly equal operative mortality. Therefore, it would seem prudent to select the operation that can be performed safely

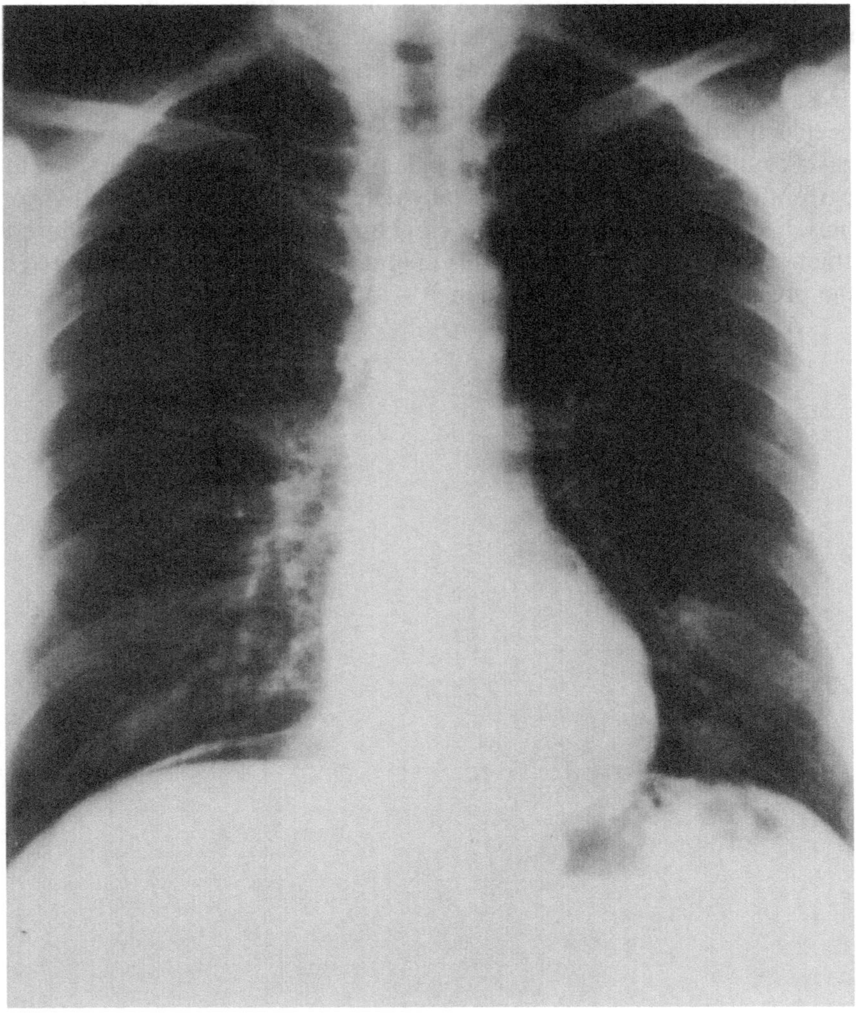

Figure 2-1

and is associated with the lowest ulcer recurrence rate. This is clearly vagotomy and antrectomy, which in most reported series is associated with an ulcer recurrence rate approximating 1%.[20] The role of parietal cell vagotomy plus omental patching of the ulcer in the treatment of perforated duodenal ulcer is currently under study. At least two small series of patients have been reported in which the immediate results were satisfactory.[24,25] However, the long-term results of the success of parietal cell vagotomy in controlling the duodenal ulcer diathesis are not yet available, and so judgment must be withheld at this time. A potential problem has been pointed out following plication of perforated duodenal ulcers, namely gastric outlet obstruction from the inflammatory reaction surrounding the perforation. This would be especially detrimental if a parietal cell vagotomy had been performed, as no complimentary emptying procedure is characteristically utilized with this operation, which is contraindicated in the presence of outlet obstruction.[26]

ANSWER: C.

2.5. Which of the following conditions is not a sequela of operations for chronic duodenal ulcer?

A. Gallstones.
B. Kidney stones.
C. Anemia.
D. Tuberculosis.
E. Gastric carcinoma.

Apart from the more commonly recognized complications of duodenal ulcer surgery such as the dumping syndrome and recurrent peptic ulceration, there are numerous other serious complications that the clinician must be aware of. Several reviews have indicated that the rate of gallstone formation following vagotomy is increased. In one study of 50 patients followed for up to 5 years, 16% of patients who had undergone vagotomy developed cholelithiasis, a rate more than four times that expected in the general population.[27] In this same study, gallbladder bile obtained from dogs after vagotomy showed a lowered phospholipid/cholesterol ratio and a decreased ability to dissolve human gallstones in vitro. In another study, 21% of patients who had undergone subtotal gastrectomy and truncal vagotomy developed gallstones subsequently, whereas only 6% of patients with subtotal gastrectomy alone developed gallstones during this same follow-up period.[28] It has been hypothesized that this tendency towards gallstone formation will be diminished by either selective vagotomy or parietal cell vagotomy.

It has long been recognized that patients who have undergone gastric resection can present with anemia many years following this operation. What is less well recognized is that vagotomy and drainage procedures can likewise predispose to comparable anemic states. In one study of 100 partial gastrectomy patients followed for an average of 8 years, anemia was found in 49%. The majority of anemic patients had combined deficiency states, including B_{12}, folate, and iron deficiencies.[29] In another study of patients followed after vagotomy and gastroenterostomy, a significant incidence of iron deficiency anemia was noted, with females being affected more commonly than males.[30]

Numerous reports, many of them from Europe, have documented an increased incidence of tuberculosis developing in patients who have undergone a partial gastrectomy for either gastric or duodenal ulcer disease.[31] In this country, a review of one large tuberculosis hospital revealed 21 patients with tuberculosis who had a previous subtotal gastrectomy. Seventeen of these patients had not had tuberculosis prior to their gastrectomy.[32] Another review spanning up to 17 years postoperatively revealed a 6.3% incidence of tuberculosis following gastrectomy.[33] A similar infection rate has been noted following vagotomy and gastroenterostomy.[30] Many authorities suspect that this tendency toward tuberculosis is caused by a nutritional deficiency state that follows gastrectomy, and this is supported by an increased incidence of tuberculosis following jejunoileal bypass for morbid obesity, a procedure that likewise induces a profound nutritional deficiency.[34]

Over 1100 cases of gastric carcinoma have been described originating in the gastric remnant following previous ulcer surgery,[35] and several studies have documented an increased incidence of cancer on long-term follow-up. In one series of 166 patients with carcinoma of the stomach, 3.6% had undergone a prior ulcer operation.[36] Another prospective study followed 74 patients after their operations for peptic ulcer. In 5.4%, cancer developed from 10 to 22 years postoperatively. This same study documented precancerous histologic alterations in the stomachs of some of the other patients.[37] In view of this association, it becomes important to investigate upper GI tract symptoms endoscopically in any patient who has previously undergone a gastric operation.

ANSWER: B.

2.6. A 42-year-old man with a chronic duodenal ulcer undergoes a vagotomy and antrectomy with a Billroth II reconstruction. Six months later, he complains of persistent epigastric pain and heartburn with frequent vomiting, associated with a 40-lb weight loss. Treatment with antacids has not helped. He is incapacitated and can no longer work. Upper gastrointestinal X rays disclose normal postoperative changes, and a gastroscopy demonstrates florid gastritis. Treatment should consists of:

A. Cholestyramine.
B. Cimetidine.
C. Conversion to a Billroth I anastomosis.
D. Roux-en-Y diversion of alkaline secretions.
E. Insertion of an isoperistaltic (Henle) jejunal segment.

The syndrome of postoperative alkaline reflux gastritis is a well-documented entity that may occur after any of the commonly employed operations for duodenal ulcer with the exception, perhaps, of parietal cell vagotomy. The usual patient will complain of abdominal discomfort unrelieved by antacids. Acid secretion will be normal or decreased, and endoscopy will document the absence of marginal ulceration and the presence of significant gastritis.[38] The pathophysiology of this condition is controversial, but there is increasing evidence that reflux of bile may be a significant factor. There is abundant experimental evidence that bile in contact with gastric mucosa renders the mucosal surface permeable to the back-diffusion of hydrogen ions and would thus cause gastritis by disrupting this normal gastric mucosal barrier. Obviously, any procedure that disrupted the normal pyloric sphincter mechanism could therefore predispose to alkaline reflux. One study that analyzed the bile concentrations in postoperative patients with and without symptoms of reflux gastritis noted that those patients who were symptomatic had a significant increase in the concentration of the secondary bile acid deoxycholic acid.[39] Other investigators have gastroscopically studied symptomatic and asymptomatic patients following duodenal ulcer surgery. Asymptomatic patients have been noted in whom there was reflux of bile with no gastritis or reflux of bile with gastritis. Symptomatic patients had reflux of bile and gastritis. The conclusions drawn from this work were that many patients had alkaline reflux following duodenal ulcer surgery but remain asymptomatic and that the mere presence of the gastroscopic finding of gastritis did not necessarily correlate with symptomatology.[40] The importance of these findings rests in the fact that any patient who suffers from upper gastrointestinal symptoms following gastric surgery should be evaluated

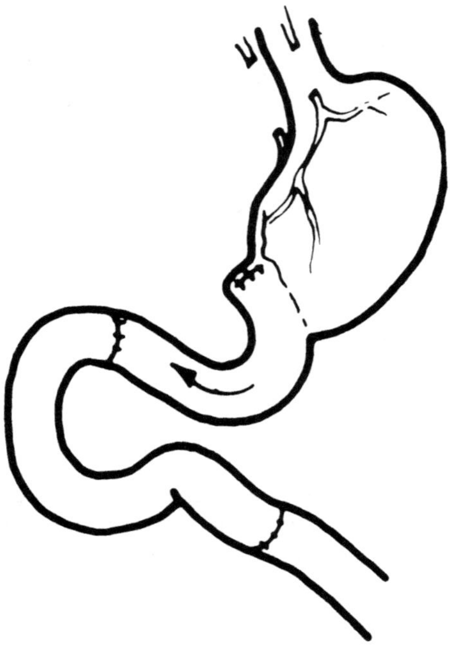

Figure 2-2

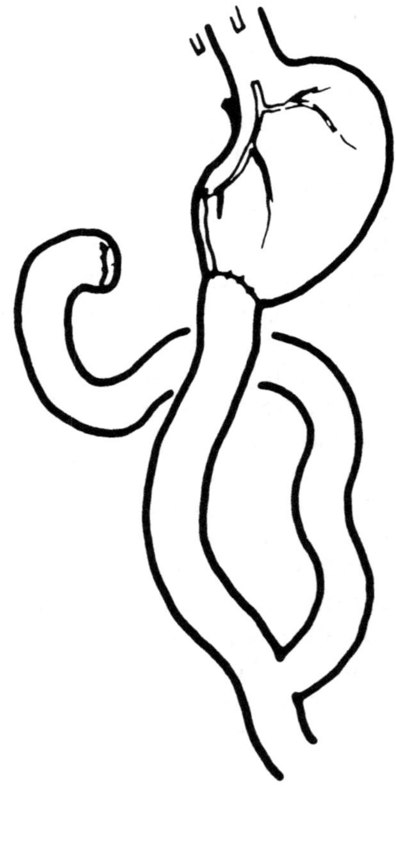

Figure 2-3

by endoscopy rather than by barium meal alone, as the latter will frequently miss significant pathology.[41]

This syndrome has been noted much more frequently in patients who underwent a Billroth II gastrectomy rather than a Billroth I reconstruction, a vagotomy and pyloroplasty, or a vagotomy and gastroenterostomy.[42] Treatment of these patients has proven difficult. It is well recognized that antacids are ineffective in controlling symptoms, as the primary problem is not hyperacidity. For this same reason, cimetidine would not be expected to help. Cholestyramine, an ion exchange resin that binds bile salts, has enjoyed anecdotal success, but has not yet been submitted to an adequate clinical trial to test its efficacy. Various surgical procedures have been attempted to correct this problem, but most have been abandoned. On the basis of several large series of patients, it would seem that the single best operation today for eliminating these symptoms is the complete diversion of alkaline secretions distally by means of a Roux-en-Y reconstruction. In performing such a procedure, it is imperative that the Roux-en-Y enteroenterostomy be at least 15 in. beyond the gastric anastomosis, thus completely eliminating the possibility of bile reflux. Utilizing this technique, the majority of patients with proven alkaline reflux can be benefited.[38,43,44] Diagrams of the Roux-en-Y diversion (Figure 2–2) and the less successful Henle loop (Figure 2–3) are shown.

ANSWER: D.

2.7. In which of the following disease states is the fasting serum gastrin level usually normal?

A. Zollinger–Ellison syndrome.
B. Gastric outlet obstruction.
C. Duodenal ulcer.
D. Retained antrum after hemigastrectomy and Billroth II reconstruction.
E. G-cell hyperplasia of the stomach.

Although the existence of a humoral stimulant of gastric acid secretion had been suspected since the turn of the century, it was not until 1964 that the hormone gastrin was isolated and purified. It has subsequently been determined that gastrin exists in several circulating forms, which differ only in amino acid composition and sequence. It would appear that the C-terminal fragment is the biologically active form. Gastrin-containing cells are called G cells and are found in the pyloric glands of the antrum and the proximal duodenum. Their concentration in the duodenum, however, is far less than that in the stomach. Measurement of serum gastrin is performed by means of a radioimmunoassay, but because of species differences and the many forms of serum gastrin, experimental results have often been contradictory, as a given immunoassay might be specific for one form of gastrin and not for another.

Gastrin release is stimulated by vagal stimuli, which act to increase acid not only by the release of gastrin but also by a direct effect on parietal cells. In addition, intragastric protein is a stimulus to gastrin release. Gastrin appears to be inhibited by the presence of acid in the gastric antrum. The actions of gastrin have been extensively studied. In pharmacologic doses, numerous actions have been described. However, it is questionable whether most of these actions occur with gastrin levels in the physiologic range. The following actions of gastrin have all been described: stimulation of water and electrolyte secretion from the stomach, pancreas, liver, and small intestine; enzyme secretion from the stomach, pancreas, and small intestine; stimulation of smooth muscle in the lower esophageal sphincter, stomach, small intestine, colon, and gallbladder; inhibition of smooth muscle in the pyloric sphincter and sphincter of Oddi; the release of hormones such as insulin; the increase in blood flow of the stomach, small intestine, and pancreas; and a trophic action on gastric and small bowel mucosa and pancreas.[45]

Elevated levels of gastrin are found in patients with pernicious anemia and atrophic gastritis. Of course, no acid hypersecretion is present in this condition. In the classic Zollinger–Ellison syndrome, caused by a gastrin-producing tumor in the pancreas, basal gastrin levels are usually elevated. Other gastrin-secreting tumors can be located also in the duodenum. Some patients with Zollinger–Ellison syndrome may have only slightly increased serum gastrin levels, and stimulation tests consisting of either calcium or secretin infusion may be necessary to elicit an augmented response. Other patients have antral G-cell hyperplasia and elevated levels of gastrin, probably caused by antral distention. In addition, if by surgical error a small amount of antral mucosa is left isolated in a duodenal stump following a Billroth II reconstruction after gastrectomy, gastrin is secreted in excess from this segment, usually leading to recurrent peptic ulceration.

Thus far, there has been found no definite link between the usual form of duodenal ulceration and elevated gastrin secretion, although there are a great deal of conflicting data on this point.[45–47]

ANSWER: C.

2.8. Which of the following is not currently regarded as a factor contributing to stress ulcer formation?

A. An alteration in gastric mucus.
B. Gastric mucosal ischemia.
C. Reflux of bile into the stomach.
D. Changes in mucosal membrane permeability.
E. Increased hydrochloric acid secretion.

The stress ulceration syndrome presents as either upper GI tract bleeding or perforation following a wide variety of stressful situations including major operations, trauma, burns, sepsis, and CNS injury or operation. The lesions can present either in the duodenum as a duodenal ulcer or in the stomach as a gastric ulcer or hemorrhagic gastritis.

The pathophysiology of this syndrome has been extensively studied both clinically and experimentally, and there is a diversity of opinion as to the sequence of events leading to this syndrome. The stomach is lined by a continuously renewed layer of gastric mucus. One study has demonstrated a decreased rate of mucus production following burn trauma in animals but no change in the chemical character of the mucus.[48] However, others have noted an altered composition of the mucus and postulate that this may be related to the development of stress ulcers.[49] Other studies have documented alterations in the amount of secretion and composition of gastric mucus following administration of aspirin or cortisone, and this has been postulated as the mechanism of drug-induced gastric injury.[50,51] Still other studies have demonstrated alterations in gastric mucus in humans following trauma.[52]

Another theory that has gained considerable support in the pathogenesis of stress ulceration is the role of gastric wall ischemia resulting from postcapillary venoconstriction or the opening of arteriovenous shunts.[53,54] Further support of this concept has been the demonstration of intestinal vasoconstriction followed by hemorrhagic intestinal necrosis after the administration of *Escherichia coli* endotoxin.[55] Other work has demonstrated that stress ulcer formation is most extensive in animals with the most extensive gastric ischemia.[56]

In addition to these factors, bile reflux into the stomach has been postulated to be important in the initiation of acute gastric ulcer and gastritis.[57–59] Corroborating this work is the finding that gastric mucosal lesions can be prevented in dogs by occluding the pylorus, thus preventing reflux.[60,61]

Perhaps the most popular theory to explain the development of stress gastritis has been the increased back-diffusion of hydrogen ion from the gastric lumen in exchange for sodium ion, leading to an autodigestion of the gastric wall.[62] A wide variety of methods have been utilized to demonstrate back-diffusion, and some of these have been unable to do so.[63,64] Other authorities feel that these differences may be methodologic in nature, but that the ability to clear a normally harmless amount of hydrochloric acid is decreased in the stress situation, and this may promote ulceration. This theory stresses that, although acid is necessary for the production of ulceration, it is not necessarily present in increased amounts.[65] This impression is supported by studies of injured patients demonstrating no clear-cut increase in the amount of acid secretion.[66] In studies of burn patients as well, no relationship between absolute levels of acid and ulcer formation has been noted.[67]

ANSWER: E.

2.9. Which of the following nonoperative treatments for stress gastritis has been associated with the best clinical results?

A. Iced saline lavage.
B. Intravenous Pitressin.
C. Intensive antacid therapy.
D. Oral cimetidine.
E. Intragastric levarterenol.

Because of the very high morbidity and mortality for various operative procedures for stress-induced gastritis, a great deal of study has been put forth to determine the ideal nonoperative management of such patients. Many modalities of treatment have been employed with varying degrees of success, but none have achieved the success reported with the instillation of large quantities of antacid into the stomach with pH monitoring. In one study, sufficient antacid buffer (Riopan) was instilled into the nasogastric tube after the stomach had been lavaged free of blood so that the resultant pH was maintained above 7.0. If the pH was lower than this, additional antacid was used during the following 15 min. Utilizing this regimen, 19 of 20 patients stopped bleeding despite the fact that they had bled an average of 4300 ml prior to antacid therapy. In each case, control of bleeding was achieved within 24 hr after complete neutralization of gastric contents. One patient did not stop bleeding and required operation; no patients rebled. Only 10 of 15 patients stopped bleeding on medical treatment with iced saline lavage and minimal quantities of antacids. The other 5 patients required operation for the control of hemorrhage, and all of these patients subsequently died.[68] In another study designed to test the efficacy of antacid titration in the prevention of stress ulceration, 100 critically ill patients were randomized between antacid titration and nasogastric suction. Only 2 of 51 patients receiving antacid prophylaxis had gastrointestinal bleeding, whereas 12 of the 49 control patients bled, a statistically significant difference. Of the 12 patients in the control group who bled, 7 were subsequently stopped with antacid treatment.[69] The main utility of intravenous Pitressin has become the control of esophageal variceal bleeding in the cirrhotic patient. Its effectiveness in other forms of upper GI tract hemorrhage is more controversial. Intra-arterial Pitressin, however, has been used with considerable success by some groups, but these results have been difficult to reproduce by others. In one study, 50 patients with gastric mucosal hemorrhage underwent angiography. Thirteen of these could not be infused with Pitressin for technical or other reasons. Of the 37 patients in whom the catheter was positioned, bleeding was controlled in 31, with rebleeding occurring in 2. Therefore, control was achieved in only 58% of patients using this modality. Despite this, this method of therapy should be considered in the poor-risk patient with stress gastritis in whom operation seems contraindicated.[70]

Another method of controlling bleeding from upper GI tract hemorrhage is the intragastric instillation of levarterenol. Perhaps 50% of the time this treatment will be successful in arresting upper GI tract hemorrhage.[71] Other methods currently being studied include gastroscopic electrocoagulation of individual bleeding points,[72] endoscopic argon-ion laser phototherapy,[73] and selective embolization of autologous clots via a distally positioned arteriographic catheter.[74]

Cimetidine, a potent drug useful in decreasing gastric acid, is currently being intensively studied in both the prevention and treatment of stress hemorrhage. Data are not yet conclusive, but it is quite possible that intravenous cimetidine may prove to be as effective as antacid treatment with pH monitoring.

ANSWER: C.

2.10. A 74-year-old man is recovering from an exploratory celiotomy for drainage of a pancreatic abscess 11 days earlier. He begins to vomit blood, and over the next 8 hr requires 6 units of blood transfused. His pulse is 120, his blood pressure 110/60, and his urine output is 60 cc in the past hour. Gastroscopy reveals multiple actively bleeding gastric ulcers. He is taken to the operating room. What is the procedure of choice to perform on this patient?

A. Vagotomy and pyloroplasty with oversewing of individual ulcers.
B. Vagotomy and antrectomy.
C. Total gastrectomy.
D. Subtotal gastrectomy.
E. Parietal cell vagotomy.

This patient presents with a typical sepsis-associated upper GI tract hemorrhage, found to be caused by multiple gastric ulcerations, a highly lethal condition with overall mortality averaging 30%–40%. Nonoperative management will be successful in the majority of cases, and as always, the decision to operate will depend upon multiple factors, but the patient's advanced age and the fact that he is still actively bleeding at the time of gastroscopy and has already required 6 units of blood all indicate that operation will be needed.

At this point, however, the surgeon is faced with numerous recommendations for optimal treatment, each of which is supported by testimony, and some by data, from the surgical literature. Vagotomy and pyloroplasty, vagotomy and antrectomy, subtotal gastrectomy, total gastrectomy, and parietal cell vagotomy all have their advocates and might be suitable under given circumstances. Each seems to have certain advantages and certain drawbacks.

Vagotomy and pyloroplasty can be performed most quickly with the lowest operative mortality, although perhaps with an increased incidence of rebleeding. Series of patients have been reported in whom this procedure has been done with a lower mortality than vagotomy and antrectomy with equal effectiveness in stopping the bleeding and equal rates of rebleeding.[75] However, other series have shown that the mortality and effectiveness for vagotomy and pyloroplasty and vagotomy and antrectomy are similar.[76] Other series comparing vagotomy and hemigastrectomy with vagotomy and pyloroplasty with oversewing of the individual bleeding points have demonstrated a clear-cut superiority for the latter, in one series with similar mortalities and only a 17% rebleeding rate.[77] A study comparing vagotomy and pyloroplasty alone with vagotomy and pyloroplasty with individual oversewing of bleeding points further noted the advantage to be derived from individual ligation of bleeding points. In the former group, 47% of patients rebled, while in the latter group this figure was 10%.[78]

Vagotomy and antrectomy, a superior operation for the long-term management of acid peptic disease culminating in duodenal ulcer, has also been advocated for stress gastritis and hemorrhage. At least one review has demonstrated that this operation can be carried out with the same mortality as vagotomy and pyloroplasty, with a rebleeding rate of only 15% compared with a rebleeding rate after vagotomy and pyloroplasty that is twice this number.[79]

Subtotal gastrectomy without vagotomy has also been used but has been associated with increased mortality rates and rebleeding in 40% to 50% of cases.[78,79] Therefore, it does not appear that this operation represents the treatment of choice in this condition. Similarly, total gastrectomy has been advocated as a definitive procedure. While it is obvious that rebleeding will not occur, it is unlikely that this operation can be performed by most practicing surgeons with the same low mortality as obtained with vagotomy and pyloroplasty. Likewise, the long-term effects of this operation on eating and digestion are more significant than the lesser procedures. It would therefore appear that this operation should be reserved for those patients who have rebled after a lesser procedure and in whom a fatal outcome is anticipated unless the bleeding can be stopped.[80] Interest in parietal cell vagotomy as treatment for hemorrhagic gastritis stems from the fact that after such a vagotomy the gastric mucosa is seen to blanch markedly in response to decreased blood flow. This operation might be shown to have some application in the future, but in view of what is presently known about the need to individually oversew larger bleeding ulcerations, and the fact that this would, of course, not be done during a parietal cell vagotomy, this operation must be considered experimental at this time.

ANSWER: A.

References

1. Boyle, J.D., Goldstein, H.: Management of pyloric obstruction. *Med. Clin. North Am.* 52:1329, 1968.
2. Kozoll, D.D., Mittelpunkt, A.L., Meyer, K.A.: Obstructing gastroduodenal ulcers: Effect of treatment on morbidity and mortality. *Arch. Surg.* 91:431, 1965.
3. Taylor, H.: The nonsurgical treatment of perforated peptic ulcer. *Gastroenterology* 33:353, 1957.
4. Jordan, P.H.: Elective operations for duodenal ulcer. *N. Engl. J. Med.* 287:1329, 1972.
5. Herrington, J.L., Sawyers, J.L., Scott, H.W.: A 25 year experience with vagotomy–antrectomy. *Arch. Surg.* 106:469, 1973.
6. Palumbo, L.T., Sharpe, W.S.: Distal antrectomy with vagectomy for duodenal ulcer: Results in 611 cases. *Ann. Surg.* 182:610, 1975.
7. Moore, F.D.: Operative treatment of duodenal ulcer: Transatlantic data and opinion. *N. Engl. J. Med.* 290:906, 1974.
8. Postlethwait, R.W.: Five year follow-up results of operations for duodenal ulcers. *Surg. Gynecol. Obstet.* 137:387, 1973.
9. Dwight, R.W., Schimmel, E.M., O'Hara, E.T., Hechtman, H.B., Williams, L.F., Vollman, R.W., Maselli, J.P., Johnson, W.C., Nabsath, D.C.: Controlled study of the surgical treatment of duodenal ulcer. *Am. J. Surg.* 129:374, 1975.
10. Eisenberg, M.M., Woodward, E.R., Carson, T.J., Dragstedt, L.R.: Vagotomy and drainage procedure for duodenal ulcer: The results of 10 years experience. *Ann. Surg.* 170:317, 1969.
11. McGregor, D.B., Savage, L.E., McVay, C.B.: Vagotomy and drainage for elective treatment of peptic ulcer. *Surg. Gynecol. Obstet.* 146:349, 1978.
12. Farmer, D.A., Harrower, H.W., Smithwick, R.H.: The choice of surgery in peptic ulcer disease. *Am. J. Surg.* 120:295, 1970.
13. Jordan, P.H.: Parietal cell vagotomy without drainage for treatment of duodenal ulcer. *Arch. Surg.* 111:370, 1976.
14. Amdrup, E., Jensen, H.-E., Johnston, D., Walker, B.E., Goligher, J.C.: Clinical results of parietal cell vagotomy (highly selective vagotomy) two to four years after operation. *Ann. Surg.* 180:279, 1974.
15. Hallenbeck, G.A., Gleysteen, J.J., Aldrete, J.S., Slaughter, R.L.: Proximal gastric vagotomy: Effects of two operative techniques on clinical and gastric secretory results. *Ann. Surg.* 184:435, 1976.
16. Wastell, C., Wilson, T, Pigott, H.: Proximal gastric vagotomy. *Proc. R. Soc. Med.* 67:1183, 1974.
17. Kronborg, O., Madsen, P.: A controlled randomized trial of highly selective vagotomy versus selective vagotomy and pyloroplasty in the treatment of duodenal ulcer. *Gut* 16:268, 1975.
18. Amdrup, E., Andersen, D., Jensen, H.-E.: Parietal cell (highly selective or proximal gastric) vagotomy for peptic ulcer disease. *World J. Surg.* 1:19, 1977.
19. Kurzweg, F.T., Danna, S.J., Daron, P.B., Williamson, J.W.: The management of perforated duodenal ulcer. *Surg. Gynecol. Obstet.* 135:365, 1972.
20. Jordan, G.L., DeBakey, M.E., Duncan, J.M.: Surgical management of perforated peptic ulcer. *Ann. Surg.* 179:628, 1974.
21. Wangensteen, S.L., Wray, R.C., Goldent, G.T.: Perforated duodenal ulcer. *Am. J. Surg.* 123:538, 1972.
22. Jarrett, F., Donaldson, G.A.: The ulcer diathesis in perforated duodenal ulcer disease. *Am. J. Surg.* 123:406, 1972.

23. Skovgaard, S.: Late results of perforated duodenal ulcer treated by simple suture. *World J. Surg.* 1:521, 1977.
24. Jordan, P.H., Korompai, F.L.: Evolvement of a new treatment for perforated duodenal ulcer. *Surg. Gynecol. Obstet.* 142:391, 1976.
25. Sawyers, J.L., Herrington, J.L.: Perforated duodenal ulcer managed by proximal gastric vagotomy and suture plication. *Ann. Surg.* 185:656, 1977.
26. Read, R.C., Thompson, B.W.: Gastric outlet obstruction after omentopexy for perforated "acute" and "chronic" duodenal ulceration. *Am. J. Surg.* 130:682, 1975.
27. Tompkins, R.K., Kraft, A.R., Zimmerman, E., Lichtenstein, J.E., Zollinger, R.M.: Clinical and biochemical evidence of increased gallstone formation after complete vagotomy. *Surgery* 71:196, 1972.
28. Sapala, M.A., Sapala, J.A., Resto Soto, A.D., Bouwman, D.L.: Cholelithiasis following subtotal gastric resection with truncal vagotomy. *Surg. Gynecol. Obstet.* 148:36, 1979.
29. Mahmud, K., Ripley, D., Swaim, W.R., Doscherholmen, A.: Hematologic complications of partial gastrectomy. *Ann. Surg.* 177:432, 1973.
30. Wheldon, E.J., Venables, C.W., Johnston, I.D.A.: Late metabolic sequelae of vagotomy and gastroenterostomy. *Lancet* 1:437, 1970.
31. Dibenedetto, A., Diamond, P., Essig, H.C.: Tuberculosis following subtotal gastrectomy. *Surg. Gynecol. Obstet.* 134:586, 1972.
32. Allison, S.T.: Pulmonary tuberculosis after subtotal gastrectomy. *N. Engl. J. Med.* 252:862, 1955.
33. Steiger, Z., Nickel, W.O., Shannon, G.J., Nedwicki, E.G., Higgins, R.F.: Pulmonary tuberculosis after gastric resection. *Am. J. Surg.* 131:668, 1976.
34. Pickleman, J.R., Evans, L.S., Kane, J.M., Freeark, R.J.: Tuberculosis after jejunoileal bypass for obesity. *J.A.M.A.* 234:744, 1975.
35. Morgenstern, L., Yamakawa, M., Seltzer, D.: Carcinoma of the gastric stump. *Am. J. Surg.* 125:29, 1973.
36. Eberlein, T.J., Lorenzo, F.V., Webster, M.W.: Gastric carcinoma following operation for peptic ulcer disease. *Ann. Surg.* 187:251, 1978.
37. Domellof, L., Eriksson, S., Janunger, K-G.: Late precancerous changes in carcinoma of the gastric stump after Billroth I resection. *Am. J. Surg.* 132:26, 1976.
38. VanHeerden, J.A., Phillips, S.F., Adson, M.A., McIlrath, D.C.: Postoperative reflux gastritis. *Am. J. Surg.* 129:82, 1975.
39. Gadacz, T.R., Zuidema, G.D.: Bile acid composition in patients with and without symptoms of postoperative reflux gastritis. *Am. J. Surg.* 135:48, 1978.
40. Berardi, R.S., Sirrospour, D., Ruiz, R., Carnes, W., Devaiah, K.A., Peterson, C., Becknell, W.E., Olivencia, J.: Alkaline reflux gastritis: A study in 40 postoperative duodenal ulcer patients. *Am. J. Surg. 132:552, 1976.*
41. Max, M.H., West, B., Knutson, C.O.: Evaluation of postoperative gastroduodenal symptoms: Endoscopy or upper gastrointestinal roentgenography? *Surgery* 86:578, 1979.
42. Bushkin, F.L., Wickbom, G., DeFord, J.W., Woodward, E.R.: Postoperative alkaline reflux gastritis. *Surg. Gynecol. Obstet.* 138:933, 1974.
43. Herrington, J.L., Sawyers, J.L., Whitehead, W.A.: Surgical management of reflux gastritis. *Ann. Surg.* 180:526, 1974.
44. Drapanas, T., Bethea, M.: Reflux gastritis following gastric surgery. *Ann. Surg.* 179:618, 1974.
45. Walsh, J.H., Grossman, M.I.: Gastrin. *N. Engl. J. Med.* 292:1324, 1975.
46. Menguy, R.: Pathophysiology of peptic ulcer. *Am. J. Surg.* 120:282, 1970.
47. Trudeau, W.L., McGuigan, J.E.: Relations between serum gastrin levels and rates of gastric hydrochloric acid secretion. *N. Engl. J. Med.* 284:408, 1971.

48. O'Neill, J.A., Ritchey, C.R., Mason, A.D., Villarreal, Y.: Effect of thermal burns on gastric mucous production. *Surg. Gynecol. Obstet.* 131:29, 1970.
49. Robert, A., Bayer, R.B., Nezamis, J.E.: Gastric mucous content during development of ulcers in fasting rats. *Gastroenterology* 45:740, 1963.
50. Menguy, R., Masters, Y.F.: Effect of cortisone on mucoprotein secretion by gastric antrum of dogs: Pathogenesis of steroid ulcer. *Surgery* 54:19, 1963.
51. Menguy, R., Desbaillets, L.: The gastric mucous barrier: Influence of protein bound carbohydrate in mucous on the rate of proteolysis of gastric mucous. *Ann. Surg.* 168:475, 1968.
52. Lucas, C.E., Sugawa, C., Friend, W., Walt, A.J.: Therapeutic implications of distributed gastric physiology in patients with stress ulcerations. *Am. J. Surg.* 123:25, 1972.
53. Nylander, G., Olerud, S.: The vascular pattern of the gastric mucosa of the rat following vagotomy. *Surg. Gynecol. Obstet.* 112:475, 1961.
54. Pruitt, B.A., Foley, F.D., Moncrief, J.A.: Curling's ulcer: A clinical pathologic study of 323 cases. *Ann. Surg.* 172:523, 1970.
55. Lillehei, R.C., MacLean, L.D.: The intestinal factor in irreversible endotoxin shock. *Ann. Surg.* 148:513, 1958.
56. Mersereau, W.A., Hinchey, E.J.: Effect of gastric acidity on gastric ulceration induced by hemorrhage in the rat utilizing a gastric chamber technique. *Gastroenterology* 64:1130, 1973.
57. Delaney, J.P., Cheng, J.W.B., Butler, B.A., Ritchie, W.P.: Gastric ulcer and regurgitation gastritis. *Gut* 11:715, 1970.
58. Menguy, R., Max, M.H.: Influence of bile on the canine gastric–antral mucosa. *Am. J. Surg.* 119:177, 1970.
59. Rhodes, J., Barnado, D.E., Phillips, S.F., Rovelstad, R.A., Hofmann, A.F.: Increased reflux of bile into the stomach of patients with gastric ulcer. *Gastroenterology* 57:241, 1969.
60. Bounous, G., Sutherland, G., McArdle, A.H., Gurd, F.N.: The prophylactic use of an "elemental" diet in experimental hemorrhagic shock and intestinal ischemia. *Ann. Surg.* 166:312, 1967.
61. Guilbert, J., Bounous, G., Gurd, F.N.: Role of intestinal chyme in the pathogenesis of gastric ulceration following experimental hemorrhagic shock. *J. Trauma* 9:723, 1969.
62. Skillman, J.J., Gould, S.A., Chung, R.S.K., Silen, W.: The gastric mucosal barrier: Clinical and experimental studies in critically ill and normal man and in the rabbit. *Ann. Surg.* 172:564, 1970.
63. Moody, F.G., Aldrete, J.: Hydrogen permeability of canine gastric secretory epithelium during the formation of acute superficial erosions. *Surgery* 70:154, 1971.
64. Ritchie, W.B., Fischer, R.P.: Studies on the pathogenesis of "stress ulcer": Electrical potential difference and ionic fluxes across canine gastric mucosa during hemorrhagic shock. *J. Surg. Res.* 3:173, 1972.
65. Silen, W.: New concepts of the gastric mucosal barrier. *Am. J. Surg.* 133:8, 1977.
66. Howard, J.M.: Gastric and salivary secretion following injury. *Ann. Surg.* 141:342, 1955.
67. O'Neill, J.A.: The influence of thermal burns on gastric acid secretion. *Surgery* 67:267, 1970.
68. Simonian, S.J., Stratoudakis, A., Lawrence, M., Mungas, J., Blackstone, M.O.: Nonsurgical control of massive acute gastric mucosal hemorrhage with antacid neutralization of gastric content. *Surg. Clin. North Am.* 56:21, 1976.
69. Hastings, P.R., Skillman, J.J., Bushnell, L.S., Silen, W.: Antacid titration in the prevention of acute gastrointestinal bleeding. *N. Engl. J. Med.* 298:1041, 1978.
70. Athanasoulis, C.A., Baum, S., Waltman, A.C., Ring, E.J., Imbembo, A., Vander Salm,

T.J.: Control of acute gastric mucosal hemorrhage: Intra-arterial infusion of posterior pituitary extract. *N. Engl. J. Med.* 290:597, 1974.
71. LeVeen, H.H., Diaz, C., Wynkoop, B.-J., Piccone, V.A., Yarnoz, M.D., Langsam, A.A., Nelson, J.H., Pedowitz, W.J., Belfasky, R.B., Falk, G.: Control of gastrointestinal bleeding. *Am. J. Surg.* 123:154, 1972.
72. Sugawa, C., Shier, M., Lucas, C.E., Walt, A.J.: Electrocoagulation of bleeding in the upper part of the gastrointestinal tract. *Arch. Surg.* 110:975, 1975.
73. Yellin, A.E., Dwyer, R.M., Craig, J.R., Bass, M., Cherlow, J.: Endoscopic argon-ion laser phototherapy of bleeding gastric lesions. *Arch. Surg.* 111:750, 1976.
74. Eisenberg, H., Steer, M.L.: The nonoperative treatment of massive pyloroduodenal hemorrhage by retracted autologous clot embolization. *Surgery* 79:414, 1976.
75. Kirtley, J.A., Scott, H.W., Sawyers, J.L., Graves, H.A., Lawler, M.R.: The surgical management of stress ulcers. *Ann. Surg.* 169:801, 1969.
76. Cody, H.S., Wichern, W.A.: Choice of operation for acute gastric mucosal hemorrhage: Report of 36 cases and review of literature. *Am. J. Surg.* 134:322, 1977.
77. Stremple, J.F., Elliot, D.W.: Hemorrhage due to diffuse erosive gastritis. *Arch. Surg.* 110:606, 1975.
78. Wilson, W.S., Gadacz, T., Olcott, C., Blaisdell, F.W.: Superficial gastric erosions: Response to surgical treatment. *Am. J. Surg.* 126:133, 1973.
79. Drapanas, T., Woolverton, W.C., Reeder, J.W., Reed, R.L., Weichert, R.F.: Experiences with surgical management of acute gastric mucosal hemorrhage: A unified concept in pathophysiology. *Ann. Surg.* 173:628, 1971.
80. Menguy, R., Gadacz, T., Zajtchuk, R.: The surgical management of acute gastric mucosal bleeding. *Arch. Surg.* 99:198, 1969.

3
PORTAL HYPERTENSION

3.1. A 60-year-old alcoholic man presents to the emergency room with hematemesis and melena. He is hypotensive and appears mildly jaundiced. Endoscopy reveals bleeding esophageal varices. Which of the following treatments should not be considered in this acutely bleeding patient?

A. Side-to-side portacaval shunt.
B. End-to-side portacaval shunt.
C. Mesocaval shunt.
D. Distal splenorenal shunt.
E. Transthoracic ligation of varices.

Many patients who bleed fram esophageal varices turn out to be poor candidates for any porta-systemic shunting procedure. In general, the presence of jaundice, significant ascites, encephalopathy, and advanced muscle wasting all indicate a poor outlook. In addition, biochemical evidence of clotting abnormalities, extreme hypoalbuminemia, and evidence of alcoholic hepatitis are likewise relative contraindications to any shunting procedure that would tend to lessen the already compromised hepatic reserve.[1] While it is recognized that ideally it would be preferable to stop the hemorrhage and medically manage these patients for a period of time, correcting clotting and nutritional abnormalities, before embarking upon an elective porta-systemic shunt, this goal is infrequently achieved, and perhaps only 10%–20% of bleeding cirrhotic patients will become eligible for an elective procedure.[2]

Because of these problems, following resuscitation and treatment of the bleeding with either a Sengstaken tube or systemic Pitressin, various operations have been advocated in the acutely bleeding patient. Orloff was able to control the hemorrhage with Pitressin in 94% of his patients and then performed an emergency portacaval shunt, usually of the side-to-side variety, with permanent control of variceal bleeding in 96% of the survivors. The operative mortality rate was approximately 50%, and the 7-year survival rate was 42%.[2] Other large series of patients have been published advocating the performance of portacaval shunt in these circumstances. The main controversies have revolved about whether an end-to-side or side-to-side shunt is preferable.[3,4] In conclusion, there is no question that portacaval shunts can bring about permanent cessation of variceal hemorrhage, but whether or not the type of shunt influences this result is moot. The major controversy has been, rather, whether a portacaval shunt or some alternative shunt should be employed. The technically easiest shunt is the interposition mesocaval shunt. This can be performed with a low operative mortality, moderate incidence of encephalopathy, and good long-term control of bleeding.[5-7]

Ligation of varices by a transthoracic approach has been advocated by various authorities. This operation brings about a prompt cessation of hemorrhage in nearly all patients but has been associated with significant mortality rates. Also, many of these patients go on to rehemorrhage in the future, and therefore have to be considered for elective porta-systemic shunting.[8,9] Survival of over 50% of patients has been documented, with the expected better results in patients with good hepatic reserve.

The distal splenorenal (Warren) shunt is gaining increasing popularity as the porta-systemic shunt of choice for the cirrhotic patient whose varices have ceased bleeding. It has not been routinely utilized for actively bleeding patients, as most groups performing these shunts have insisted upon an extensive preoperative investigation of these patients, including liver function tests, liver biopsies, and portal angiography. Also, because this shunt is technically more difficult to construct that the other forms of portasystemic shunts, its usefulness in the acutely bleeding patient is limited.

ANSWER: D.

3.2. Which of the following problems does not accompany the use of a Sengstaken–Blakemore tube inserted for balloon tamponade of bleeding esophageal varices?

A. Aspiration.
B. Asphyxia.
C. Esophageal rupture.
D. Rebleeding upon balloon deflation.
E. Vagal-induced bradycardia.

Unfortunately, none of the operative or nonoperative methods of stopping hemorrhage from esophageal varices are uniformly effective and free of lifethreatening complications. Emergency porta-systemic shunting, direct ligation of the esophageal varices, transendoscopic injection of sclerosing agents into varices, systemic Pitressin, and balloon tamponade all have been used successfully by certain groups.

Balloon tamponade using a Sengstaken–Blakemore tube or a modification of it has the advantage of ready availability and simplicity. Basically, the tube consists of a rounded gastric balloon that impinges on the cardia of the stomach and a longer and flatter esophageal balloon that when inflated fits the contour of the esophagus. After insertion into the stomach, the gastric balloon is blown up and traction is applied on the tube as it exits from the nose. This upward pressure helps tamponade any gastric varices and also fixes the tube in place. Following inflation of the esophageal balloon, bleeding ceases in 80%–90% of the patients.[10,11] In most protocols, the balloon is left inflated 24–48 hr and then deflated and left in place a further 24 hr. At this time, the tube is removed if bleeding has not recurred. Bleeding recurs perhaps 20%–30% of the time, necessitating reinflation of the balloon.[12]

Complications from use of the tube, however, have been noted frequently. Esophageal laceration or perforation from overdistention of the balloon, aspiration of gastric contents or blood, and asphyxia from deflation of the gastric balloon and riding up of the esophageal balloon to occlude the airway have all been described. Several series report approximately a 9% rate of major complications resulting from the use of the tube.[10,12] However, the most critical report of the potential dangers associated with the Sengstaken–Blakemore tube came from Conn and Simpson, who noted major complications in over one third of patients and a mortality rate of approximately 20%. These authors concluded that balloon tamponade should be used only when other methods of treatment had failed.[13] However, it is likely that these figures are exaggerated and could be lowered by rigid adherence to a prescribed protocol. However, as any one physician rarely sees many of these patients, experience is likely to be limited, and it would prove difficult to gain the expertise necessary to achieve these optimal results.

ANSWER: E.

3.3. Which of the following side effects is not noted during the infusion of Vasopressin (Pitressin) for the control of bleeding esophageal varices?

A. Decreased cardiac output.
B. Tachycardia.
C. Hypertension.
D. Cardiac arrhythmias.
E. Angina pectoris.

Vasopressin is a potent vasoconstrictor that has been found to be very effective in arresting hemorrhage from bleeding esophageal varices. Its mechanism of action appears to be the vasoconstriction of prehepatic splanchnic vessels, resulting in a reduced flow into the portal venous system and therefore a reduced portal venous pressure.[14,15] The drug has been administered as an IV bolus, as an IV infusion, and by selective infusion into the superior mesenteric artery via an arteriogram catheter. When a bolus is utilized, 20 units of vasopressin are injected. When an infusion is utilized, 0.4 units/min is infused until the bleeding ceases; this is followed by a 24-hr infusion of 0.2 units/min and a further 24-hr infusion of 0.1 unit/min. Data are somewhat conflicting with regard to the effectiveness of these various regimens. In one study, approximately 50% of variceal bleeders were stopped with intra-arterial administration and an intravenous infusion.[14] Orloff and colleagues have noted greater than 90% effectiveness for the drug when administered as an IV bolus, and Nussbaum and colleagues noted that intra-arterial administration was 97% effective in their carefully done study.[2,16]

Regardless of the route of infusion, vasopressin definitely reduces portal venous pressure and portal blood flow.[17] Because of the problems of intra-arterial infusion, including the need for special equipment and personnel, delay in administering the drug, and complications caused by the arteriographic catheter, attention has focused on the relative effectiveness and complication rates of the various routes of administration. Vasopressin causes a significant decrease in coronary blood flow and cardiac output along with a bradycardia and hypertension. Cardiac arrhythmias can be noted in patients with underlying coronary artery disease, and angina and myocardial infarction can be precipitated by administration of the drug.[18] Several studies have demonstrated that the cardiovascular effects and the effects on the portal circulation are equal with intra-arterial administration or constant IV infusion of the drug.[17,19] There are, however, conflicting data regarding side effects secondary to the two intravenous routes of administration. Some studies have demonstrated that cardiovascular abnormalities are decreased utilizing vasopressin as an infusion,[15] while other studies have maintained that a bolus of the drug yields fewer complications, presumably because a smaller total dose is used.[20] However, the consensus at this time appears to favor the continuous IV infusion of the drug. For those patients who manifest significant cardiovascular complications, there is a suggestion that administration of isoproterenol administered along with the vasopressin can eliminate many of the cardiovascular effects.[18]

ANSWER: B.

3.4. The chief advantage of the distal splenorenal (Warren) shunt appears to be:

A. A decreased incidence of postoperative encephalopathy.
B. A shortened operating time.
C. Technical ease of the operation.
D. Improvement of hypersplenism.
E. The absence of postoperative ascites.

Because of dissatisfaction with conventional porta-systemic shunting procedures in terms of patient survival, incidence of rebleeding, and incidence of postoperative liver failure and encephalopathy, Warren introduced the selective distal splenorenal shunt. The purpose of this shunt is to decompress the gastroesophageal varices by shunting blood from them selectively through the short gastric vessels into the spleen, from which porta-systemic decompression is accomplished by a splenorenal shunt. An equally important goal is felt to be maintenance of portal vein perfusion to the liver to avoid postoperative liver failure and encephalopathy. It was hypothesized that ideally this procedure should grant the best of both worlds, namely protection against further rebleeding and maintenance of liver function.

To a large degree, these expectations have been borne out. Angiographically documented shunt patency rates are approximately 95% in 58 patients reported by Warren.[21] In addition, varices disappear in most patients as determined by upper GI tract examinations,[21] but in one other study of 26 patients the varices persisted but were of smaller size.[22] Additionally, pre- and postoperative wedged hepatic vein pressures have been measured and found to be similar, indicating maintenance of portal perfusion.[21] In a study of 24 patients with hematologic evidence of hypersplenism, it was noted that the white blood cell count rose an average of 1000 cells/mm^3, while the platelet count increased by more than 40,000 platelets/mm^3.[23]

However, factors limiting the widespread acceptance of the distal splenorenal shunt have been a fear of an excessive operative mortality rate and the alleged excessive difficulty of the procedure. Warren himself noted the deaths of 7 of his first 12 patients, a 58% surgical mortality rate, but his current operative mortality rate is about 7%.[21] Another series of 66 patients undergoing an elective shunt had no deaths within 30 days and a high postoperative survival of patients.[24] There is no doubt that it is a technically more difficult shunt than some of its competitors and that at least initially in any series of patients, the operating times are prolonged.

The shunt does accomplish its aims, however. Rebleeding has been uncommon, being noted in only 3.7% of one series.[22] Warren himself has noted that rebleeding can occur and for this reason regards portal-azygous disconnection an integral part of the procedure. He has had no patient rebleed who had a patent shunt.[25] Encephalopathy has been noted significantly less frequently with this shunt. In one randomized study comparing distal splenorenal shunt with mesocaval shunts, encephalopathy was seen much less commonly after the former operation.[26] Postoperative ascites has been noted in the majority of patients. In his study of over 100 patients treated by this shunt, Warren noted easily controlled ascites in many patients. However, six patients were difficult to manage, and three of these eventually required insertion of a LeVeen peritoneo-jugular shunt.[27]

On a more negative note, Vang has noted more difficulties with the Warren shunt. Of 25 patients whom he treated, 10 died from liver failure, 6 rebled, and hypersplenism was not improved. Only two of his patients were without encephalopathy.[28] Therefore, it is obvious that further long-range studies are needed to verify the results of this shunting procedure, but at this time it appears that it may well be the procedure of choice for the patient who has suffered a variceal hemorrhage, has easily controllable ascites, and can be prepared for an elective operation.

ANSWER: A.

3.5. A 9-year-old boy with documented portal vein thrombosis has had two esophageal variceal hemorrhages in the past 4 years. He presents with melena and orthostatic hypotension. After 2 units of transfused blood, his vital signs are stable and the bleeding has ceased. Proper management at this time should consist of:

A. Splenectomy.
B. Portacaval shunt.
C. Continued observation.
D. Distal splenorenal shunt.
E. Splenorenal shunt.

This child presents with esophageal varices secondary to portal vein obstruction. These children usually have normal liver function, and some give a history of an antecedent omphalitis as the probable etiology of the venous thrombosis. Splenomegaly is the rule, and pancytopenia is frequently noted. Several large series of such patients have been published, but there is no current consensus as to treatment recommendations.[29-31]

A number of general trends seem to be evolving, however, and these can guide the clinician called upon to care for one of these children. Portasystemic shunts have proven very difficult to fashion, probably because of the small caliber of the veins in children. This has led to shunt thrombosis and rebleeding in approximately 50% of these children.[29,31] Other procedures such as splenectomy alone, splenic transposition into the chest, esophagogastrectomy, and variceal ligations all have been tried with a uniform lack of success. In general, it has been noted that repetitive variceal hemorrhage is the rule, and that these hemorrhages are rarely sufficiently severe to endanger the life of the child. Most will stop spontaneously, although some will require balloon tamponade or Pitressin administration. One series of 69 children with portal vein occlusion has been published in which the group suffered 338 variceal hemorrhages. Fifty-three of these children underwent 164 operations, pointing out the difficulties in definitive surgical treatment of this condition. The only deaths in the series were in the operated group. Sixteen other children suffered multiple hemorrhages but underwent no operation, and there were no deaths in this group.[29]

On the basis of these data, it would seem that the wisest course of action in the child who has normal liver function and a portal vein thrombosis with secondary variceal hemorrhage would be transfusion during the acute hemorrhage, with surgery reserved only for those children who fail to stop bleeding. The operation of choice is debatable, but in at least two series a mesocaval shunt has proven to be more satisfactory than any other form of porta-systemic decompression.[29,31]

ANSWER: C.

3.6. A 23-year-old woman who has been taking birth control pills for 3 years presents with a 1-month history of increasing abdominal pain and ascites. Hepatomegaly is present and liver function tests are abnormal. The test most likely to yield a definite diagnosis in this patient would be:

A. Liver scan.
B. Pancreas scan.
C. Hepatic arteriogram.
D. Endoscopic retrograde pancreatography.
E. Inferior vena cavagram.

A Budd–Chiari syndrome is confirmed; treatment should consist of:

A. Anticoagulants.
B. Diuretics and salt restriction.
C. End-to-side portacaval shunt.
D. Side-to-side portacaval shunt.
E. LeVeen shunt.

The clinical disorder caused by occlusion of the hepatic venous outflow with or without inferior vena cava obstruction is known as the Budd–Chiari syndrome. Over 500 cases have been documented in the medical literature. The disease is idiopathic in the majority of patients, but various entities such as polycythemia vera, tumorous invasion of the inferior vena cava and hepatic veins, ingestion of oral contraceptives, trauma, sickle cell anemia, and leukemia have been noted.[32] In addition, membranous obstruction of the inferior vena cava just below the level of the diaphragm has been reported frequently from Japan, and appears to be a common cause of the syndrome in that country.[33]

The clinical course of the syndrome may be rapid or chronic, leading to death from liver failure within a matter of weeks or death from liver failure with or without esophageal varices months to years later. Most series document the usual fatal outcome of this entity.[32,34] Many patients with this disease are not diagnosed until autopsy is performed, but with the availability of good-quality inferior vena cavagrams with selective hepatic venous injections, the diagnosis can be made with certainty in the majority of cases. The incidence of inferior vena cava occlusion accompanying hepatic vein thrombosis is much higher in Japan,[33] whereas series of patients from the United States have shown approximately 20% of patients to have this accompanying problem.[35] It is important to document the presence of caval obstruction, however, as attempts to perform portacaval shunts will be doomed to failure if this abnormality exists.[32,36]

Treatment of this condition has proven to be most difficult. There are scattered reports of successful treatment using only diuretics and salt restriction with or without anticoagulation, but these results seem quite inconstant. A recent series of six patients treated by side-to-side portacaval shunt noted excellent long-term results in five of these patients, with a disappearance of all clinical signs and symptoms and restoration of hepatic morphological changes towards normal.[32] The same authors induced hepatic venous obstruction in dogs, and once again noted a successful outcome in those dogs treated with side-to-side portacaval shunt. In view of this, it would appear at this time that any partially-diverting shunt such as a side-to-side portacaval shunt or a mesocaval shunt, either direct or as an H-graft would be acceptable. The other treatment that might prove successful is the LeVeen peritoneo-jugular shunt. This has been used in at least 18 reported patients with Budd–Chiari syndrome, with successful results in 17.[32] Other treatments such as splenic transposition into the left pleural space[37] and streptokinase therapy during the acute phase of the illness have been attempted,[38–39] but experience with such methods is limited at this time, and it would appear that until more data is available, side-to-side portacaval shunt is the treatment of choice.

ANSWERS: E; D.

3.7. A 46-year-old alcoholic man who has had three documented bouts of acute pancreatitis presents to the emergency room vomiting blood. Endoscopy reveals esophageal and gastric varices. Hemorrhage continues despite intravenous Pitressin administration, and celiotomy is performed. A normal liver is noted, along with a markedly enlarged spleen and a dilated gastroepiploic vein. Treatment should consist of:

A. Distal splenorenal shunt.
B. Splenorenal shunt.
C. Portacaval shunt.
D. Splenectomy.
E. Mesocaval shunt.

This patient presents with the classic findings suggestive of portal hypertension secondary to extrahepatic left-sided venous occlusion. Classically, splenic vein thrombosis follows an episode of pancreatitis. This leads to alternate venous collaterals from the spleen via the short gastric and gastroepiploic vessels, leading to gastric and esophageal varices. Although documentation of this entity has been sparse, it is obvious that it is more common than is usually appreciated. In one study of 20 patients with chronic pancreatitis studied by splenoportography, 9 patients had splenic vein thrombosis. Five of these patients had neither splenomegaly nor GI bleeding at the time of the report.[40] Despite its rarity, recognition of this syndrome is most important because the proper treatment of such patients consists merely of splenectomy. This will decompress the localized gastric and esophageal varices and rebleeding will not occur. Failure to appreciate this might lead one to perform a portacaval shunt, with the ensuing failure to decompress the localized gastric and splenic varices and ultimate rebleeding.[41,42] Figure 3-1 illustrates the occluded splenic vein and resulting collaterals that give rise to varices.

ANSWER: D.

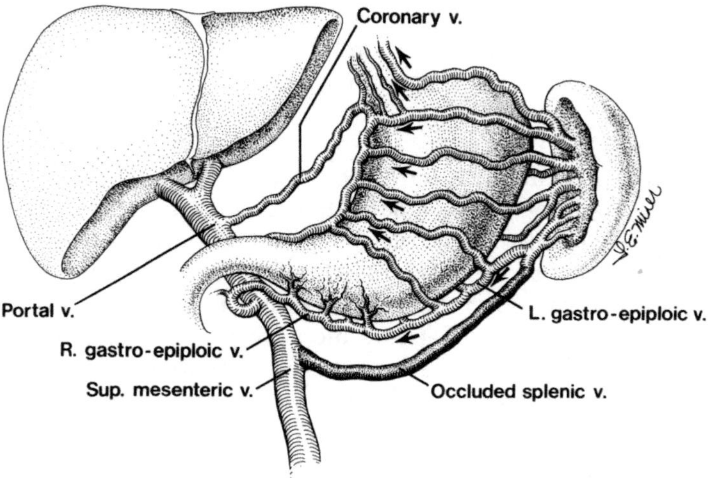
Coronary v.
Portal v.
R. gastro-epiploic v.
Sup. mesenteric v.
L. gastro-epiploic v.
Occluded splenic v.

Figure 3-1

3.8. A 45-year-old alcoholic patient has tense ascites and is unable to get out of bed because of it. On a low-salt diet and diuretics, he loses no weight. Laboratory tests are as follows: hemoglobin, 12.0 g%; WBC, 6400 cells/mm^3; prothrombin time, normal; bilirubin, 2.3 mg%; BUN, 70 mg%; and creatinine, 3.6 mg%. Treatment should consist of:

A. Distal splenorenal shunt.
B. Mesocaval shunt.
C. LeVeen peritoneo-jugular shunt.
D. End-to-side portacaval shunt.
E. Side-to-side portacaval shunt.

This man presents with intractable ascites that is diet- and diuretic-resistant. The outlook for such patients is poor, with most of them dying within weeks to months of the onset of treatment.[43] As a consequence of the liver failure and ascites, decreased renal perfusion and increased salt retention occur, leading to the hepato-renal syndrome. Diuretics tend to worsen this condition by leading to increasing dehydration and prerenal azotemia. LeVeen recently described a peritoneo-jugular shunt that has been quite successful in controlling the ascites. Basically, the shunt consists of a one-way valve placed in the peritoneal cavity, with an exit tube that is tunneled subcutaneously in a cephalad direction and then inserted into the superior vena cava via either the internal or external jugular veins. The valve is opened whenever the intra-abdominal pressure exceeds central venous pressure by 3 to 5 cm of water.[43,44]

Once the shunt is in place and functioning, a rapid reduction in weight and abdominal girth occurs, accompanied by a markedly increased urinary output and urinary sodium clearance. Along with this, the BUN and creatinine decrease, as does the hematocrit, owing to hemodilution.[43,45] In addition, the serum aldosterone level decreases following shunt insertion, and it has been assumed that increased aldosterone and perhaps renin levels are partially responsible for this syndrome.[43,46]

Not all patients with intractable ascites are candidates for LeVeen shunt insertion, however. Shunt placement is contraindicated in those patients who have infected ascitic fluid or severe congestive heart failure that is not reversible by standard medications. Heart failure would tend to raise the central venous pressure to such a high level that a pressure gradient could never be achieved. In addition, the patient with active alcoholic hepatitis or a bilirubin level of over 10 mg% owing to hepatocellular dysfunction is a poor candidate, because most of these patients will lapse into liver failure postoperatively and die.[43] Many complications have been noted following LeVeen shunt insertion, and these should be looked for. A disseminated intravascular coagulation picture has been noted in some patients, manifested by a hemorrhagic diathesis.[43,47] Treatment of this complication consists of occluding the shunt tubing, administering fresh frozen plasma, and in certain cases instituting heparin therapy. If the problem perists or recurs when the shunt is reopened, most likely the shunt will have to be removed. Other complications include congestive heart failure from the fluid overload. This can usually be treated with digitalis and diuretic preparations. Ascitic leaks at the abdominal insertion site and infected shunts can also occur; in the latter instance, removal of the shunt will be necessary. In addition to these problems, perhaps 25% or more of patients with shunts will have some form of shunt malfunction owing either to malpositioning of the venous portion in the right antrium or superior vena cava, or to kinking or clotting of the tube. However, despite all these problems, the LeVeen peritoneo-venous shunt represents a unique and successful solution to a previously fatal problem. Several series of patients have now been followed for over two years following LeVeen shunts, and they continue to do well.[43,44]

ANSWER: C.

References

1. Orloff, M.J., Duguay, L.R., Kosta, L.D.: Criteria for selection of patients for emergency portacaval shunt. *Am. J. Surg.* 134:146, 1977.
2. Orloff, M.J., Charters, A.C., Chandler, J.G., Condon, J.K., Grambort, D.E., Modafferi, T.R., Levin, S.E., Brown, N.B., Sviokla, S.C., Knox, D.G.: Portacaval shunt as emergency procedure in unselected patients with alcoholic cirrhosis. *Surg. Gynecol. Obstet.* 141:59, 1975.
3. Bismuth, H., Franco, D., Hepp, J.: Portal-systemic shunt in hepatic cirrhosis: Does the type of shunt decisively influence the clinical result? *Ann. Surg.* 179:209, 1974.
4. Turcotte, J.G., Wallin, V.W., Child, C.G.: End-to-side versus side-to-side portacaval shunts in patients with hepatic cirrhosis. *Am. J. Surg.* 117:108, 1969.
5. Drapanas, T., LoCicero, J., Dowling, J.B.: Hemodynamics of the interposition mesocaval shunt. *Ann. Surg.* 181:523, 1975.
6. Graziano, J.L., Sullivan, H.J.: Portal decompression: Clinical experience with the "H" graft. *Ann. Surg.* 178:209, 1973.
7. Reichle, F.A., Fahmy, W.F., Golsorkhi, M.: Prospective comparative clinical trial with distal splenorenal and mesocaval shunts. *Am. J. Surg.* 137:13, 1979.
8. Ottinger, L.W., Moncure, A.C.: Transthoracic ligation of bleeding esophageal varices in patients with intrahepatic portal obstruction. *Ann. Surg.* 179:35, 1974.
9. Wirthlin, L.S., Linton, R.R., Ellis, D.S.: Transthoracoesophageal ligation of bleeding esophageal varices: A reappraisal. *Arch. Surg.* 109:688, 1974.
10. Hermann, R.E., Traul, D.: Experience with the Sengstaken–Blakemore tube for bleeding esophageal varices. *Surg. Gynecol. Obstet.* 130:879, 1970.
11. Pitcher, J.L.: Safety and effectiveness of the modified Sengstaken–Blakemore tube: A prospective study. *Gastroenterology* 61:291, 1971.
12. Bauer, J.J., Kreel, I., Kark, A.E.: The use of the Sengstaken–Blakemore tube for immediate control of bleeding esophageal varices. *Ann. Surg.* 179:273, 1974.
13. Conn, H.O., Simpson, J.A.: Excessive mortality associated with balloon tamponade of bleeding varices: A critical reappraisal. *J.A.M.A.* 202:587, 1967.
14. Johnson, W.C., Widrich, W.C., Ansell, J.E., Robbins, A.H., Nabseth, D.C.: Control of bleeding varices by vasopressin. *Ann. Surg.* 186:369, 1977.
15. Thomford, N.R., Sirinek, K.R.: Intravenous vasopressin in patients with portal hypertension: Advantages of continuous infusion. *J. Surg. Res.* 18:113, 1975.
16. Nussbaum, M., Younis, M.T., Baum, S., Blakemore, W.S.: Control of portal hypertension: Selective mesenteric arterial infusion of vasopressin. *Arch. Surg.* 108:342, 1974.
17. Sirinek, K.R., Thomford, N.R., Pace, W.G.: Adverse cardiodynamic effects of vasopressin not avoided by selective intra-arterial administration. *Surgery* 81:723, 1977.
18. Sirinek, K.R., Thomford, N.R.: Isoproterenol in offsetting adverse effects of vasopressin in cirrhotic patients. *Am. J. Surg.* 129:130, 1975.
19. Barr, J.W., Lakin, R.C., Rosch, J.: Similarity of arterial and intravenous vasopressin on portal and systemic hemodynamics. *Gastroenterology* 69:13, 1975.
20. Johnson, W.C., Widrich, W.C., Ansell, J.E., Robbins, A.H., Nabseth, D.C.: Control of bleeding varices by vasopressin: A prospective randomized study. *Ann. Surg.* 186:369, 1977.
21. Warren, W.D., Salam, A.A., Hutson, D., Zeppa, R.: Selective distal splenorenal shunt: Technique and results of operation. *Arch Surg.* 108:306, 1974.
22. Hutson, D.G., Pereiras, R., Zeppa, R., Levi, J.U., Schiff, E.R., Fink, P.: The fate of esophageal varices following selective distal splenorenal shunt. *Ann. Surg.* 183:496, 1976.

23. Hutson, D.G., Zeppa, R., Levi, J.U., Schiff, E.R., Livingstone, A.S., Fink, P.: The effect of distal splenorenal shunt on hypersplenism. *Ann. Surg.* 185:605, 1977.
24. Zeppa, R., Hutson, D.G., Bergstresser, P.R., Levi, J.U., Schiff, E.R., Fink, P.: Survival after distal splenorenal shunt. *Surg. Gynecol. Obstet.* 145:12, 1977.
25. Welch, C.E., Malt, R.A.: Abdominal surgery. *N. Engl. J. Med.* 300:765, 1979.
26. Reichle, R.A., Fahmy, W.F., Golsorkhi, M.: Prospective comparative clinical trial with distal splenorenal and mesocaval shunts. *Am. J. Surg.* 137:13, 1979.
27. Warren, W.D.: Ascites and portasystemic shunts. *Am. J. Surg.* 135:607, 1978.
28. Vang, J., Simert, G., Hansson, J.A., Thylen, S., Bengmark, S.: Results of a modified distal splenorenal shunt for portal hypertension. *Ann. Surg.* 185:224, 1977.
29. Fonkalsrud, E.W., Myers, N.A., Robinson, M.J.: Management of extrahepatic portal hypertension in children. *Ann. Surg.* 180:487, 1974.
30. Pinkerton, J.A., Holcomb, G.W., Foster, J.H.: Portal hypertension in childhood. *Ann. Surg.* 175:870, 1972.
31. Voorhees, A.B., Price, J.B.: Extrahepatic portal hypertension. *Arch Surg.* 108:338, 1974.
32. Orloff, M.J., Johansen, K.H.: Treatment of Budd–Chiari syndrome by side-to-side portacaval shunt: Experimental and clinical results. *Ann. Surg.* 188:494, 1978.
33. Yamamoto, S., Yokoyama, Y., Takeshige, K., Iwatsuki, S.: Budd–Chiari syndrome with obstruction of the inferior vena cava. *Gastroenterology* 54:1070, 1968.
34. Parker, R.G.F.: Occlusion of the hepatic veins in man. *Medicine* 38:369, 1959.
35. Thompson, R.B.: Thrombosis of the hepatic veins. *Arch. Intern. Med.* 80:602, 1947.
36. Ludwick, J.R., Markel, S.F., Child, C.G.: Chiari's disease: A clinicopathological study. *Arch. Surg.* 91:697, 1965.
37. Strauch, G.O.: Supradiaphragmatic splenic transposition: A successful option in the treatment of Chiari's disease. *Am. J. Surg.* 119:379, 1970.
38. Malt, R.A., Dalton, J.C., Johnson, R.E., Gurewich, V.: Side-to-side portacaval shunt versus nonsurgical treatment of Budd–Chiari syndrome. *Am. J. Surg.* 136:387, 1978.
39. Warren, R.L., Schlant, R.C., Wenger, N.K., Galambos, J.T.: Treatment of Budd–Chiari syndrome with streptokinase. *Gastroenterology* 62:200, 1972.
40. Rignault, D., Mine, J., Moine, D.: Splenoportographic changes in chronic pancreatitis. *Surgery* 63:571, 1968.
41. Salam, A.A., Warren, W.D., Tyras, D.H.: Splenic vein thrombosis: A diagnosable and curable form of portal hypertension. *Surgery* 74:961, 1973.
42. Turrill, F.L., Mikkelsen, W.P.: "Sinistral" (left sided) extrahepatic portal hypertension. *Arch. Surg.* 99:365, 1969.
43. LeVeen, H.H., Wapnick, S.: Peritoneovenous shunt for ascites. *Surg. Annu.* 10:191, 1978.
44. Reinhardt, G.F., Stanley, M.M.: Peritoneovenous shunting for ascites. *Surg. Gynecol. Obstet.* 145:419, 1977.
45. Wapnick, S., Grosberg, S., Kinney, M., LeVeen, H.H.: LeVeen continuous peritoneo-jugular shunt: Improvement of renal function in ascitic patients. *J.A.M.A.* 237:131, 1977.
46. Berkowitz, H.D., Mullen, J.L., Miller, L.D., Rosato, E.F.: Improved renal function and inhibition of renin and aldosterone secretion following peritoneovenous (LeVeen) shunt. *Surgery* 84:120, 1978.
47. Lerner, R.G., Nelson, J.C., Corines, P., delGuercio, L.R.M.: Disseminated intravascular coagulation: Complication of LeVeen peritoneo-venous shunts. *J.A.M.A.* 240:2064, 1978.

4
PANCREATICO-BILIARY PROBLEMS

4.1. A 64-year-old previously healthy woman presents to the emergency room with a 2-day history of increasing abdominal pain, nausea, and vomiting. Her temperature is 38.4°C; abdominal exam discloses a tender right upper quadrant mass with local peritoneal signs present. A white blood cell count is 16,400 cells/mm^3, and a serum bilirubin level is 1.8 mg%. An abdominal ultrasound study discloses gallstones. Treatment should consist of:

A. Medical treatment with intravenous fluids, nasogastric tube, and antibiotics only.
B. Medical treatment with intravenous fluids, nasogastric tube, and antibiotics, followed by operation in 4–7 days.
C. Medical treatment with intravenous fluids, nasogastric tube, and antibiotics, followed by operation in 6–8 weeks.
D. Immediate cholecystostomy.
E. Cholecystectomy following initial resuscitative measures.

This question addresses the proper management of an elderly patient with acute cholecystitis. One of the first problems confronting the clinician dealing with a patient with a right upper quadrant inflammatory process is that of diagnosis. Many conditions, such as acute pancreatitis, pyelonephritis, appendicitis, and hepatitis, can be confused with the clinical picture of cholecystitis, making some test for acute cholecystitis imperative.[1] At the present time, two diagnostic studies are easily performed in the emergency situation and have very high diagnostic accuracy. The first is ultrasonography of the gallbladder, which will demonstrate stones in at least 90% of cases. This test can be completed within a half hour in an unprepared patient and because of this is the initial diagnostic procedure of choice in the patient suspected of harboring acute cholecystitis.[2] Another test that has shown promise in the diagnosis of acute cholecystitis is cholescintigraphy, utilizing a radioactive material excreted by the liver (e.g. BIDA, PIPIDA scan). Failure to visualize the gallbladder, coupled with excretion of the radioactive material into the bile ducts, will indicate acute cholecystitis in over 95% of patients.[3]

Results of treatment of patients with acute cholecystitis depend upon the patient population treated. In elderly or diabetic patients, medical treatment with intravenous fluid, nasogastric tube, and antibiotics will often fail, necessitating emergency operation at a later time, with a much higher mortality rate. One series of patients with acute cholecystitis disclosed that one third of medically treated patients failed to improve and had to undergo emergency surgery. Most deaths in this series occurred in such patients rather than in those operated upon promptly.[4] Another study looking at acute cholecystitis in the elderly noted that 38 out of 39 patients over the age of 60 had failed medical management, and in this group, empyema or gangrene of the gallbladder and subsequent liver or subphrenic abscess was common.[5]

Because of these factors, most patients who have a definite diagnosis of acute cholecystitis should undergo volume resuscitation and treatment with antibiotics followed by operation within 24 hr. This will obviate the problem of those patients who fail to get better, lead to overall decreased length of hospitalization and hospital morbidity, and eliminate the problem of recurrent acute cholecystitis during an arbitrary 6- to 8-week waiting period. Mortality rates consistently below 1% can be anticipated with this early operative approach.[6] Cholecystostomy can be used in certain elderly or poor-risk patients with acute cholecystitis and will reliably tide them over the period of acute inflammation. However, the majority of these patients will require cholecystectomy later, and therefore this procedure cannot be regarded as definitive. It should be used in those patients who are too ill to undergo a general anesthetic and if possible should be performed under local anesthesia.[7] In the present case, the patient, although elderly, was in good health previously, and there are therefore no contraindications to cholecystectomy.

ANSWER: E.

4.2. A 68-year-old woman with a history of diabetes mellitus, requiring 20 units of NPH insulin daily, and a myocardial infarction 3 years previously is admitted to the coronary care unit with an acute myocardial infarction. Three days later, she is hemodynamically stable but begins to complain of right upper quadrant pain and abdominal distention. Within 24 hr her temperature is 38.6°C, and her white blood cell count is 14,200 cells/mm^3. Examination discloses right upper quadrant tenderness and guarding, along with a tender, palpable mass. An abdominal ultrasound and biliary excretion scan are carried out and are shown as Figures 4-1 and 4-2. Treatment should consist of:

A. Percutaneous transhepatic intubation of the biliary tract.
B. Antibiotics and nasogastric suction.
C. Cholecystostomy under local anesthesia.
D. Cholecystostomy under general anesthesia.
E. Cholecystectomy.

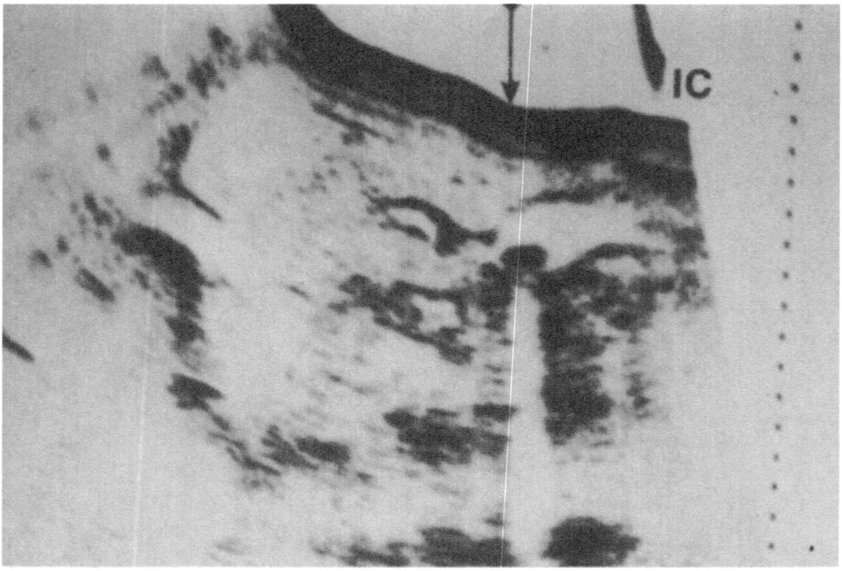

Figure 4-1

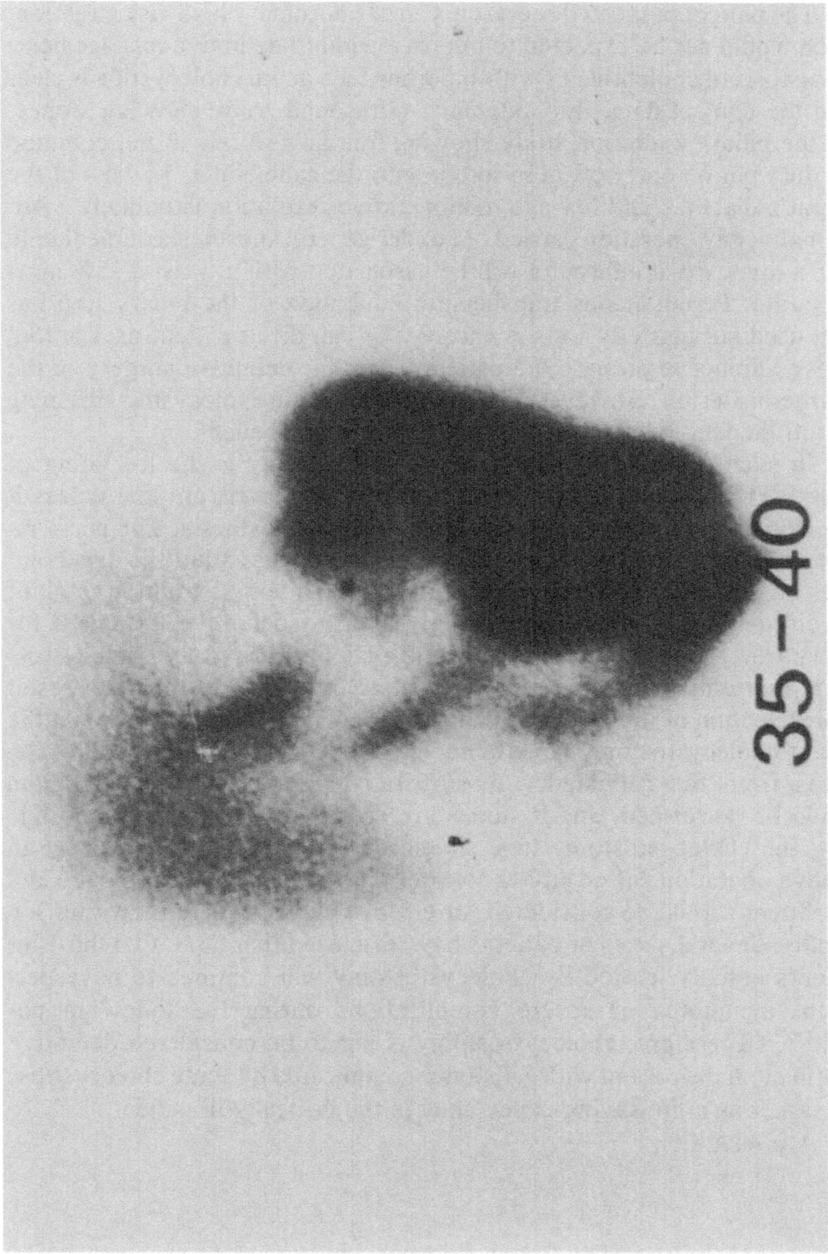

Figure 4-2

The patient presented represents an extraordinary high-risk situation, which would not be expected to improve without definitive management. A diagnosis of cholelithiasis with superimposed acute cholecystitis is clear from the clinical data, the abdominal ultrasound study showing stones, and the biliary excretion study showing free flow of bile in the common bile duct but no entry of radioisotope into the gallbladder. In view of the patient's diabetes and her age, nonoperative resolution is unlikely.[5] Additionally, any operation carried out under general anesthesia immediately after a myocardial infarction will be associated with at least a 25% mortality rate. Percutaneous transhepatic intubation of the biliary tree has been used successfully for the chronically jaundiced patient as a preoperative adjunct to prepare the patient better for definitive surgery of the obstructing lesion. However, in a patient with acute cholecystitis, draining the intrahepatic biliary tree will not result in any benefit.

In such a high-risk patient, a cholecystostomy is the treatment of choice. The advantages of cholecystostomy, however, are lost unless it is performed as a planned operation under local anesthesia. The performance of cholecystostomy after general anesthesia has all of the disadvantages of general anesthesia in the critically ill patient in addition to all of the disadvantages of cholecystostomy as a nondefinitive treatment for biliary tract disease.[8] In most series of patients treated by cholecystostomy, mortality rates have ranged from 20% to 40%, mainly as a result of preselection of the most critically ill patients for this procedure. At the time of cholecystostomy, an attempt should be made to remove all of the stones from the gallbladder. Postoperatively, a tube cholecystogram should be performed, and if stones are present within the common bile duct, the cholecystostomy tube should be left in place, followed by an elective operation.[7] If no stones are present, the tube can be removed and the patient should be considered for elective cholecystectomy within 3–6 months. Several series of patients have disclosed that up to two thirds of patients initially treated by cholecystostomy will continue to have persistent symptoms or severe complications during the follow-up period.[7,9,10] Therefore, cholecystostomy is not to be considered definitive treatment in the patient with gallstones complicated by acute cholecystitis, but rather as a life-saving expediency in the critically ill patient.

ANSWER: C.

4.3. A 76-year-old woman presents to the hospital with right upper quadrant pain, a temperature of 39.8°C, and clinical jaundice. Her pulse is 96 and blood pressure is 130/94. After 24 hr of intravenous fluid administration and treatment with a cephalosporin antibiotic, her temperature is 38.4°C, and her abdominal pain is unchanged. The white blood cell count is 18,200 cells/mm^3, and the serum bilirubin level is 6.8 mg%. An abdominal ultrasound discloses multiple gallstones. Treatment at this time should consist of:

A. Addition of gentamicin and clindamycin to antibiotic coverage.
B. Cholecystectomy.
C. Cholecystectomy and common bile duct exploration.
D. Cholecystostomy under local anesthesia.
E. Cholecystostomy under general anesthesia.

The diagnostic triad of pain, fever, and jaundice indicates that this patient has acute ascending cholangitis, presumably on the basis of common bile duct stones secondary to her documented gallstones. This syndrome of infection in the biliary tree is most often due to stone disease, but may be due to other partial or complete biliary obstructions from tumor, stricture, or pancreatitis. In most series of patients, stone disease accounts for over 60% of all cases of ascending cholangitis.[11]

The gram-negative aerobic bacteria are the most common organisms that are isolated from infected bile, making one of the cephalosporin drugs a good first-line antibiotic of choice in a patient with ascending cholangitis. *Bacteroides fragilis* is seen uncommonly in the biliary tree, and then usually only in the presence of prior biliary operations or biliary intestinal anastomoses.[12,13] In one series, *B. fragilis* was isolated in only 2% of all cultures taken of infected biliary trees.[14]

The disease tends to occur mainly in the elderly, and mortality rates of 20%–60% are usual. The majority of patients with ascending cholangitis will promptly respond to antibiotic therapy, and, after this, appropriate diagnostic tests can be carried out, followed by operative treatment.[11] One variant of the disease, which has been labeled acute suppurative ascending cholangitis, consists of pain, fever, and jaundice, along with hypotension and CNS depression. In these instances, nonoperative treatment alone is universally fatal, and after rapid fluid and antibiotic resuscitation, operation should be carried out promptly.[15,16] At the time of operation, the gallbladder should be removed and the common bile duct explored and any stones removed. Following this, a T tube is placed. Cholecystostomy alone is often not sufficient treatment for ascending cholangitis, as the common bile duct will not be decompressed.[12,16]

ANSWER: C.

4.4. A 30-year-old obese woman injures her back and receives X rays in an emergency room. Calcified gallstones are noted, and careful questioning of the patient fails to elicit any history of abdominal pain, jaundice, or significant indigestion. Which of the following courses of management should be recommended to this patient?

A. Observation only.
B. Operation when the first gallbladder symptoms occur.
C. Cholecystectomy.
D. Chenodeoxycholic acid.
E. Weight reduction, low fat and high fiber diet.

Clinicians are commonly presented with the clinical problem of a patient who has truly asymptomatic gallstones. Approximately 15%–20% of the adult population of the United States harbor gallstones,[17] and the morbidity and mortality from gallbladder disease are a major public health problem. Unfortunately, for the clinician advising a patient with asymptomatic gallstone disease, there are a certain percentage of patients, perhaps 30% or 40%, who will remain asymptomatic throughout their lifetime and whose gallstones will be discovered only at autopsy. Because of this, many physicians have adopted a wait-and-see attitude.

This attitude is probably unwise for a variety of reasons. Several studies have been carried out in which a long-term follow-up of patients with asymptomatic gallstones was carried out. In one study of 781 patients followed for up to 11 years, over 35% of patients developed severe complications or symptoms requiring surgery.[18] Obviously, had the follow-up been longer, this figure could only have increased. Another study of patients followed for from 5 to 20 years disclosed approximately 50% of patients developing severe symptoms or complications.[19]

Operative mortality rates for elective cholecystectomy in patients under the age of 50 approximate 0.2%. This is contrasted with similarly aged patients who undergo cholecystectomy for acute cholecystitis with operative mortality rates of 1% to 3%. These figures rise sharply with advancing age, so that over the age of 60, acute cholecystitis is a grave condition and mortality rates of 5%–7% are noted. In view of the fact that those patients who will develop severe symptoms cannot be predicted on the basis of age, type of gallstone, or gallbladder function,[20] and that perhaps 30% of patients will develop acute cholecystitis as their first symptom,[21] a strong argument can be made for elective surgery in the asymptomatic patient. Surely, if the patient has diabetes mellitus this is mandatory because of the markedly increased incidence of complications in this group of patients.[20]

Reliance on adjuncts such as weight reduction and a low-fat or low-fiber diet, although theoretically appealing, have not been demonstrated to reduce the future incidence of symptomatic gallbladder disease.[22,23] Treatment with oral chenodeoxycholic acid can dissolve radiolucent gallstones in some cases, but radiopaque gallstones are not amenable to treatment by this means.[24]

ANSWER: C.

4.5. Which of the following is not a contraindication to treatment with oral chenodeoxycholic acid in a patient with proven gallstones?

A. History of liver disease.
B. Radiolucent stones.
C. Radiopaque stones.
D. Frequent biliary colic.
E. Inflammatory bowel disease.

Chenodeoxycholic acid is a human bile acid that renders the bile of patients with increased saturation of cholesterol more unsaturated. This property has given rise to its potential usefulness as an agent to be used in the dissolution of cholesterol gallstones. In several published studies, patients with radiolucent cholesterol gallstones have been treated with varying amounts of oral chenodeoxycholic acid, and the size and number of their gallstones monitored by oral cholecystography. In one study, two thirds of patients with radiolucent gallstones who were treated for 6 months or longer showed a disappearance or a decrease in size of their gallstones. The remainder of the patients were noted to have no change. Eleven patients with radiopaque gallstones and seven patients with non-visualized gallbladders derived no benefit.[24] Another study disclosed a poor response rate in patients with large solitary gallstones, gallbladders that visualize poorly on oral cholecystography, and radiopaque gallstones. The response in those patients with radiolucent stones was dose related, and doses over 15 mg/kg per day were required to achieve an effect.[25] In both of these studies, gallstones recurred after varying intervals of time following cessation of treatment.

Side effects have been limited to diarrhea and mild liver function test abnormalities, but liver biopsies of patients taking this drug have shown no consistent abnormalities.[24,25] To study further the toxicity of these drugs, they were administered to pregnant and nonpregnant baboons in one study. Both mother and infant baboons were noted to have significant hepatic histological abnormalities. The significance of these findings is currently unclear.[26]

At the present time, the National Cooperative Gallstone Study is attempting to determine the safety and efficacy of this drug. The protocol includes patients 21 through 79 years of age with radiolucent gallstones without biliary colic or cholecystitis within the previous month. Women must be unable to bear children or be more than 40 years old and using a contraceptive device. Other exclusions in this study are patients with any history of liver disease, gastric ulcer, or inflammatory bowel disease.

What the ultimate usefulness of this drug will prove to be is unclear at this time. When one considers that the drug must be given constantly for many years and that those patients presenting acutely with intractable biliary colic or acute cholecystitis are not suitable candidates, the clinician will be left with a rather small subgroup of patients with relatively asymptomatic radiolucent stones who will be suitable candidates for treatment. However, even in these circumstances, whether or not it will prove wise to place patients with a 20- to 30-year life expectancy on a drug that they will have to take constantly for many years will remain a moot point.

ANSWER: B.

4.6. A 72-year-old woman in otherwise excellent health is 20 years post-cholecystectomy and presents with right upper quadrant pain, fever, and jaundice. Antibiotic treatment results in prompt improvement and a subsequent intravenous cholangiogram and abdominal ultrasound demonstrate a 2.5-cm-diameter common bile duct with multiple 3-mm stones within it. Treatment should consist of:

A. Choledochoduodenostomy.
B. Roux-en-Y choledochojejunostomy.
C. Transduodenal sphincteroplasty.
D. Choledochotomy, stone extraction, and T tube insertion.
E. Endoscopic papillotomy.

This woman is presenting with ascending cholangitis secondary to common bile duct obstruction, presumably on the basis of recurrent common bile duct stones. In general, when common bile duct stones are detected within two years of cholecystectomy, they are regarded as retained or overlooked at the time of the initial operation. At times later than this, surgeons tend to regard them as primary common duct stones. Several factors account for the formation of common bile duct stones in the postcholecystectomy patient. There is some evidence that lithogenic bile persists in the gallstone patient even after cholecystectomy.[27] In addition, in many instances either a functional or anatomic partial obstruction exists at the ampulla, resulting in bile stasis, sludging, and stone formation. Although various surgeons would undoubtedly disagree on the optimal treatment in such a patient, choledochoduodenostomy is a safe and simple procedure with minimal long-term side effects.[28,29] In one series of 175 cases followed over an 18-year period, only two cases of subsequent cholangitis were recognized, attesting to the long-term safety and efficacy of this procedure.[30] A Roux-en-Y choledochojejunostomy would accomplish the same end but is technically more complicated and therefore hardly justifiable. In the situation in which a dilated common bile duct is not present, a transduodenal sphincteroplasty should be carried out. Some surgeons regard choledochoduodenostomy and sphincteroplasty as equal operations, and in experienced hands morbidity and mortality rates are similar. There is some evidence that with the passage of time, careful follow-up will disclose perhaps as many as half of the patients treated with sphincteroplasty developing recurrent symptoms.[31]

Most surgeons would regard choledochotomy, stone extraction, and T tube insertion as an inadequate procedure because of the presumed high incidence of recurrent stone formation. However, one series of 22 patients followed for approximately 5 years showed only 4 of 22 patients with recurrent stones.[32] With longer follow-up, this percentage of recurrences would be expected to increase, but the evidence would indicate that in certain very poor-risk patients, stone extraction alone might be sufficient treatment.

In recent years, endoscopic papillotomy has been advocated as a nonoperative means of common bile duct stone extraction.[33–36] The procedure is carried out through an endoscope. After visualization and cannulation of the ampulla, a knife or sphincterotome is inserted, and a sphincterotomy carried out, thus enlarging the ampullary opening. An international review of this procedure was carried out in 1978 with a 90% success rate, a 1.4% mortality rate, a 7% major complication rate, and a 2.3% incidence of patients requiring emergency surgery after the papillotomy. Therefore at this time, although the procedure remains promising, more experience is required before its role in the management of patients with common bile duct stones can be determined.

ANSWER: A.

4.7. A 42-year-old woman has gallstones and common bile duct stones. She undergoes cholecystectomy, common bile duct exploration with stone removal, and insertion of an 18 French T tube. On the seventh postoperative day, a T tube cholangiogram is performed. The result is shown as Figure 4-3. Management of this patient should consist of:

A. Removal of the T tube.
B. Reoperation and choledochotomy.
C. Extraction of the stone through the T tube.
D. Instillation of bile salts or heparin through the T tube.
E. Endoscopic papillotomy.

Even utilizing intraoperative cholangiography, the surgeon will be faced with the problem of retained common bile duct stones in 3%–6% of patients. [37,38] This fact makes it mandatory to perform postoperative T tube cholangiography on every patient before T tube removal. Numerous methods are presently available for managing the patient with retained common bile duct stones. Implicit in this is general agreement that stone extraction is necessary to prevent future episodes of cholangitis or obstructive jaundice and also the fact that no one technique is clearly superior nor universally applicable to all patients. Various substances have been advocated for instillation through the T tube in hopes of dissolving gallstones. Heparin has been utilized in this regard with some success, as have bile salts.[39–42] There are potential disadvantages to both these techniques. Both require in-hospital treatment for many days plus repeated cholangiograms. In addition, there is clinical and experimental evidence that bile salts may be toxic to the bile duct epithelium, leading to potential liver damage or bile duct strictures. The most widely used method for removing retained common duct stones in which a T tube has been left in the patient is biliary stone extraction through the T tube tract. This method depends upon the presence of a large caliber T tube (14–18 French) and a relatively straight tract from the T tube site to the skin. After a waiting period of 4–8 weeks in which a well-formed fibrous tract develops, the T tube is removed and a stone grasping basket is inserted under fluoroscopic control. Success rates of over 95% have been reported.[43] A newer method that has been described is endoscopic sphincterotomy after cannulation of the ampulla of Vater. However, the success and morbidity rates utilizing this technique are inferior to those obtained with trans-T-tube extraction, and the long-term effects of sphincterotomy are unknown.[34–36]

ANSWER: C.

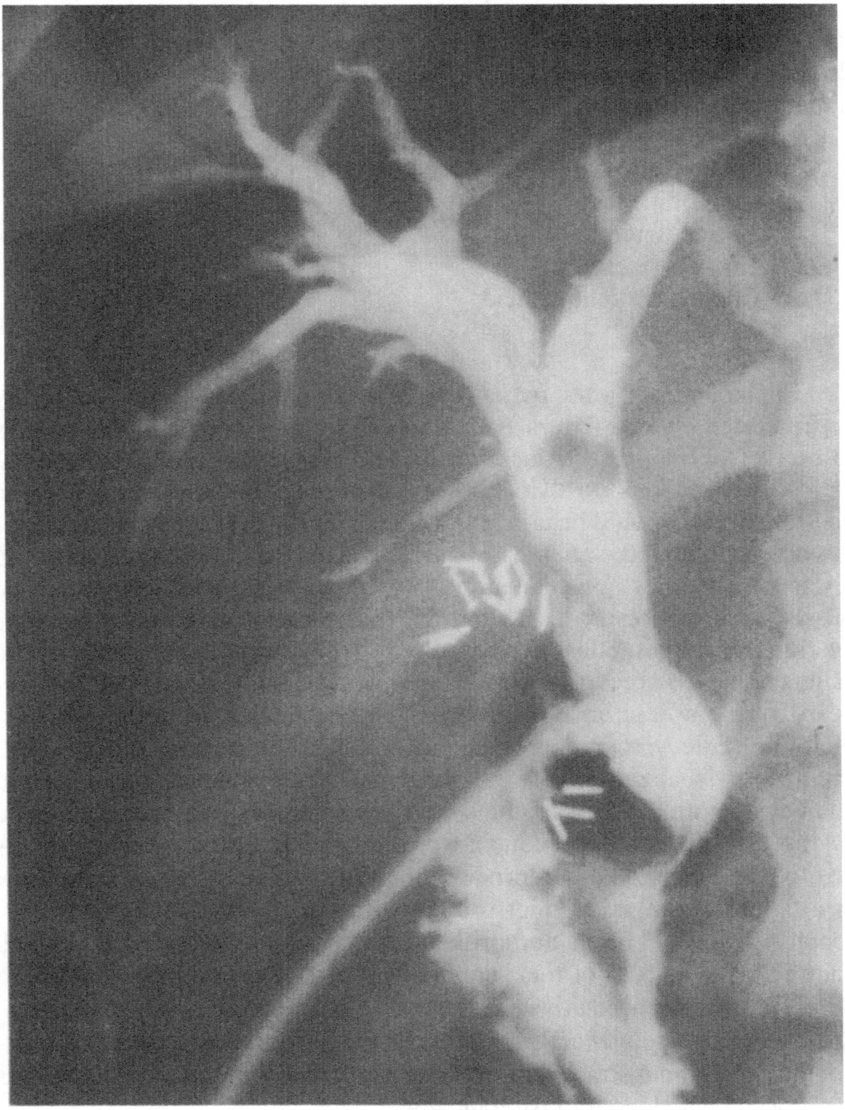

Figure 4-3

4.8. A 27-year-old woman gives a 7-month history of right upper quadrant colicky pain radiating to the back. The pain is brought on by eating and lasts 1½–3 hr. She has lost 14 lb during this period. An upper GI tract X ray, oral cholecystogram, abdominal ultrasound, and cholecystokinin (CCK) cholecystogram are shown as Figures 4-4 through 4-8. A duodenal drainage study discloses a few cholesterol crystals. Treatment of this patient should consist of:

A. Endoscopic papillotomy (sphincterotomy).
B. Cimetidine.
C. Anticholinergic drugs.
D. Cholecystectomy.
E. Chenodeoxycholic acid.

Clinicians caring for patients with abdominal pain will occasionally be frustrated by a patient, usually a young woman, who has what sounds to be typical biliary colic, and yet on oral cholecystography and abdominal ultrasound has no evidence of gallstones. In such a patient, two additional tests should be utilized to document the presence of gallbladder disease. Although the abdominal ultrasound and oral cholecystogram will disclose gallstones approximately 95% of the time, tiny stones can be missed by either test.[44,45] In addition, there is another group of patients who do not harbor gallstones and often on histologic examination of the gallbladder give no evidence of chronic cholecystitis. These patients appear to have a functional disorder of the gallbladder. In both instances, the CCK cholecystogram or duodenal drainage studies can be diagnostic. Following visualization with gallbladder contrast material, as in an oral cholecystogram, CCK is administered intravenously in a blinded fashion so that the patient does not know when she is receiving the drug. A positive test consists of a reproduction of the patient's colicky symptoms or a failure of the gallbladder to contract normally on sequential fluoroscopic views.[46–49] Some authorities feel that all normal gallbladders will contract at least 50% of their volume within 30 min; therefore failure to do so represents a positive CCK test.[46,47] In one series of 12 patients, CCK preoperatively exactly reproduced the patient's pain, whereas postoperatively, administration of the drug elicited no symptoms. All patients had normal gallbladders histologically.[49]

Duodenal drainage consists of fluoroscopically placing a tube opposite the ampulla, followed by the oral administration of magnesium sulfate, a potent choleretic drug. Aspiration of bile is performed. The first bile, which has been called A bile, consists of clear bile from the liver and bile

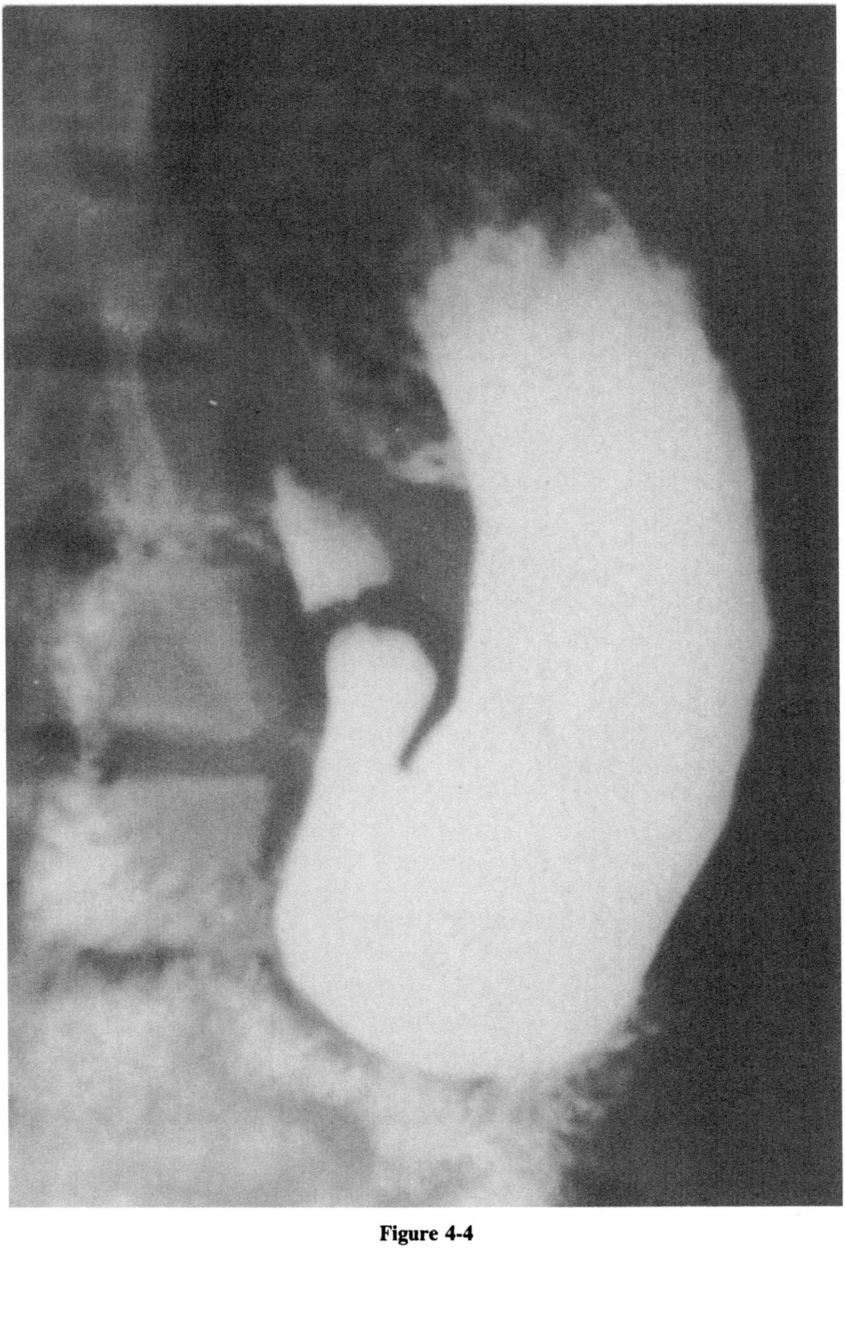

Figure 4-4

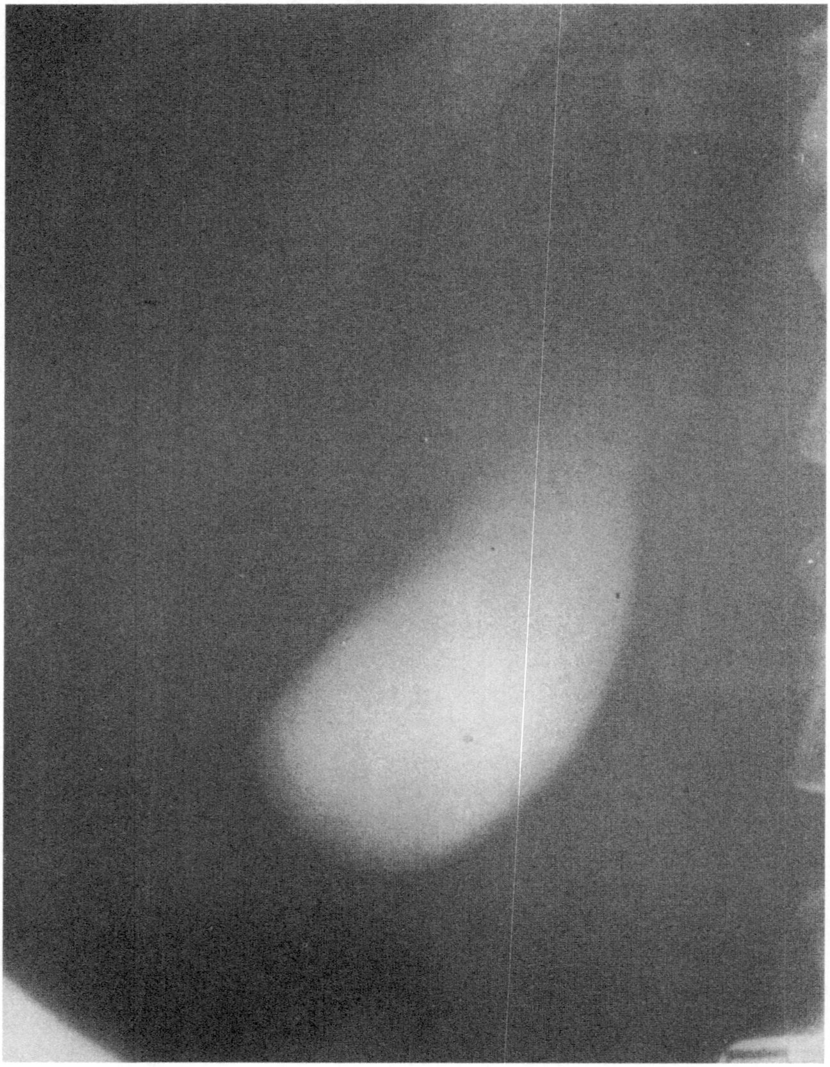

Figure 4-5

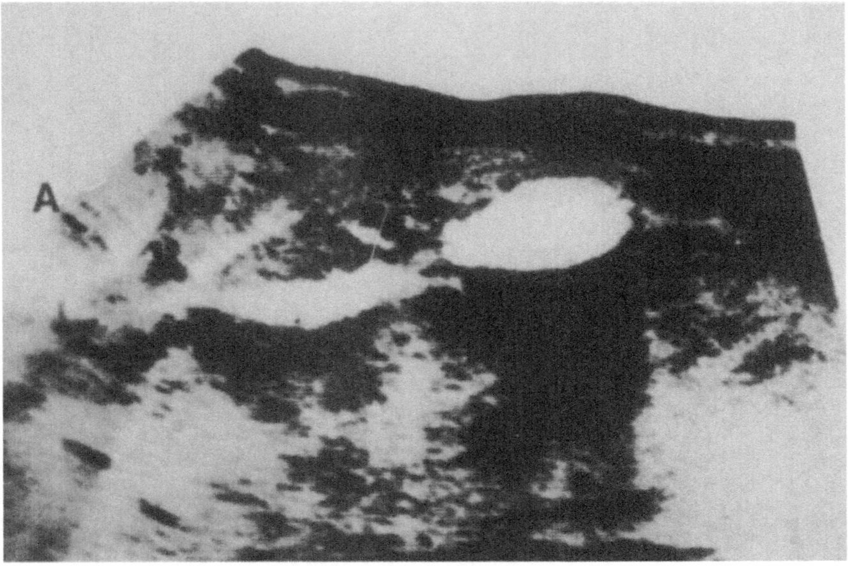

Figure 4-6

duct. Following this, the gallbladder contracts and darker B bile is obtained. This is then examined for cholesterol crystals or white blood cells.[47,50]

In the patient with typical biliary colic, if either one of these tests is positive, cholecystectomy can be performed with excellent assurance that the patient's symptoms will subside postoperatively. However, even if these tests are negative, a young woman with *typical* biliary colic (as opposed to any vague upper abdominal pain following eating) may be considered for operation, as may any patient who has recurrent attacks of "idiopathic" pancreatitis. The results of operation in both these groups of patients will be gratifying if careful selection criteria are utilized. In the patient presented, both the duodenal drainage study and CCK cholecystogram were positive, making cholecystectomy the treatment of choice. Chenodeoxycholic acid, although it has been shown to dissolve cholesterol gallstones, has not been used in the various cholecystopathy syndromes. Antacid drugs would be of no benefit, and endoscopic papillotomy is utilized for retained or recurrent common bile duct stones.

ANSWER: D.

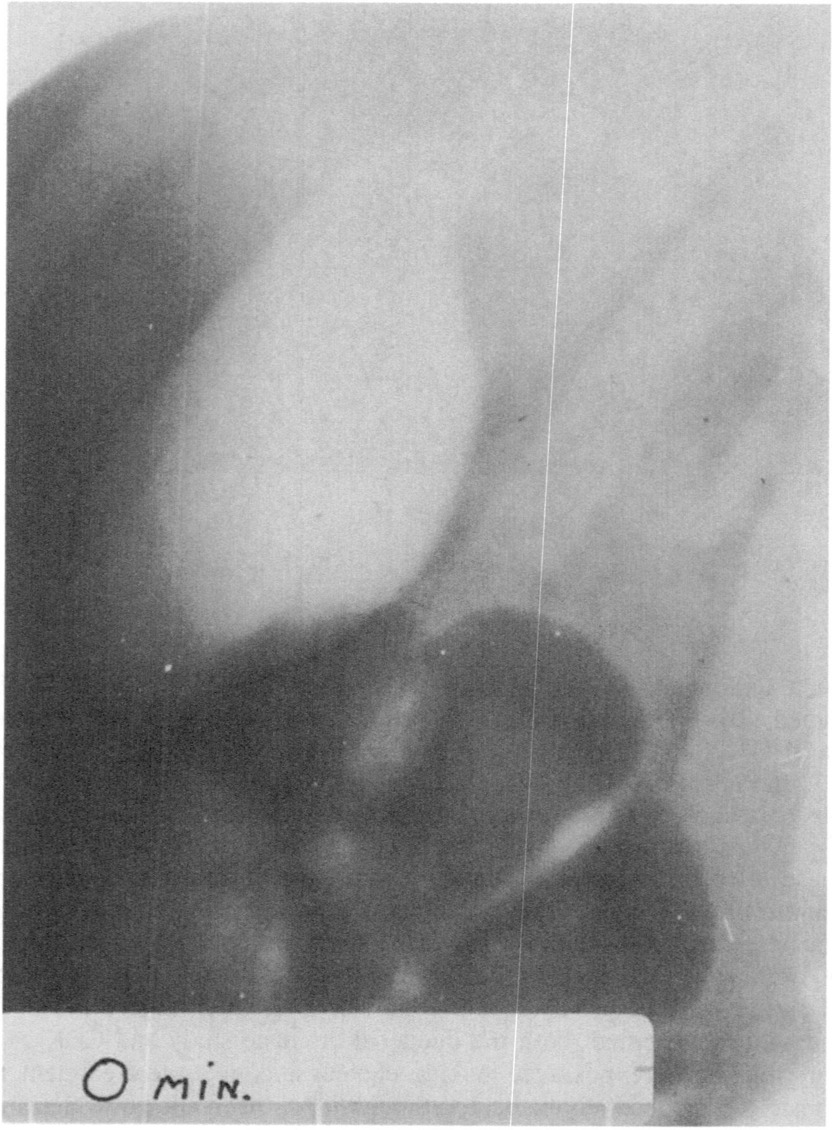

Figure 4-7

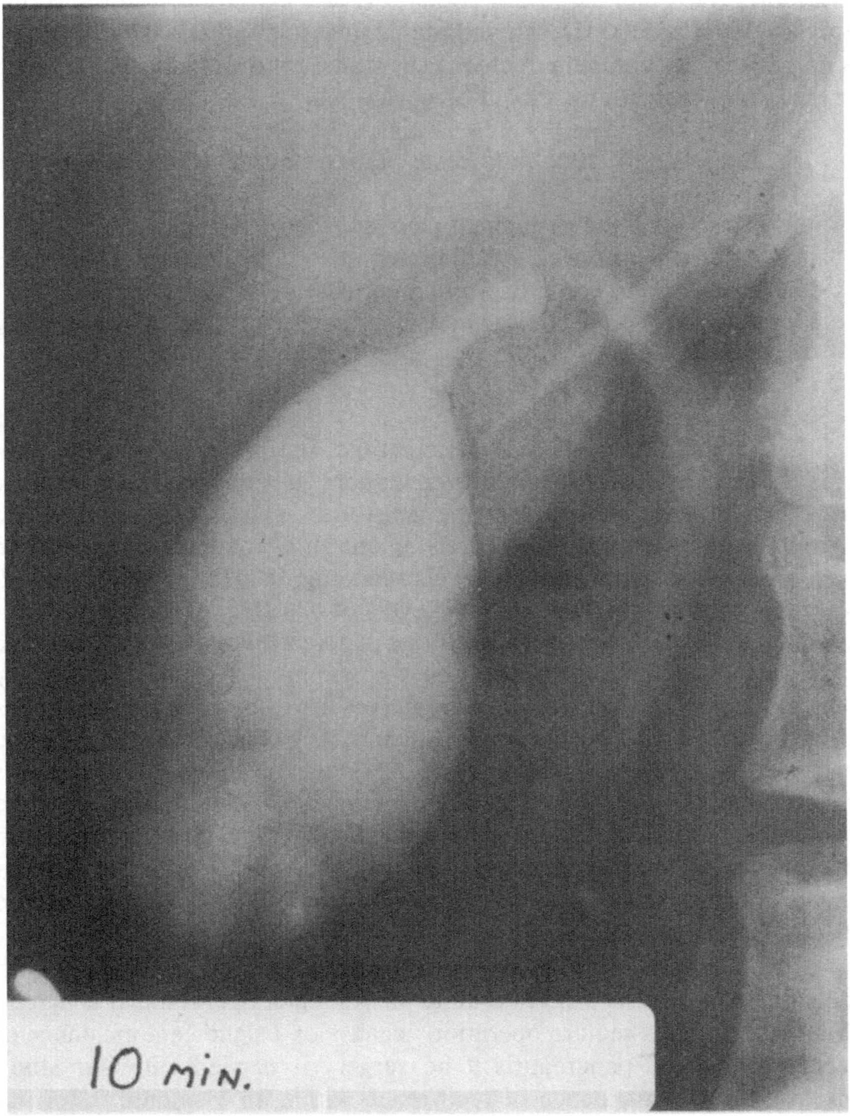

Figure 4-8

4.9. A 48-year-old woman presents to the hospital with a 12-hr history of severe epigastric pain and vomiting. Her temperature is 37.8°C, and she has marked tenderness in the epigastrium with evidence of peritoneal irritation. The white blood cell count is 12,400 cells/mm^3, and the serum amylase level is 3200 IU. An abdominal ultrasound discloses gallstones, a normal-caliber common duct without stones, and a mildly swollen pancreas. Cholecystectomy should be performed:

A. Immediately after fluid resuscitation and antibiotic therapy are instituted.
B. As soon as the abdominal pain subsides.
C. After a 4- to 6-week waiting period.
D. After a 3- to 6-month waiting period.
E. As soon as all clinical and laboratory evidence of pancreatitis subsides.

This patient has gallstone pancreatitis. The presence of acute pancreatitis in a nonalcoholic patient who harbors gallstones can almost surely be assumed to be the result of the gallstones. This is confirmed by the extremely high serum amylase levels. In one study, patients with gallstone pancreatitis had serum amylase levels averaging 1800 IU, while those with alcoholic pancreatitis had amylase levels of 800 IU.[51] It is now well accepted that the pathogenesis of gallstone pancreatitis relates to the passage of stones from the gallbladder into the common duct with temporary pancreatic duct obstruction. Several studies have shown that these stones could be recovered from the stools in at least 90% of patients with gallstone pancreatitis, whereas the finding of such stones in the stools of patients with alcoholic pancreatitis is quite uncommon.[52,53] In addition, operative cholangiograms have demonstrated a much higher incidence of reflux into the pancreatic duct in patients with gallstone pancreatitis, leading to the conclusion that this may also be a factor in the genesis of the disease.[53,]

The main area of controversy concerning the care of a patient with gallstone pancreatitis centers around the timing of operation. It is agreed that these patients require operation because of a significant incidence of recurrence of the pancreatitis if no surgery is carried out. One study disclosed a 33% incidence of recurrence within an 11-month follow-up period.[55] Another study disclosed a 48% recurrence of the pancreatitis, and one half of these cases recurred within 30 days of the initial attack.[56] These data not only indicate the need for surgery, but also would tend to influence one not to recommend an arbitrary waiting period following hospital discharge after the initial attack. Early operation during the initial phase of the attack is likewise associated with increased morbidity and mortality rates,[55] and therefore the wisest course of action is a definitive course of nonoperative management as long as the patient's condition is improving. Following subsidance of all signs, symptoms, and laboratory evidence of pancreatitis, elective operation can then be undertaken on the same hospitalization with minimal morbidity. Early operation is reserved for those patients whose clinical condition is deteriorating, who have increasing jaundice with or without sepsis, or who pose a diagnostic problem and might harbor some other acute abdominal process.

At the time of operation, a cholecystectomy and operative cholangiogram should be performed. Common bile duct exploration is not necessary unless stones are noted on the cholangiogram or palpated within the common bile duct. This recognizes the fact that most patients with gallstone pancreatitis will spontaneously pass their common duct stones, and no more than 25% will harbor stones within the duct at the time of operation.[57]

ANSWER: E.

4.10. Which of the following factors is not associated with an increased mortality in patients with acute pancreatitis?

A. Serum calcium concentration less than 7 mg%.
B. Renal failure.
C. P_{O_2} less than 60 torr.
D. Hypotension.
E. Serum amylase greater than 1000 IU.

Despite many advances in patient monitoring and fluid and electrolyte management, approximately 10% to 15% of patients admitted with the diagnosis of acute pancreatitis will succumb to the complications of the disease regardless of the cause of the pancreatitis.[58] In its most severe form, the disease manifests itself as multiple organ system failure, very often associated with pancreatic necrosis and sepsis.[59] The most virulent form of the disease has been called hemorrhagic pancreatitis and is associated with a dropping hematocrit and gross retroperitoneal hemorrhage. In one series of patients with hemorrhagic pancreatitis, all 30 patients who were not operated upon died, whereas nine out of 21 patients operated upon (43%) survived.[60]

It is obvious, then, that there is a subgroup of patients with acute pancreatitis who will require some form of operative intervention, and numerous prognostic factors have been sought as a guide for management. Hypotension, tachycardia, fever, and the presence of an abdominal mass on admission have all been shown to correlate with increased mortality in this condition, along with hypotension, hypocalcemia, renal failure, or respiratory failure.[58] Despite the agreement that there are some patients with acute pancreatitis who inexorably progress to death, there is no uniformity of opinion as to the proper surgical management. Recommendations range from peritoneal lavage, either instituted via the percutaneous route or with tube placement at the time of celiotomy, to radical surgical debridement of the pancreas and peripancreatic tissues.[61–65] However, probably the most widely used treatment today for the patient who manifests evidence of sepsis and multiple organ system failure and who is not responding to conservative management is exploratory celiotomy with sump and penrose drainage of the pancreas and retroperitoneum, along with a cholecystostomy to decompress the biliary tract and a gastrostomy for nasogastric decompression and suction, coupled with the use of a feeding jejunostomy for maintenance of nutrition. Utilizing this treatment, as many as three quarters of these patients have been salvaged from what was previously a uniformly fatal disorder.[66–68]

ANSWER: E.

4.11. Two weeks following an attack of acute alcoholic pancreatitis, a 25-year-old man develops a tender visible mass in the epigastrium. His temperature is 37.4°C, and the mass appears to be 8 cm in diameter. His white blood cell count is 9200 cells/mm^3, and an abdominal ultrasound discloses a 5-cm fluid collection adjacent to the pancreatic head. Treatment should consist of:

A. Drainage with sump drains.
B. Drainage with Penrose drains.
C. Observation of the mass.
D. Pancreatic cystgastrostomy.
E. Roux-en-Y pancreaticocystjejunostomy.

The development of a peripancreatic mass subsequent to an attack of acute pancreatitis may signify the development of a hematoma, pseudocyst, phlegmon, or pancreatic abscess. Depending upon the clinical circumstances, each of these will be treated differently, and therefore diagnostic measures must be undertaken to elucidate the nature of such masses. Recently, an abdominal ultrasound has been shown to be the most useful test for following serial changes in retroperitoneal fluid collections. The test is easily performed, noninvasive, and can accurately delineate even very small masses. In other instances, the use of abdominal CAT scanning, arteriography, or endoscopic retrograde pancreatography can be beneficial.[69]

Not all masses will require operation, and the incidence of true resolution of confirmed pseudocysts is difficult to ascertain. In certain series in the literature, it has been noted that pancreatic swellings or phlegmons were noted to disappear, but this is not tantamount to resolution of a true pseudocyst.[70] However, resolution of pseudocysts has been documented in from 8% to 20% of patients in well studied series.[71–73] Complications, however, are common during the observation of pseudocysts, occurring in from 30% to 40% of patients.[71,73,74] These complications include the development of obstructive jaundice, GI tract obstruction, rupture of the pseudocyst either into the peritoneal cavity or into adjacent viscera, and hemorrhage into the pseudocyst, usually from erosion of a major vessel. This last complication is associated with a mortality rate of at least 60%.[71]

For those patients with documented pseudocysts who do not manifest any evidence of complications, observation is the treatment of choice. In some of these patients, spontaneous resolution will occur; in others, a 4- to 7-week period is allowed to elapse, during which time the walls of the pseudocyst become thick and mature thus allowing internal drainage procedures to be attempted. In most instances, spontaneous resolution cannot be expected to take place after 7 weeks.[74] For those patients who manifest any of the complications during the period of observation, operation is indicated. Usually, external drainage procedures will be required, and this will often result in a temporary pancreatic fistula.

Internal drainage procedures, consisting of a cystgastrostomy, cystduodenostomy, and Roux-en-Y cystjejunostomy, are associated with complete resolution of the cysts in the majority of cases. Up to 15% of pseudocysts can recur after internal drainage,[72] and a certain number of patients will suffer from postoperative hemorrhage into the pseudocyst. However, this latter problem has probably been overstated in the past, with one recent series of patients noting less than a 2% incidence of hemorrhage following internal drainage.[75]

ANSWER: C.

4.12. Which of the following is not a common complication of pancreatic abscess?

A. Pancreatic fistula.
B. Recurrent abscess.
C. Upper GI tract hemorrhage.
D. Renal and pulmonary failure.
E. Intra-abdominal hemorrhage.

Pancreatic abscess is one of the most grave complications of acute pancreatitis, occurring in 6%–8.5% of patients with acute pancreatitis.[76,77] This complication occurs an average of 15 days after the onset of acute pancreatitis[78] and is seen far more commonly in association with postoperative pancreatitis than with alcoholic or biliary pancreatitis. In one series, 39% of patients with postoperative pancreatitis developed a pancreatic abscess, whereas only 3%–6% of patients with biliary and alcoholic pancreatitis suffered this complication.[78]

The signs and symptoms of the condition are those of any localized intra-abdominal infection, and the usual gram-negative organisms are responsible. If not treated operatively, death is certain. With operation, mortality rates of 20%–40% may be expected.[76–78] As with any patient with sepsis, multiple system failure, including pulmonary, renal, cardiac, and hepatic failure, is frequently noted. In addition, patients with pancreatic abscess have a very high incidence of hemorrhagic complications. Both upper GI tract and intra-abdominal hemorrhages are seen frequently. In one series, 23 of 63 patients had sustained major hemorrhage; 15 of these were upper GI tract hemorrhages and 11 were intra-abdominal hemorrhage secondary to local vessel erosion.[78] The other complication noted frequently is that of recurrent pancreatic abscess. Because of the nature of the abscess process and the proximity to many vital structures, a radical debridement and drainage of the pancreas is often not possible, and a limited debridement and drainage must be relied upon. Recurrence of pancreatic abscess requiring reoperation is noted in approximatley one third of patients. The optimal treatment, therefore, of a patient suspected of harboring a pancreatic abscess combines early diagnosis with appropriate broad spectrum antibiotic coverage and early operation with debridement of as much devitalized tissue as possible, followed by radical sump drainage of the pancreas and lesser sac. Most of these patients will require total parenteral nutrition, as resumption of alimentation is unlikely within several weeks. In addition, prompt reoperation should be carried out if there is any evidence of smoldering or recurrent infection.

ANSWER: A.

4.13. Two weeks following an attack of acute alcoholic pancreatitis, a 34-year-old man develops massive abdominal swelling. Paracentesis reveals clear yellow fluid with 20 white blood cells/mm^3, an amylase content of 860 IU, and a total protein level of 3.1 g%. An abdominal ultrasound discloses a 4-cm cyst at the junction of the pancreatic head and body. Three weeks later, the patient is afebrile but has difficulty eating because of the abdominal swelling. Treatment should consist of:

A. LeVeen peritoneojugular shunt.
B. Continued observation.
C. Subtotal pancreatectomy.
D. Roux-en-Y pancreaticocystjejunostomy.
E. Puestow procedure (longitudinal pancreaticojejunostomy).

In any alcoholic patient who develops ascites, or in any patient with a history of pancreatitis who develops ascites, the possibility of pancreatic ascites must be considered. By definition, pancreatic ascites consists of ascitic accumulations with a total protein content of greater than 2.5 g% and an elevated amylase concentration. A history of pancreatitis is customary, but not seen in all patients.[79] The serum amylase concentration is only inconstantly elevated.[80] Approximately one third of these patients will also manifest a left pleural effusion,[81,82] and in the majority of cases a pancreatic cyst is present that has ruptured into the free peritoneal cavity creating an irritative peritoneal reaction with an exudation of fluid.[82] In those cases without a demonstrable pancreatic pseudocyst, direct rupture of a pancreatic duct is noted.

Diagnosis is established by paracentesis, with abdominal ultrasound utilized to localize the location of the cyst. In addition, the performance of endoscopic retrograde pancreatography can be invaluable in localizing cysts and ruptured ducts.[82]

A few patients will improve on supportive management only. In one series, 1 out of 4 such cases was cured nonoperatively, but 2 of the remaining 3 patients died during the treatment period.[82]

In another series, 10 out of 22 patients were successfully treated nonoperatively. The remaining 12 patients represented failures of medical management, and of these 4 patients died.[81] Therefore, it would appear that although the initial treatment of the patient with pancreatic ascites using intravenous therapy and total parenteral nutrition may be promising, if the condition does not show evidence of improvement operation should be considered. As in the treatment of uncomplicated pancreatic pseudocysts, sufficient time should be allowed to permit maturation of the cyst walls so that an internal anastomosis via a Roux-en-Y pancreatico-cystjejunostomy can be carried out. For those cysts in the tail of the pancreas, distal pancreatectomy will suffice. A LeVeen shunt would not be indicated, as this would circulate amylase-rich peritoneal fluid throughout the circulation. A Puestow procedure is used for those patients with chronic pancreatitis and pancreatic ductal dilatation. Subtotal pancreatectomy would needlessly sacrifice too great an amount of functioning pancreatic tissue.

ANSWER: D.

4.14. A 48-year-old alcoholic man gives a 3-year history of progressive abdominal pain, increased by eating but now occurring constantly. He has lost 32 lb in the previous year and has been hospitalized for 70 days during that period. Serum amylase concentration is normal; abdominal X rays and an endoscopic retrograde pancreatogram are shown as Figures 4-9 and 4-10. An oral cholecystogram and upper GI tract X ray are normal. Treatment at this time should consist of:

A. Sphincteroplasty.
B. Splanchnic block.
C. Longitudinal pancreaticojejunostomy (Puestow procedure).
D. Subtotal pancreatectomy.
E. Distal pancreaticojejunostomy (Duval procedure).

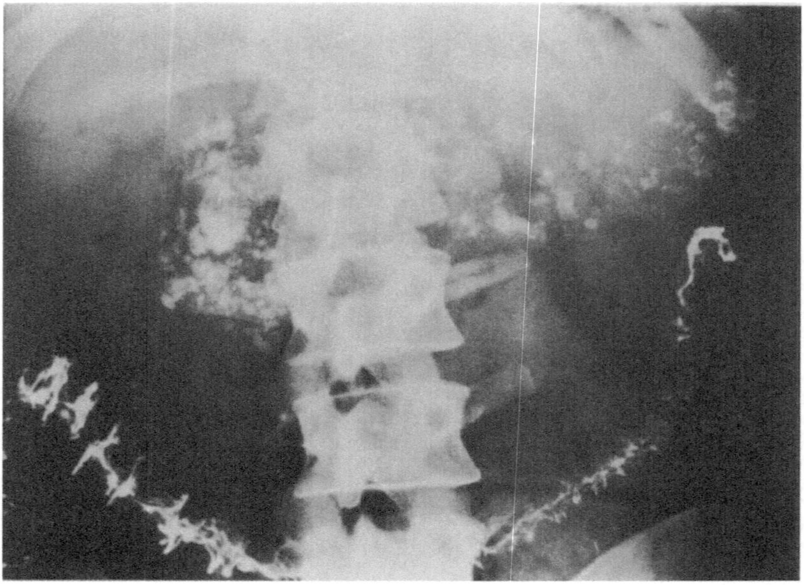

Figure 4-9

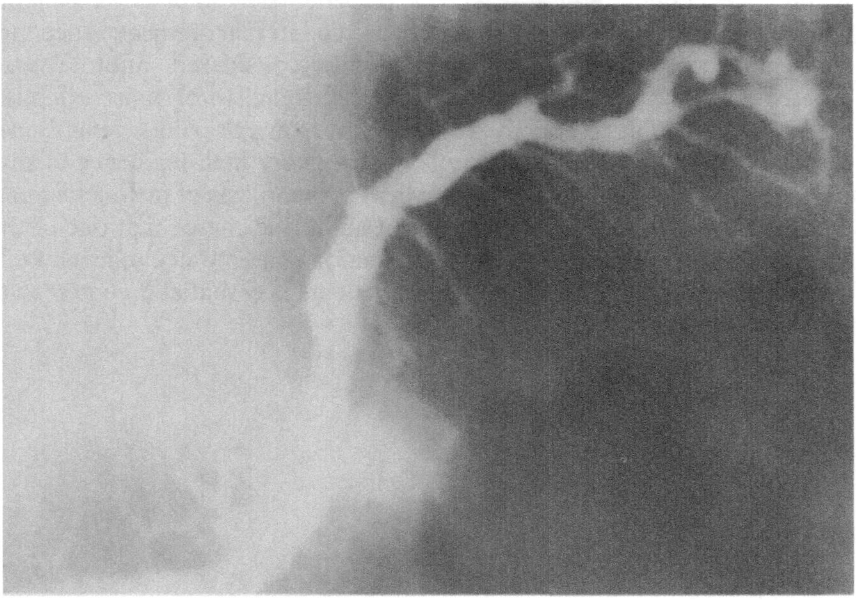

Figure 4-10

This man has progressive chronic pancreatitis, as evidenced by the pancreatic calcifications and typical endoscopic retrograde cholangiopancreatography (ERCP) findings demonstrating ductal dilatation. Some of these patients will also manifest evidence of diabetes mellitus and pancreatic insufficiency. Prior to any decision regarding operative treatment, ERCP should be carried out.[83] This study will differentiate those patients who have a fibrotic strictured pancreatic duct from those with a dilated pancreatic duct, with or without pancreaticolithiasis.

Historically, many operations have been utilized to relieve the nearly constant pain from which these patients suffer. Splanchnic nerve blockade or celiac ganglionectomy are no longer performed for this condition. Furthermore, transduodenal sphincteroplasty is now obsolete in the management of chronic pancreatitis, and indeed the only indication for biliary tract surgery in these patients is the presence of concomittant gallstones or common bile duct stones.[84,85]

For those patients with a dilated ductal system, internal drainage into a defunctionalized Roux-en-Y loop is feasible. It has been found that short pancreaticojejunostomies are generally not helpful.[86] Longitudinal pancreaticojejunostomy draining 80% or more of the pancreatic ductal system is, however, effective in at least 80% of patients.[84,87] For those patients without major pancreatic ductal dilatation, no internal drainage procedure is feasible, and resectional therapy must be considered. Subtotal pancreatectomy (80%–95% resection) has been found to be more effective than a 50%–80% pancreatic resection,[85] but although pain is reliably decreased, subtotal pancreatectomy leads to a very high incidence of diabetes mellitus and significant steatorrhea.[88] Regardless of the ductal anatomy and the method of treatment, most authorities agree that one of the major prognostic indicators is the continuation of heavy alcoholic intake.[89] Therefore, selection of well-motivated patients is essential if good results are to be obtained.

ANSWER: C.

References

1. Halasz, N.A.: Counterfeit cholecystitis: A common diagnostic dilemma. *Am. J. Surg.* 130:189, 1975.
2. Cintora, I., Ben-Ora, A., MacNeil, R., Gilsdorf, R.B.: Cholecystosonography for the decision to operate when acute cholecystitis is suspected. *Am. J. Surg.* 138:818, 1979.
3. Weissman, H.S., Frank, M.S., Bernstein, L.H., Freeman, L.M.: Rapid and accurate diagnosis of acute cholecystitis with 99MTC-HIDA cholescintigraphy. *Am. J. Roentgenol. Radium Ther. Nucl. Med.* 132:523, 1979.
4. Wright, H.K., Holden, W.D.: The risks of emergency surgery for acute cholecystitis. *Arch. Surg.* 81:341, 1960.
5. Morrow, D.J., Thompson, J., Wilson, S.E.: Acute cholecystitis in the elderly. *Arch. Surg.* 113:1149, 1978.
6. Hinchey, E.J., Elias, G.L., Hampson, L.G.: Acute cholecystitis. *Surg. Gynecol. Obstet.* 120:475, 1965.
7. Glenn, F.: Cholecystostomy in the high risk patient with biliary tract disease. *Ann. Surg.* 185:185, 1977.
8. Gingrich, R.A., Awe, W.C., Boyden, A.M., Petersen, C.G.: Cholecystostomy in acute cholecystitis: Factors influencing morbidity and mortality. *Am. J. Surg.* 116:310, 1968.
9. Hays, D.M., Glenn, F.: The fate of the cholecystostomy patient. *J. Am. Geriatr. Soc.* 3:21, 1955.
10. Malmstrom, P., Olsson, A.M.: Cholecystostomy for acute cholecystitis. *Am. J. Surg.* 126:397, 1973.
11. Saharia, P.C., Cameron, J.L.: Clinical management of acute cholangitis. *Surg. Gynecol. Obstet.* 142:369, 1976.
12. Saik, R.P., Greenburg, A.G., Farris, J.M., Peskin, G.W.: Spectrum of cholangitis. *Am. J. Surg.* 130:143, 1975.
13. Bourgault, A.M., England, D.M., Rosenblat, J.E., Forgacs, P., Bieger, R.C.: Clinical characteristics of anaerobic bactibilia. *Arch. Intern. Med.* 139:1346, 1979.
14. Keighley, M.R.B., Drysdale, R.B., Quoraishi, A.H., Burdon, D.W., Alexander-Williams, J.: Antibiotic treatment of biliary sepsis. *Surg. Clin. North Am.* 55:1379, 1975.
15. Dow, R.W., Lindenauer, S.M.: Acute obstructive suppurative cholangitis. *Ann. Surg.* 169:272, 1969.
16. Hinchey, E.J., Couper, C.E.: Acute obstructive suppurative cholangitis. *Am. J. Surg.* 117:62, 1969.
17. Shaffer, E.A., Small, D.M.: Gallstone disease: Pathogenesis and management. *Curr. Probl. Surg.* 13:7, 1976.
18. Wenckert, A., Robertson, B.: The natural course of gallstone disease. *Gastroenterology* 50:376, 1966.
19. Lund, J.: Surgical indications in cholelithiasis: Prophylactic cholecystectomy elucidated on the basis of long-term followup on 526 nonoperated cases. *Ann. Surg.* 151:153, 1960.
20. Peskin, G.W.: The treatment of silent gallstones. *Surg. Clin. North Am.* 53:1063, 1973.
21. Method, H.L., Mehn, W.H., Frable, W.J.: "Silent" gallstones. *Arch Surg.* 85:338, 1962.
22. Pomare, E.W., Heaton, K.W., Low-Beer, T.S., Espiner, H.J.: The effect of wheat bran upon bile salt metabolism and upon the lipid composition of bile in gallstone patients. *Digestive Diseases* 21:521, 1976.
23. Bennion, L.J., Grundy, S.M.: Risk factors for the development of cholelithiasis in man. *N. Engl. J. Med.* 299:1161, 1978.

24. Iser, J.H., Dawling, R.H., Mok, H.Y.I., Bell, G.D.: Chenodeoxycholic acid treatment of gallstones. *N. Engl. J. Med.* 293:378, 1975.
25. Thistle, J.L., Hofmann, A.F., Ott, B.J., Stephens, D.H.: Chenotherapy for gallstone dissolution. *J.A.M.A.* 239:1041, 1978.
26. McSherry, C.K., Morrissey, K.P., Swarm, R.L., May, P.S., Niemann, W.H., Glenn, F.: Chenodeoxycholic acid induced liver injury in pregnant and neonatal baboons. *Ann. Surg.* 184:490, 1976.
27. Kaminski, D.L., Barner, H.B., Codd, J.E., Wolfe, B.M.: Evaluation of the results of external choledochoduodenostomy for retained, recurrent, or primary common duct stones. *Am. J. Surg.* 137:162, 1979.
28. Stuart, M., Hoerr, S.O.: Late results of side-to-side choledochoduodenostomy and of transduodenal sphincterotomy for benign disorders. *Am. J. Surg.* 123:67, 1972.
29. Madden, J.L., Chung, J.Y., Kandalaft, S., Parekh, M.: Choledochoduodenostomy: An unjustly maligned surgical procedure. *Am. J. Surg.* 119:45, 1970.
30. Degenshein, G.A.: Choledochoduodenostomy: An 18 year study of 175 consecutive cases. *Surgery* 76:319, 1974.
31. Nardi, G.: Discussion of a paper by Hayes, M.A., Cahow, C.E.: A technique for pancreatico biliary sphincteroplasty. *Am. J. Surg.* 137:470, 1979.
32. Saharia, P.C., Zuidema, G.D., Cameron, J.L.: Primary common duct stones. *Ann. Surg.* 185:598, 1977.
33. Siegel, J.H.: Endoscopic management of choledocholithiasis and papillary stenosis. *Surg. Gynecol. Obstet.* 148:747, 1979.
34. Safrany, L.: Duodenoscopic sphincterotomy and gallstone removal. *Gastroenterology* 72:338, 1977.
35. Safrany, L.: Endoscopic treatment of biliary tract diseases: An international study. *Lancet* 2:983, 1978.
36. Liguory, C., Loriga, P.: Endoscopic sphincterotomy: Analysis of 155 cases. *Am. J. Surg.* 136:609, 1978.
37. Burhenne, H.J.: Complications of nonoperative extraction of retained common duct sontes. *Am. J. Surg.* 131:260, 1976.
38. Hall, R.C., Sakiyalak, P., Kim, S.K., Rogers, L.S., Webb, W.R.: Failure of operative cholangiography to prevent retained common duct stones. *Am. J. Surg.* 125:51, 1973.
39. Gardner, B.: Experiences with the use of intra choledocho heparinized saline for the treatment of retained common duct stones. *Am. J. Surg.* 177:240, 1973.
40. Gardner, B., Dennis, C.R., Patti, J.: Current status of heparin dissolution of gallstones. *Am. J. Surg.* 130:293, 1975.
41. Pitt, H.A., Cameron, J.L.: Sodium cholate dissolution of retained biliary stones: Mortality rate following intrahepatic infusion. *Surgery* 85:457, 1979.
42. Mack, E., Saito, C., Goldfarb, S., Carlson, G.L., Hofmann, A.: Local toxicity of T-tube infused cholate in the rhesus monkey. *Surg. Forum* 28:408, 1977.
43. Burhenne, H.J., Richards, V., Mathewson, C., Westdahl, P.R.: Nonoperative extraction of retained biliary tract stones requiring multiple sessions. *Am. J. Surg.* 128:288, 1974.
44. Andersson, A., Bergdahl, L.: Disease of the gallbladder in patients with normal cholecystograms. *Am. J. Surg.* 132:322, 1976.
45. Demuth, W.E.: Cholecystectomy following a normal cholecystogram. *Am. Surg.* 35:653, 1969.
46. Freeman, J.B., Cohen, W.N., DenBesten, L.: Cholecystokinin cholangiography and analysis of duodenal bile in the investigation of pain in the right upper quadrant of the abdomen without gallstones. *Surg. Gynecol. Obstet.* 140:371, 1975.
47. Freeman, J.B., Olson, C.M.: Refinements in the detection of gallbladder disorders. *Contemp. Surg.* 13:9, 1978.

48. Nathan, M.H., Newman, A., Murray, D.J.: Normal findings in oral and cholecystokinin cholecystography. *J.A.M.A.* 240:2271, 1978.
49. Valberg, L.S., Jabbari, M., Kerr, J.W., Curtis, A.C., Ramchand, S., Prentice, R.S.A.: Biliary pain in young women in the absence of gallstones. *Gastroenterology* 60:1020, 1971.
50. Humphries, T.J., Cloutier, C.T.: The value of duodenal bile examination in the evaluation of persistent pain in the upper part of the abdomen. *Surg. Gynecol. Obstet.* 147:177, 1978.
51. Paloyan, D., Simonowitz, D.: Diagnostic considerations in acute alcoholic and gallstone pancreatitis. *Am. J. Surg.* 132:329, 1976.
52. Acosta, J.M., Ledemsa, C.L.: Gallstone migration as a cause of acute pancreatitis. *N. Engl. J. Med.* 290:484, 1974.
53. Kelly, T.R.: Gallstone pancreatitis. *Arch. Surg.* 109:294, 1974.
54. Taylor, T.V., Rimmer, S.: Pancreatic duct reflux in patients with gallstone pancreatitis. *Lancet* 1:848, 1980.
55. Ranson, J.H.C.: The timing of biliary surgery in acute pancreatitis. *Ann. Surg.* 189:654, 1979.
56. Paloyan, D., Simonowitz, D., Skinner, D.B.: The timing of biliary tract operations in patients with pancreatitis associated with gallstones. *Surg. Gynecol. Obstet.* 141:737, 1975.
57. Kelly, T.R.: Gallstone pancreatitis: Pathophysiology. *Surgery* 80:488, 1976.
58. Jacobs, M.L., Daggett, W.M., Civetta, J.M., Vasu, M.A., Lawson, D.W., Warshaw, A.L., Nardi, G.L., Bartlett, M.K.: Acute pancreatitis: Analysis of factors influencing survival. *Ann. Surg.* 185:43, 1977.
59. Feller, J.H., Brown, R.A., Toussaint, G.P.M., Thompson, A.G.: Changing methods in the treatment of severe pancreatitis. *Am. J. Surg.* 127:196, 1974.
60. Jordan, G.L., Spjut, H.J.: Hemorrhagic pancreatitis. *Arch. Surg.* 104:489, 1972.
61. Bolooki, H., Gliedman, M.L.: Peritoneal dialysis in treatment of acute pancreatitis. *Surgery* 64:466, 1968.
62. Rosato, E.F., Mullis, W.F., Rosato, F.E.: Peritoneal lavage therapy in hemorrhagic pancreatitis. *Surgery* 74:106, 1973.
63. Ranson, J.H.C., Rifkind, K.M., Turner, J.W.: Prognostic signs and nonoperative peritoneal lavage in acute pancreatitis. *Surg. Gynecol. Obstet.* 143:209, 1976.
64. Norton, L., Eiseman, B.: Near total pancreatectomy for hemorrhagic pancreatitis. *Am. J. Surg.* 127:191, 1974.
65. White, T.T., Heimbach, D.M.: Sequestrectomy and hyperalimentation in the treatment of hemorrhagic pancreatitis. *Am. J. Surg.* 132:270, 1976.
66. Warshaw, A.L., Imbembo, A.L., Civetta, J.M., Daggett, W.M.: Surgical intervention in acute necrotizing pancreatitis. *Am. J. Surg.* 127:484, 1974.
67. Lawson, D.W., Daggett, W.M., Civetta, J.M., Corry, R.J., Bartlett, M.K.: Surgical treatment of acute necrotizing pancreatitis. *Ann. Surg.* 172:605, 1970.
68. Blackburn, G.L., Williams, L.F., Bistrian, B.R., Stone, M.S., Phillips, E., Hirsch, E., CLowes, G.H.A., Gregg, J.: New approaches to the management of severe acute pancreatitis. *Am. J. Surg.* 131:114, 1976.
69. Sugawa, C., Walt, A.J.: Endoscopic retrograde pancreatography in the surgery of pancreatic pseudocysts. *Surgery* 86:639, 1979.
70. Bradley, E.L., Clements, L.J.: Spontaneous resolution of pancreatic pseudocysts: Implications for timing of operative intervention. *Am. J. Surg.* 129:23, 1975.
71. Sankaran, S., Walt, A.J.: The natural and unnatural history of pancreatic pseudocysts. *Br. J. Surg.* 62:37, 1975.
72. Frey, C.F.: Pancreatic pseudocysts: Operative strategy. *Ann. Surg.* 188:652, 1978.

73. Bradley, E.L., Clements, J.L., Gonzalez, A.C.: The natural history of pancreatic pseudocysts: A unified concept of management. *Am. J. Surg.* 137:135. 1979.
74. Martin, E.W., Catalano, P., Cooperman, M., Hecht, C., Carey, L.C.: Surgical decision making in the treatment of pancreatic pseudocysts. *Am. J. Surg.* 138:821, 1979.
75. VanHeerden, J.A., ReMine, W.H.: Pseudocysts of the pancreas. *Arch. Surg.* 110:500, 1975.
76. Frey, C.F., Lindenauer, S.M., Miller, T.A.: Pancreatic abscess. *Surg. Gynecol. Obstet.* 149:722, 1979.
77. Ranson, J.H.C., Spencer, F.C.: Prevention, diagnosis and treatment of pancreatic abscess. *Surgery* 82:99, 1977.
78. Miller, T.A., Lindenauer, S.M., Frey, C.F., Stanley, J.C.: Pancreatic abscess. *Arch. Surg.* 108:545, 1974.
79. Cameron, J.L., Brawley, R.K., Bender, H.W., Zuidema, G.D.: The treatment of pancreatic ascites. *Ann. Surg.* 170:668, 1969.
80. Smith, R.B., Warren, W.D., Rivard, A.A., Amerson, J.R.: Pancreatic ascites: Diagnosis and management with particular reference to surgical techniques. *Ann. Surg.* 177:538, 1973.
81. Cameron, J.L., Kieffer, R.S., Anderson, W.J., Zuidema, G.D.: Internal Pancreatic fistulas: Pancreatic ascites in pleural effusions. *Ann. Surg.* 184:587, 1976.
82. Sankaran, S., Walt, A.J.: Pancreatic ascites recognition and management. *Arch. Surg.* 111:430, 1976.
83. Mullens, J.E.: Endoscopic retrograde cholangiopancreatography (ERCP) in the diagnosis of chronic pancreatitis. *Surgery* 84:308, 1978.
84. Way, L.W., Gadacz, T., Goldman, L.: Surgical treatment of chronic pancreatitis. *Am. J. Surg.* 127:202, 1974.
85. White, T.T., Slavotinek, A.H.: Results of surgical treatment of chronic pancreatitis. *Ann. Surg.* 189:217, 1979.
86. White, T.T., Hart, M.J.: Pancreaticojejunostomy versus resection in the treatment of chronic pancreatitis. *Am. J. Surg.* 138:129, 1979.
87. Prinz, R.A., Kaufman, B.H., Folk, F.A., Greenlee, H.B.: Pancreaticojejunostomy for chronic pancreatitis: 2 to 21 year follow-up. *Arch. Surg.* 113:520, 1978.
88. Frey, C.F., Child, C.G., Fry, W.: Pancreatectomy for chronic pancreatitis. *Ann. Surg.* 184:403, 1976.
89. Traverso, L.W., Tompkins, R.K., Urrea, P.T., Longmire, W.P.: Surgical treatment of chronic pancreatitis. *Ann. Surg.* 190:312, 1979.

5
BOWEL OBSTRUCTION

5.1. A 73-year-old woman presents to the emergency room with a 4-day history of crampy abdominal pain, distention, and obstipation. Examination discloses a tympanitic abdomen with high-pitched bowel sounds and with no tenderness or peritoneal signs present. The temperature is 37.4°C and the white blood cell count is 6300 cells/mm^3. Abdominal X rays and a barium enema are performed and are shown as Figures 5-1 and 5-2. Proctoscopy reveals a fungating neoplasm 22 cm from the anus. Treatment should consist of:

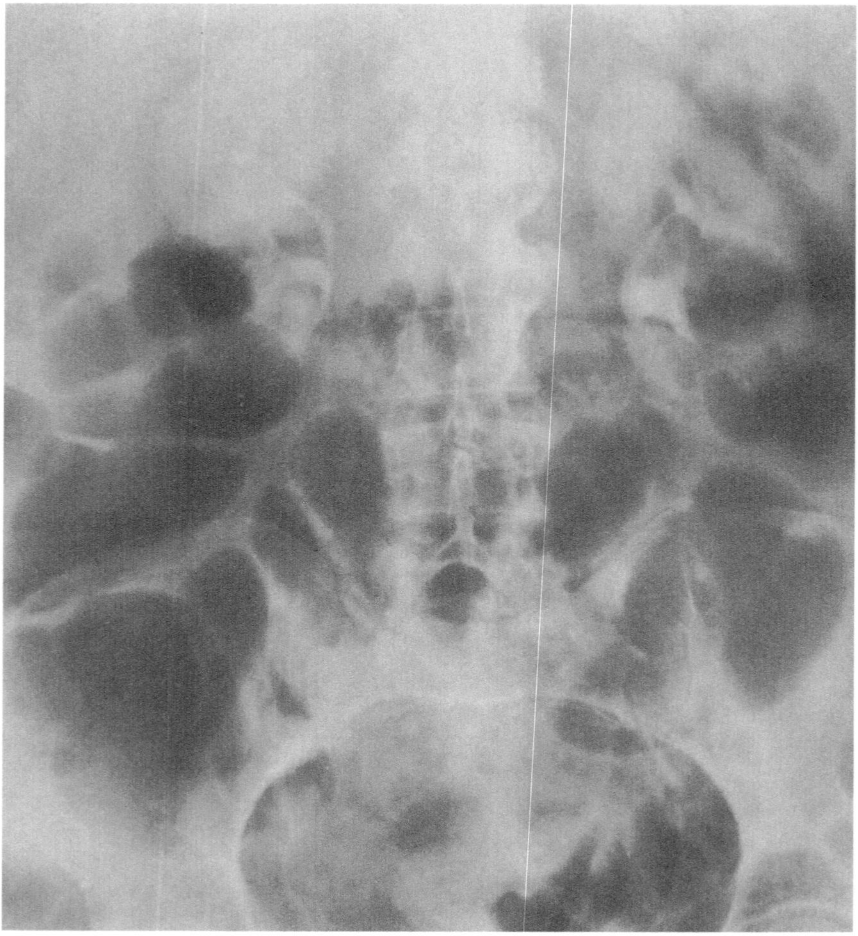

Figure 5-1

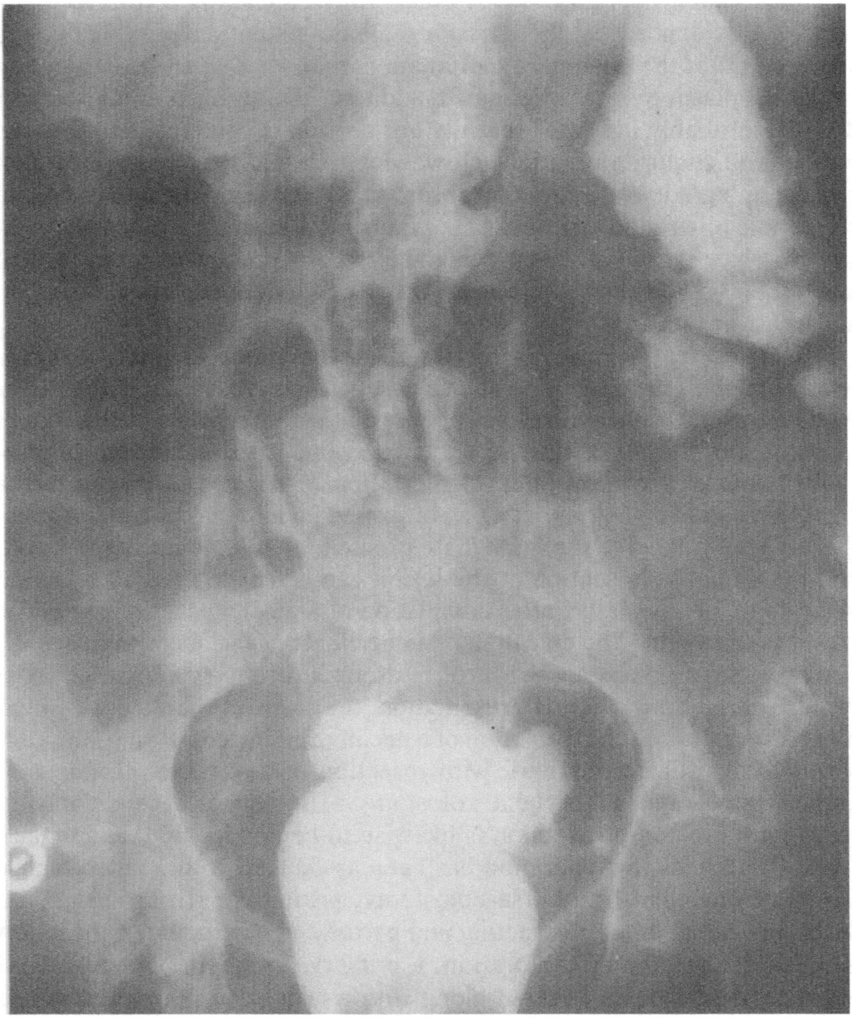

Figure 5-2

A. Insertion of a rectal tube.
B. Cecostomy.
C. Celiotomy, sigmoid resection, and anastomosis.
D. Celiotomy, sigmoid resection, and end sigmoid colostomy.
E. Transverse colostomy.

This patient has an obvious obstructing carcinoma of the rectosigmoid, as evidenced by the massive colonic distention proximally, the sharp cutoff of the column of barium on barium enema, and confirmation of the neoplasm by proctoscopy. In addition, the absence of a history of diarrhea probably indicates that the obstruction is complete and that the patient will require operation. However, it should be remembered that clinical antegrade obstruction is absent in 50% of patients with complete retrograde obstruction demonstrated on barium enema.[1] It is usually possible to place those patients in whom diarrhea is present on a mechanical and antibiotic bowel preparation and do a subsequent one-stage resection and anastomosis.

In the situation presented, immediate operation is indicated after resuscitation of the patient. In such a case, primary resection of the tumor with or without anastomosis is probably a more extensive operation than is justified in these critically ill patients. If there is no evidence of peritonitis from either perforation of the lesion or rupture of the cecum, a right transverse colostomy can be performed under local or general anesthesia. This will solve the immediate problem of colonic decompression, and the definitive resection of the lesion can be carried out as a second stage 10 to 14 days later, after completion of a mechanical and antibiotic bowel preparation. The colostomy can be closed subsequent to this.[2,3] If, however, there is any evidence of peritonitis or any suspicion of cecal rupture at the time of initial presentation, the surgeon should not content himself merely with the formation of a decompressing colostomy. Instead, a celiotomy will be required, with resection of any perforated or gangrenous area, and subsequent colostomy. The use of a cecostomy to relieve a left-colon obstruction is likewise to be condemned, as in many series of patients this operation has been associated with a much higher mortality rate than transverse colostomy, presumably from inadequate decompression.[2] If an obstructing and perforated carcinoma of the colon is noted at the time of exploration, a primary resection of the involved intestine should be carried out along with a wide swath of mesentery to remove regional lymph nodes. An end sigmoid colostomy and an oversewing of the rectal stump completes the procedure. Even though the prognosis of the patient with a perforated colon carcinoma is poor, it is still possible to salvage some of these patients with a standard cancer procedure. If an actual or impending rupture of the cecum is present, a tube cecostomy should be performed. If this is not feasible, the cecum should be exteriorized as a cecostomy. In left-colon obstructions, the cecum tends to rupture first, as it is the thinnest and most distensible portion of the colon. Perforation rarely occurs below a radiologic cecal diameter of 9 cm, and therefore the clinician must realize that in managing a patient with a cecum greater than this size, operation must be considered early to prevent this grave complication.[4]

Malignant obstructions of the transverse colon pose a more difficult problem. Although primary resection and anastomosis may be successfully performed in some cases, it would seem safer to perform a resection and formation of an end ileostomy and mucous fistula with restoration of bowel continuity at a later time. However, owing to the potential lymphatic drainage of this area to both the left and right sides of the colon, a proper cancer operation in this area entails subtotal colectomy. Malignant obstructions of the right colon are well handled by resection and primary anastomosis.[2] Less commonly in large-bowel obstruction, a concomitant small-bowel obstruction will be seen owing to adherence of small intestine to an area of obstructing inflammation in the colon. Proper management in this situation depends upon the formation of a right transverse colostomy to relieve the colon obstruction, along with the insertion of a long intestinal tube for the small-bowel obstruction. With resolution of the inflammatory mass, the small-bowel obstruction will resolve, and the patient can be managed as an uncomplicated large bowel obstruction. Attempts to perform an exploratory celiotomy in this situation and manually free the small bowel obstruction from the inflammatory mass are hazardous, as they can result in a breakdown of the walled-off inflammatory process, thus creating the need for an emergency left hemicolectomy.

ANSWER: E.

5.2. A 74-year-old woman with no previous abdominal symptoms and a history of two myocardial infarctions is brought to the emergency room complaining of severe abdominal pain that began abruptly 3 hr earlier. She is writhing in pain on the examining table, and her pulse is 88 and irregular. Her abdominal examination discloses only mild tenderness diffusely. Bowel sounds are hypoactive, and no peritoneal signs are present. Her temperature is 37.4°C, and the white blood cell count and serum amylase concentration are normal. Four views of the abdomen are reported as normal. The test most likely to lead to a correct diagnosis in this patient is:

A. Barium enema.
B. CAT scan.
C. Intravenous pyelogram.
D. Arteriogram.
E. Intravenous cholangiogram.

One of the most catastrophic acute abdominal conditions results from interruption of the mesenteric blood supply to the intestines with resultant intestinal ischemia and gangrene. The reported mortality rates for this condition range from 60% to 100%. Several different disease processes can affect the mesenteric vessels and cause interruption of blood supply. Most common among these are a superior mesenteric artery embolus or thrombosis.

The clinical picture associated with these conditions can be subtle. Pain is an early and significant complaint, being severe and noncrampy and seemingly out of proportion to the abdominal examination. Striking elevations in temperature and white blood cell count can be noted. Vomiting can be seen, as can diarrhea, which soon becomes bloody. The serum amylase concentration can be modestly elevated, sometimes leading to confusion with acute pancreatitis. Emboli to the superior mesenteric artery generally occur in patients with atrial fibrillation, a previous myocardial infarction with an associated mural thrombus, or as a result of proximal atherosclerotic plaques that are broken off and embolized downstream. Thrombosis of the mesenteric artery occurs solely in those patients with progressive narrowing of the artery from atherosclerotic disease. In any patient thought to have a mesenteric vascular occlusion, arteriography should be performed immediately, for it is obvious that only with early resuscitation followed by arteriography and immediate operation can the uniformly poor results obtained in these patients be improved.[5–8] The differentiation between the two varieties can generally be made by arteriography. An embolus tends to lodge more distally in the mesenteric arteries, sparing the most proximal jejunal branches, whereas the thrombosis tends to involve the root of the mesenteric artery, and therefore the entire small intestine and part of the large intestime become ischemic.[6]

In the treatment of an embolus to the superior mesenteric artery, the first task is to deal with the arterial occlusion. By mobilizing the right colon downward into the left, the origin of the superior mesenteric artery can be identified and a Fogarty catheter utilized to perform an embolectomy. Following repair of the vessel, 15 or 20 min should be allowed in order to observe the previously ischemic intestine. Although it is well recognized that the presence of normal color and distal arterial pulsations does not necessarily signal bowel viability, it will often be noted that previously dusky and cyanotic bowel will regain a nearly normal color following revascularization, and this intestine can usually be safely retained.[7] If, however, at the end of the observation period the bowel remains nonviable, primary resection and anastomosis is indicated. In certain cases, the differentiation of viable from nonviable intestine may prove impossible, and in such circumstances a second-look operation should be performed 12 to 18 hr later. It should be emphasized that the decision for the second-look operation should be made at the time of the original operation. It is important not to gauge the need for the second procedure on the basis of the patient's clinical course following initial surgery, as this can often be misleading. Resection of the gangrenous intestine alone with no attempt at revascularization will result in a fatal outcome in virtually all cases.[7]

The more common entity, superior mesenteric artery thrombosis, superimposed on a chronically atherosclerotic vessel, is even more lethal than a mesenteric embolism. The preoperative management of these patients is identical to that of patients with embolus, and the need for early celiotomy is essential. Approximately half of these patients will give a prodrome of increasing postprandial abdominal pain coming on weeks to months before the onset of the acute occlusion. If these patients are seen and diagnosed at this time, intestinal revascularization can be carried out before intestinal ischemia results. Once again, primary attention must be paid to the vessel occlusion. After the route of the mesenteric vessel has been exposed, bypass of the occlusion is recommended, utilizing either autogenous saphenous vein or a 6- to 8-mm Dacron graft from the aorta to the mesenteric artery just distal to the occlusion. Endarterectomy has been attempted, but the technical aspects of the procedure in this area are quite difficult and the results uniformly poor. The graft will generally result in some return of evidence of intestinal viability, and the appropriate bowel resection can then be carried out if indicated. Again, the need for a second-look operation must be decided upon at this time. In both superior mesenteric artery embolus and thrombosis, the role of postoperative anticoagulation remains controversial.

ANSWER: D.

5.3. A 62-year-old woman with myeloid metaplasia undergoes splenectomy. On the seventh postoperative day she is afebrile, and her platelet count is 840,000/mm^3. Over a 24-hr period, she develops severe diffuse abdominal pain and vomiting. Her temperature is 38.6°C, and her abdomen is diffusely tender but not rigid. Peritoneal signs are present. She passes a watery stool, which is positive for occult blood. Her white blood cell count is 28,400 cells/mm^3, and her serum amylase content is 140 IU. Four views of the abdomen disclose only a nonspecific ileus pattern. Treatment should consist of:

A. Fluid resuscitation, nasogastric suction, and antibiotics.
B. Celiotomy and closure of perforated duodenal ulcer.
C. Drainage of left subphrenic abscess.
D. Celiotomy and bowel resection.
E. Celiotomy, embolectomy, and bowel resection.

The key to the management of this patient lies in the awareness of the entity of mesenteric venous occlusion and resultant small-bowel gangrene. This entity is much less common than mesenteric arterial occlusions from embolus or thrombosis, but early diagnosis is critical, as many of these patients are salvageable with early operation owing to the fact that segmental bowel gangrene can occur in this condition, unlike the more diffuse bowel gangrene noted in acute arterial occlusions.[5,9] This condition is seen in patients with hypercoagulable states and also in those with cirrhosis and portal hypertension leading to stagnation of mesenteric venous flow.

A peripheral issue in this instance is the role of the splenectomy and the resultant postsplenectomy thrombocytosis in predisposing to the mesenteric occlusion. Although there are many case reports of patients with postsplenectomy thrombocystosis who have sustained thromboembolic complications, most prospective studies have not been able to note such an assocation.[10-12] However, two recent reports appear to indicate that although the patient without hematologic disease who undergoes splenectomy is not at increased risk of developing thromboembolic complications, those patients with myeloproliferative disorders who undergo splenectomy have an increased risk of thrombosis and perhaps should receive anticoagulants or antiplatelet drugs postoperatively.[13,14]

ANSWER: D.

5.4. A 72-year-old mentally retarded man presents to the emergency room with a 2-day history of abdominal pain, distention, and vomiting. Examination reveals tympany and high-pitched bowel sounds. No peritoneal signs are present. The patient's temperature is 37.6°C, and the white blood cell count is 14,000 cells/mm^3. A supine abdominal X ray and barium enema are shown as Figures 5-3 and 5-4. The patient should next undergo:

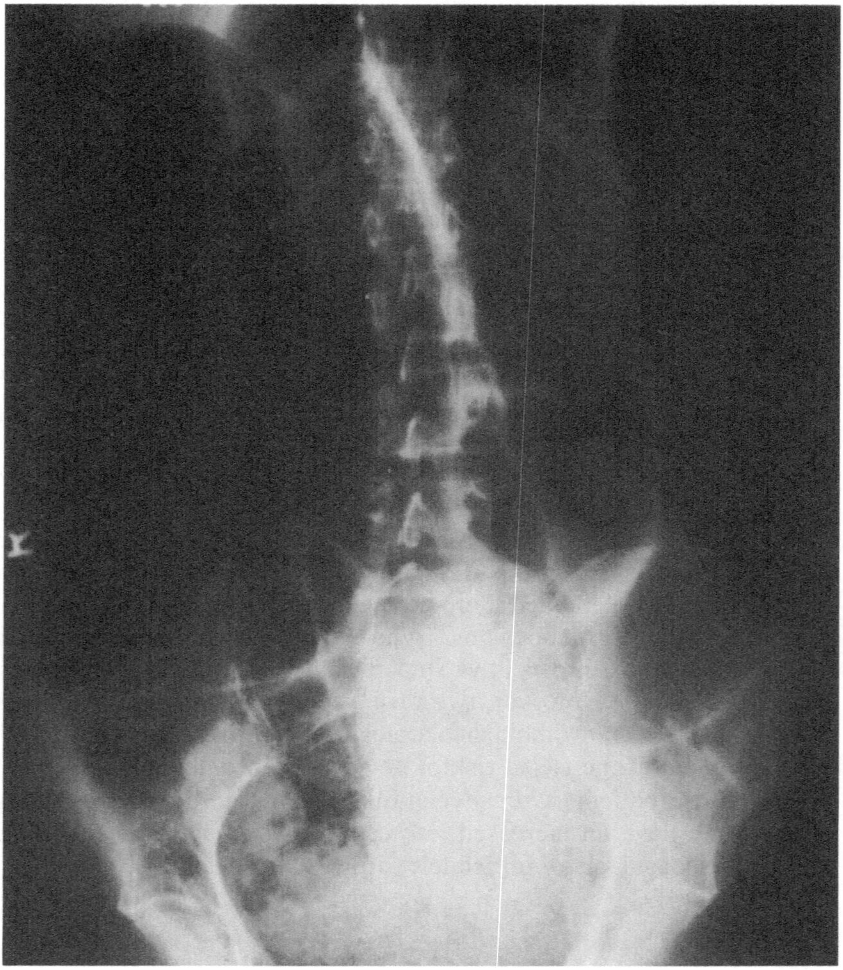

Figure 5-3

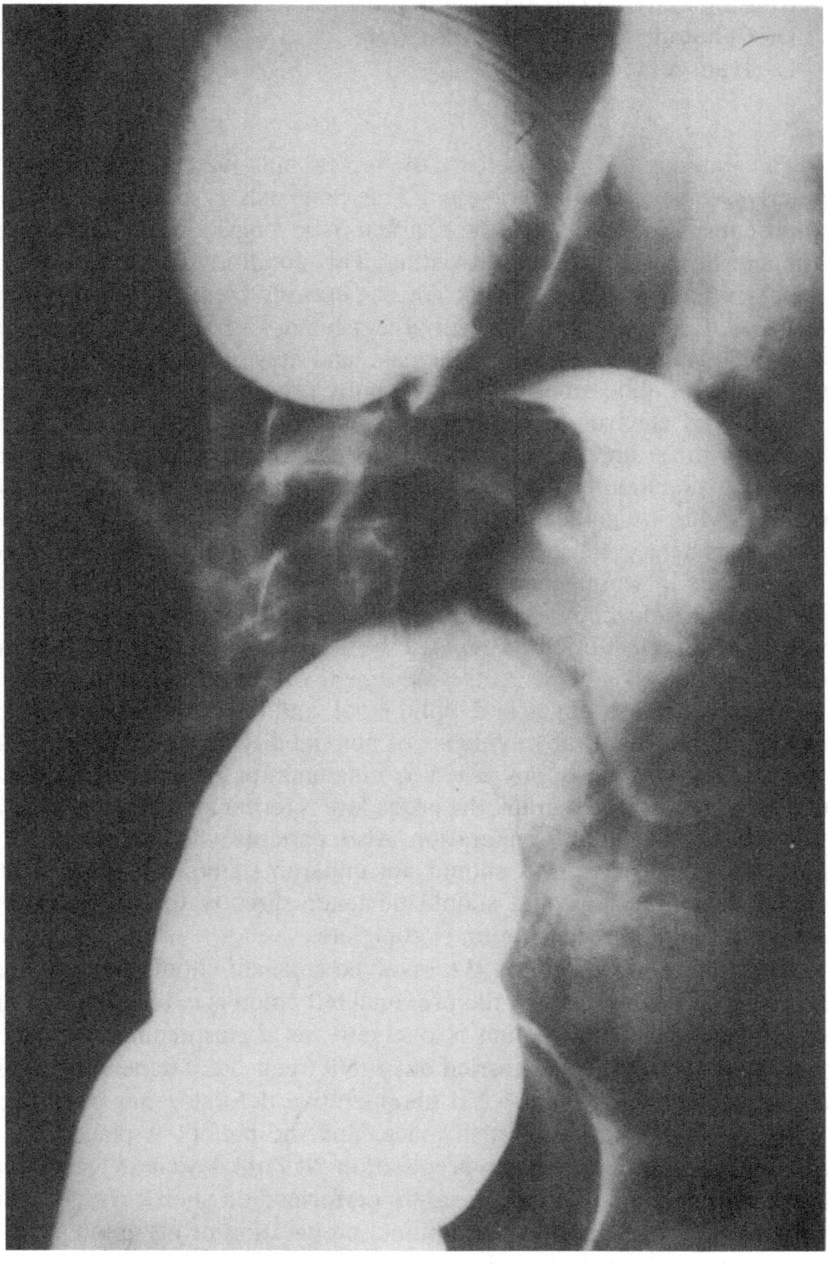

Figure 5-4

A. High-pressure barium enema.
B. Sigmoidoscopy.
C. Celiotomy and sigmoid detorsion.
D. Celiotomy and sigmoid resection.
E. Transverse colostomy.

The abdominal X ray discloses the typical massive colonic distention regularly seen in sigmoid volvulus. This diagnosis is confirmed by the barium enema, which shows the characteristic "bird's-beak" deformity at the site of the rectosigmoid twisting. This condition occurs mainly in the elderly and, for reasons that are not entirely clear, in the mentally retarded. Often these patients will give a history of similar episodes of abdominal distention and pain in the past, and they present clinically with abrupt onset of abdominal pain with rapidly progressive distention.

Fluid and electrolyte abnormalities are often profound in this condition, and these imbalances, coupled with the general debility and decreased cardiopulmonary reserve seen in this group of patients, yield a condition with a significant mortality.[15] Once the diagnosis of sigmoid volvulus has been confirmed, nonoperative reduction should be attempted in all patients in whom there is no evidence of ischemic or gangrenous bowel. A sigmoidoscopy is performed, and once the point of obstruction is reached, a well lubricated rectal tube is passed through the twisted area. In perhaps 80% of cases, this treatment will be effective, giving rise to an immediate rush of gas and liquid stool, and the rectal tube can then be left in place.[16–18] If any evidence of nonviability of the colon is noted at the time of sigmoidoscopy, such as inflammation or ulceration of the mucosa or blood in the rectum, the procedure is terminated and the patient is immediately prepared for operation. Also, patients who present initially with evidence of peritonitis should not undergo sigmoidoscopy and attempted decompression and should be taken directly to the operating room when volume resuscitation is complete.

At the time of celiotomy, the involved segment should be detorsed and resected. Following this, the proximal left colon is exteriorized as an end colostomy and the rectum is oversewn as a Hartmann procedure. Reanastomosis can then be carried out 4 to 8 weeks later depending upon the condition of the patient.[3,19] If nonoperative detorsion has been successful, the rectal tube is left in place, and the patient is placed on a mechanical and antibiotic colon preparation. Several days later, resection and primary anastomosis can be safely performed on such a patient who is fully resuscitated and has had optimal preparation of his colon.

If operation is not carried out, the volvulus will recur in 55%–90%

of patients.[16,18] It must be remembered that sigmoid colopexy is an inadequate operation, frequently followed by recurrence of the sigmoid volvulus, and therefore no definitive treatment less than sigmoid resection will suffice.[3,19] However, in certain patients who are extremely elderly or debilitated, it may prove wiser not to perform an elective resection and accept the risk of recurrence. In many of these patients, the mere fact that one episode of volvulus has been successfully reduced probably increases the chances that any subsequent attack can likewise be nonoperatively managed.

ANSWER: B.

5.5. A 48-year-old man gives a 3-day history of progressive abdominal pain, vomiting, and distention. On examination, his abdomen is tympanitic with high-pitched bowel sounds and left upper quadrant tenderness. His temperature is 37.8°C, and the white blood cell count is 12,800 cells/mm^3. Abdominal X rays and a barium enema are taken and are shown as Figures 5-5, 5-6, and 5-7. The patient should undergo immediate:

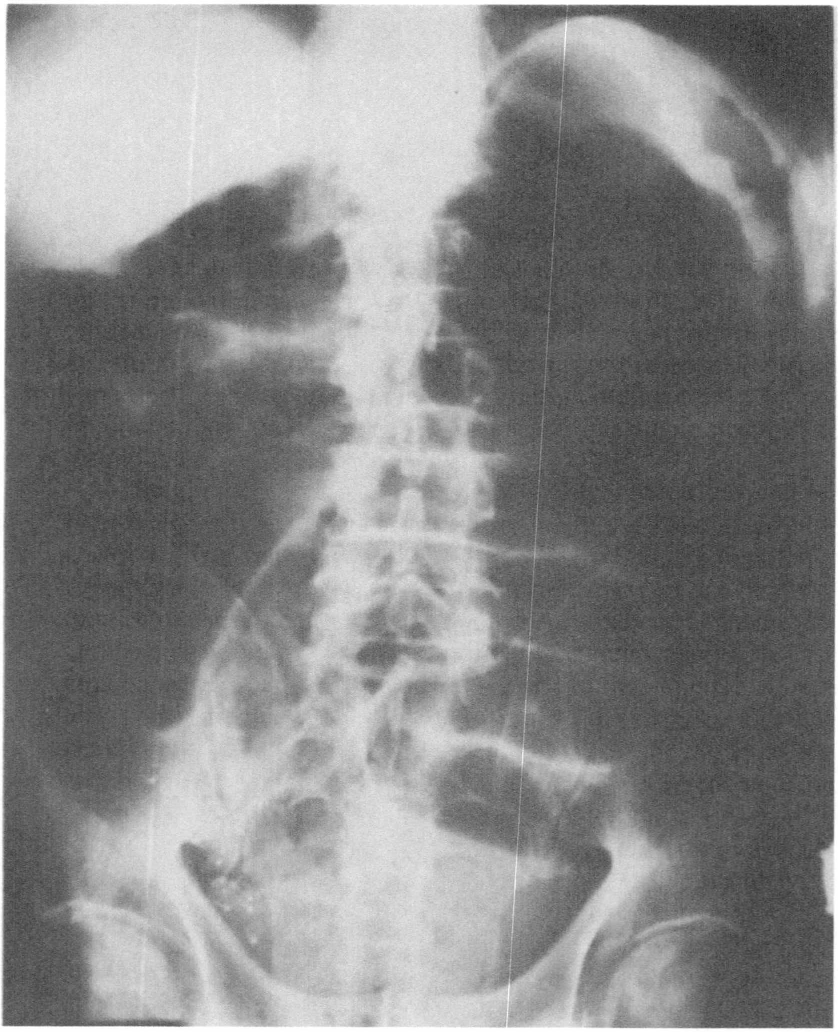

Figure 5-5

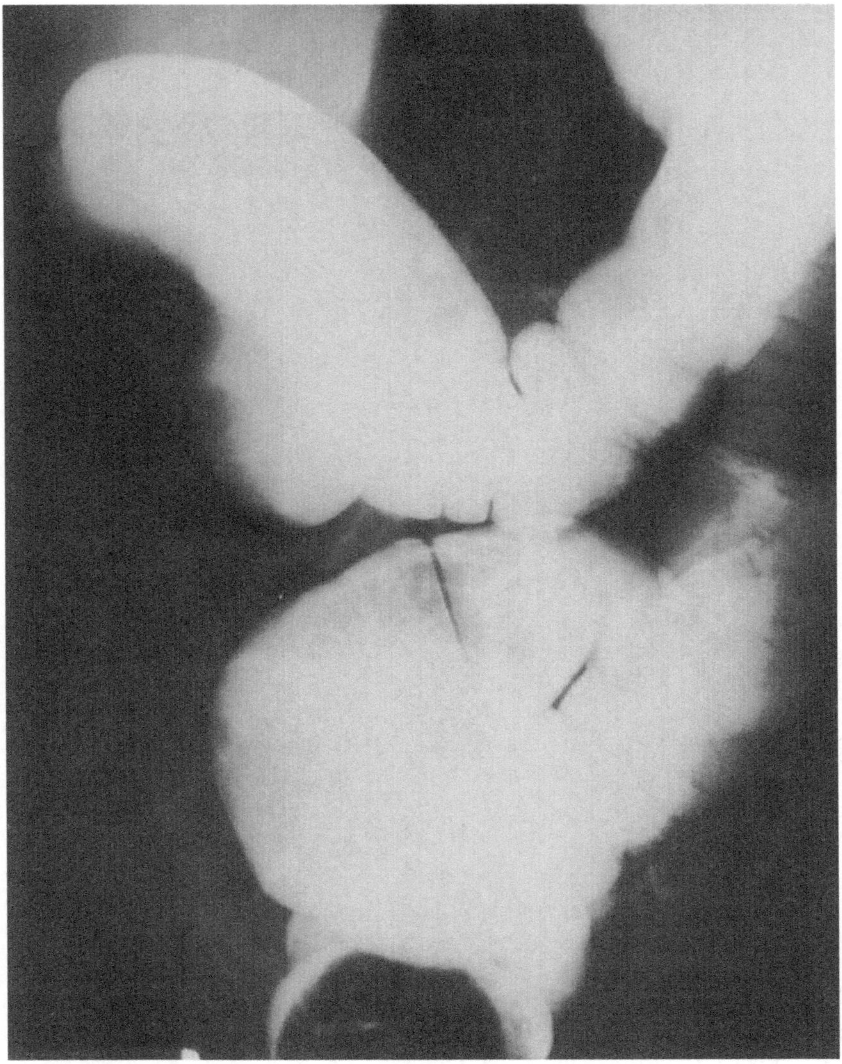

Figure 5-6

A. Cecostomy.
B. Transverse colostomy.
C. Celiotomy and cecal detorsion.
D. Hydrostatic barium enema.
E. Ileostomy.

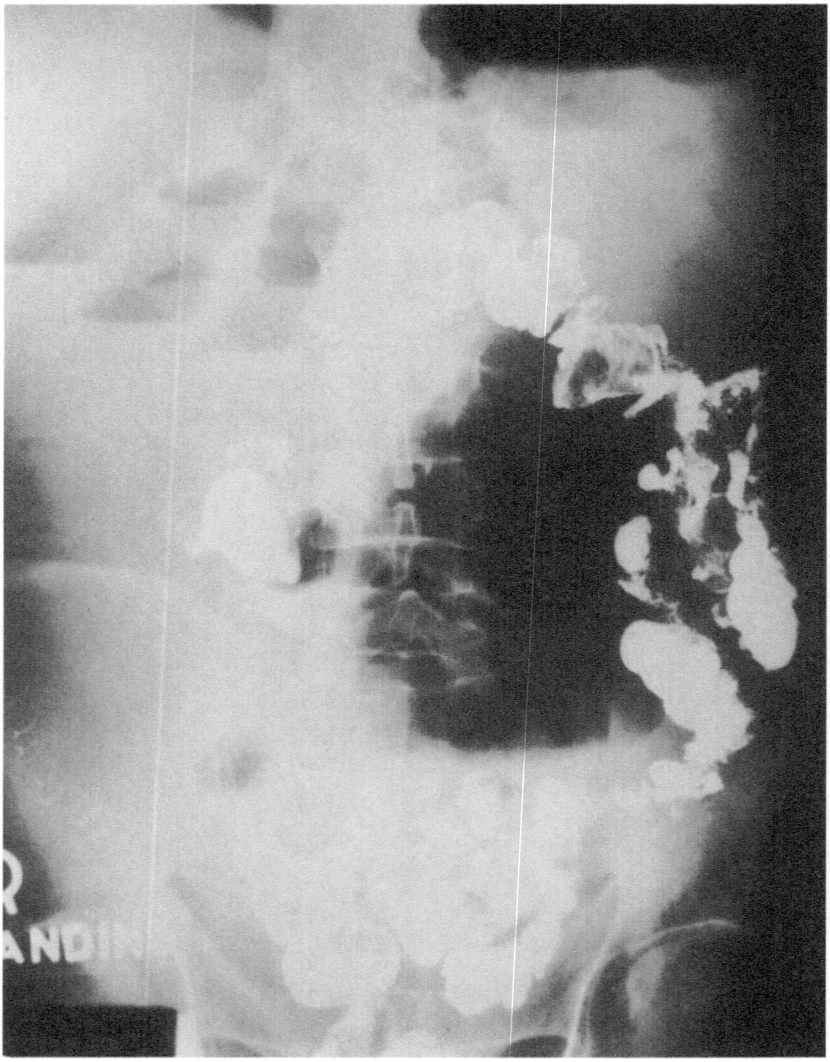

Figure 5-7

The supine abdominal X ray discloses a large gas-filled loop of bowel in the left upper quadrant. The situation becomes quite clear upon study of the barium enema, which shows a distinct cutoff of the column of barium at the ascending colon. The postevacuation view shows some residual dilated small-bowel loops in the right upper quadrant, but the pathognomonic massively dilated cecal gas shadow in the left side of the abdomen confirms the diagnosis.

The signs and symptoms of cecal volvulus are indistinguishable from those of sigmoid volvulus or from the other forms of large-bowel obstruction. The diagnosis can usually be suspected on the basis of abdominal X rays, and is then confirmed by barium enema. Following volume resuscitation, these patients must be operated upon immediately because of the risk of cecal gangrene and perforation. A transverse midabdominal incision offers the advantages of good access to the area plus a low incidence of postoperative complications. Detorsion of the involved cecum has proven to be an inadequate operation, as recurrence of the cecal volvulus is likely.[20] There is, however, considerable controversy regarding the roles of cecostomy, cecopexy, and cecal resection.[3,21] If the cecum is definitely viable with no evidence of serosal splitting or patchy gangrene, a tube cecostomy can be performed. In addition, a long peritoneal flap can be elevated along the right paracolic gutter, and this can be sutured to the ascending colon with nonabsorbable suture material.[20] These steps will prevent recurrence of the volvulus. However, if the cecum is nonviable or possesses areas of patchy gangrene or serosal splitting, a right hemicolectomy with primary ileotransverse colostomy should be carried out. Although an occasional cecal volvulus will detorse during the course of a barium enema, recurrence is so common that this cannot be regarded as a form of therapy.

ANSWER: C.

5.6. A 42-year-old woman underwent an abdominal hysterectomy 4 years previously. She presents to the emergency with a 3-hr history of severe, constant, noncrampy midabdominal pain radiating to the back. She has vomited three times and passed no gas or stool since the pain began. Her pulse is 120. Her temperature is 37.6°C. Her abdomen is very tender around the umbilicus and guarding is present throughout. Peritoneal signs are present and bowel sounds are hypoactive. The white blood cell count is 12,400 cells/mm^3 and the serum amylase is 80 IU. Abdominal X rays are normal. Treatment should consist of:

A. Laparoscopy.
B. Insertion of a long intestinal tube.
C. Immediate appendectomy.
D. Nasogastric tube, anticholingeric drugs, and antibiotics.
E. Immediate celiotomy.

Any patient who has had a previous abdominal operation must be suspected of having intestinal obstruction at any time in the future when they present with abdominal pain. In this instance, the presence of an acute onset of severe pain radiating to the back is highly suggestive of a strangulation obstruction of the small intestine. This is further confirmed by the presence of local tenderness, tachycardia, leukocytosis, and fever.

The above history represents a rather classical presentation of an acute strangulation obstruction of small intestine. However, many cases present in a much more subtle fashion, making the differentiation between simple and strangulation obstruction most difficult. Because of the lack of consistent criteria to differentiate these two varieties of bowel obstruction, early operation after a period of volume resuscitation and nasogastric suction has been advocated in all cases of bowel obstruction.[22,23] Reliance on predetermined criteria indicating nonviability of intestine has proven quite misleading. In one series of patients with strangulation obstruction, 70% of patients had no fever, 42% had no leukocytosis or tachycardia, and X rays indicated a strangulation obstruction in only 10%.[23] Other authors have pointed out that normal X rays are seen frequently in strangulation obstruction, as the closed loop rapidly fills up with fluid, giving a normal appearance to the abdominal roentgenogram before any evidence of bowel dilatation appears.[22,24]

In view of these difficulties, any patient with an abdominal scar or an incarcerated external hernia who presents with any signs or symptoms of bowel obstruction should be rapidly volume-repleted and treated with nasogastric suction. If any signs of nonviable intestine are present—such as local tenderness, fever, tachycardia, or leukocytosis—prompt operation should be carried out. If none of these signs are present, it may be assumed that a simple obstruction is present and continued nonoperative management may be successful. In one series of 238 patients, it was noted that no patient had dead bowel if all of these signs were absent. If one sign was present, some patients had dead bowel; if more than one sign was present, the chances of this occurrence increased significantly.[25]

ANSWER: E.

5.7. A 26-year-old man undergoes an appendectomy for a perforated acute appendicitis. No nasogastric tube is utilized, and the patient begins to vomit on the third postoperative day. He is afebrile and has a white blood cell count of 7800 cells/mm^3. X rays of the abdomen disclose distended small intestine, and a barium upper GI tract study with a small bowel follow-through is performed, one film of which is shown as Figure 5-8. The patient should not be treated with:

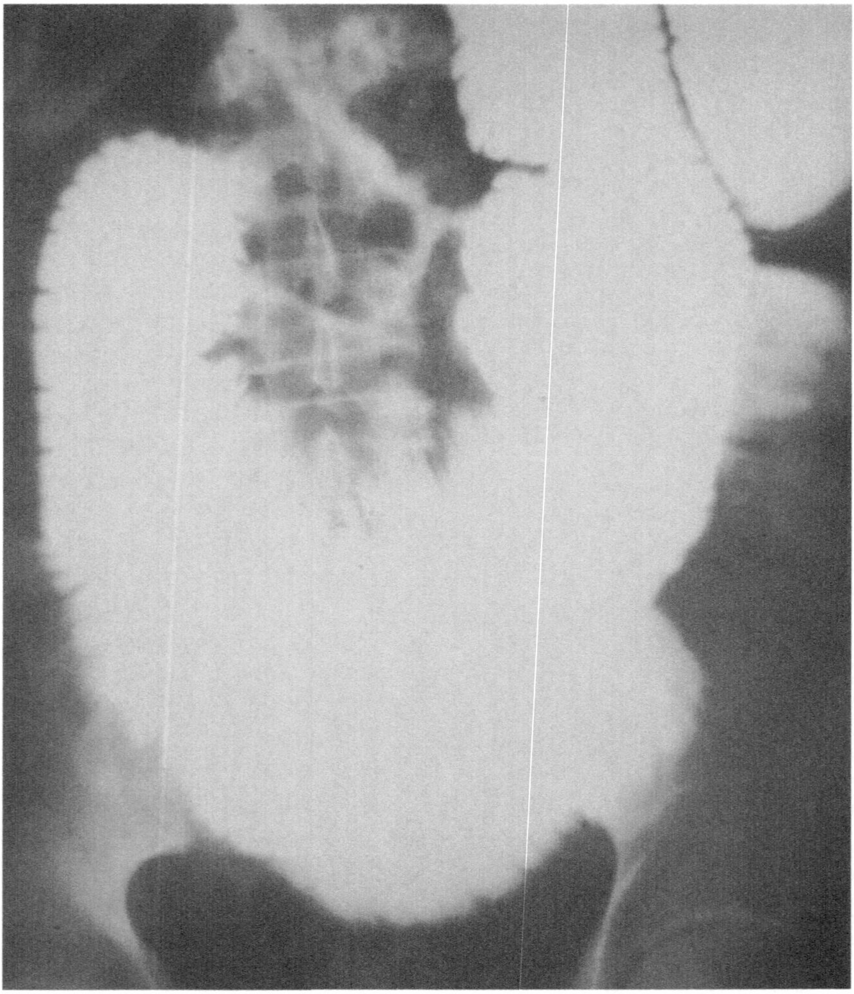

Figure 5-8

A. Metoclopramide.
B. Nasogastric tube.
C. Long intestinal tube.
D. Operation.
E. Urecholine.

This patient represents a common postoperative problem, namely the development of a symptom complex caused by either an adynamic ileus or a mechanical small bowel obstruction. It is often difficult to differentiate the two, as both will present with abdominal distention, high-pitched bowel sounds, vomiting, and obstipation. Differentiation can generally be made in such a case by utilizing an upper GI tract barium study. In the case presented, this clearly shows a markedly distended small bowel loop with no passage of barium beyond a point of fixed obstruction.

The management of such a patient is controversial. Urecholine has been utilized in the treatment of patients with postvagotomy gastric atony with some success, but its usefulness in paralytic ileus or mechanical obstruction is not documented.[26] A more promising pharmacologic approach has been the use of metoclopramide, which has been shown to stimulate the peristaltic activity of duodenum and small bowel.[27] However, this drug would not be expected to benefit a patient with a mechanical obstruction. There are many advocates of the use of nasogastric tubes and long intestinal tubes in such a situation. Although a nasogastric tube will prevent vomiting and suction off most upper GI contents, it is possible that the successful passage of a long intestinal tube will allow more direct decompression of the inflamed obstructed area, leading to a decrease in local edema and resolution of the obstruction. This potential advantage is, of course, somewhat negated by the disadvantages of having to use two intestinal tubes, one for the intestine and the other to suction the stomach so that gastric dilitation does not occur, and of having to expend the time and effort to successfully insert the long intestinal tube.

In several series of postoperative intestinal obstructions, the conclusion has been reached that immediate operation is indicated in most instances.[28,29] However, many of these studies have failed to differentiate between complete and incomplete small bowel obstructions, and operation has been carried out promptly without a trial of nonoperative management. Surely, if any evidence of ischemic intestine is present, immediate operation is indicated. In the absence of such signs, it is probably safe to undertake several days of long intestinal tube suction in the hope

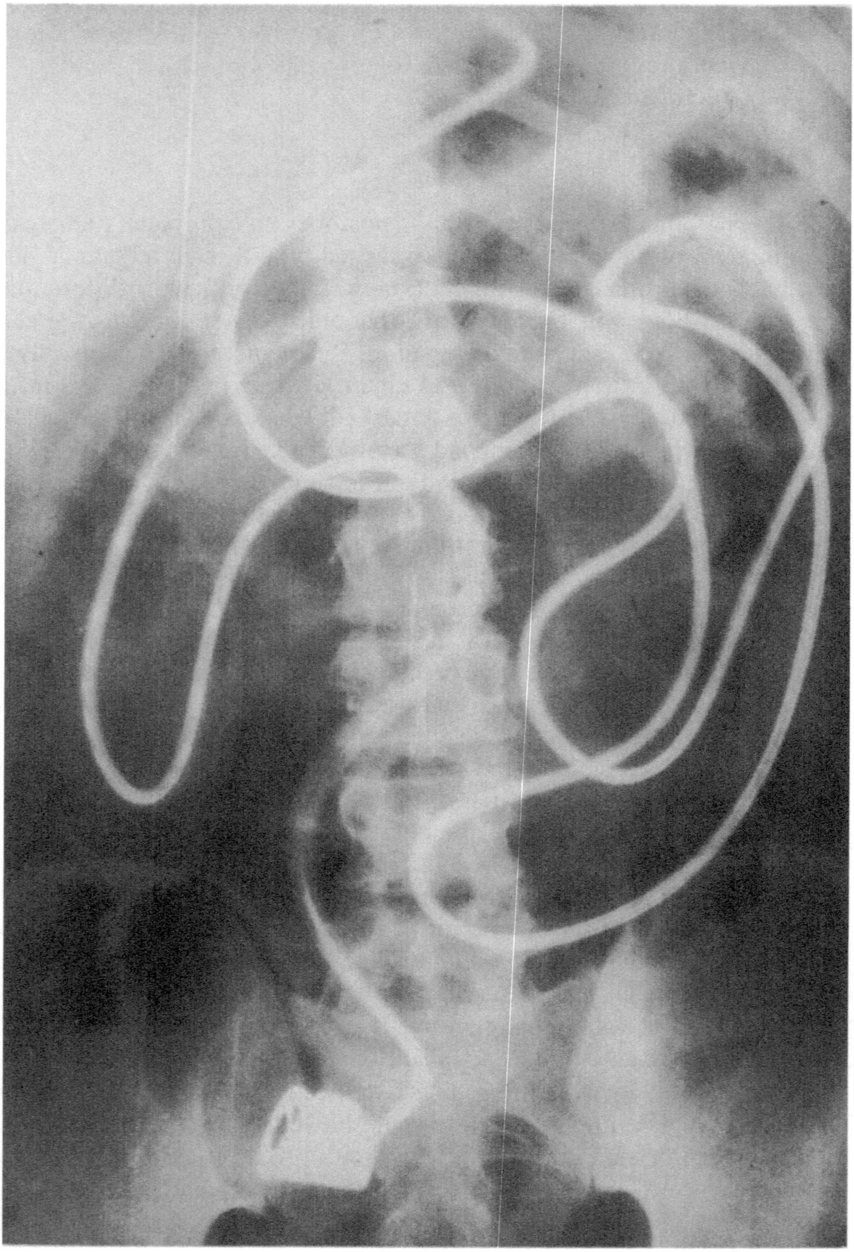

Figure 5-9

that the obstruction is caused by soft inflammatory adhesions that will resolve with adequate suction. In the patient presented, a long intestinal tube was successfully passed, and the obstruction was completely resolved after about 7 days of therapy (see Figure 5-9).

ANSWER: C.

5.8. A 73-year-old woman presents to the emergency room with a 4-day history of progressive crampy abdominal pain, distention, and vomiting. This is her first such attach, although she has suffered from "indigestion" for years. Twenty-six years ago she underwent an uncomplicated abdominal hysterectomy. She appears dehydrated, and her temperature is 37.8°C. Her abdomen is diffusely tender without peritoneal signs. The white blood cell count is 14,200 cells/mm^3. The serum amylase content is 310 IU. A supine abdominal X ray is shown as Figure 5-10. Treatment should consist of:

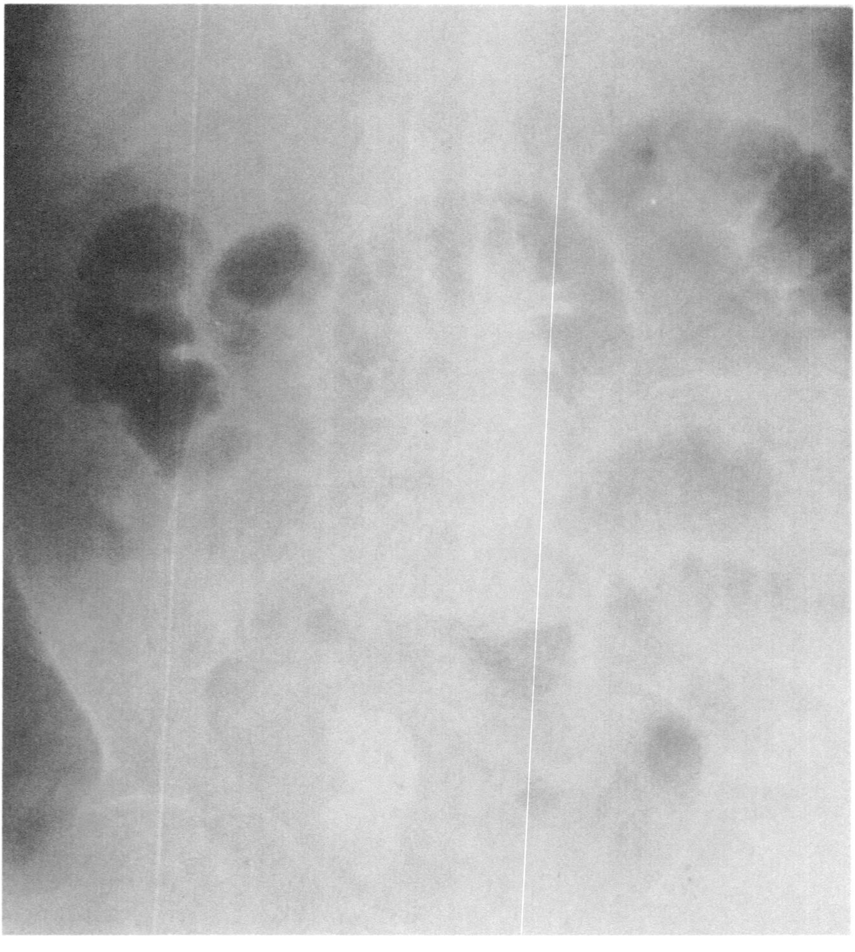

Figure 5-10

A. Volume resuscitation and antibiotics.
B. Celiotomy and lysis of adhesions.
C. Celiotomy and appendectomy.
D. Cystoscopy.
E. Celiotomy and enterolithotomy.

This elderly woman presents with signs and symptoms suggestive of a mechanical small bowel obstruction. The history of a previous laparotomy makes adhesions a likely cause, but examination of the supine abdominal X ray discloses two radiopaque densities in the lower abdomen. Proper management will depend upon the recognition of the significance of previous attacks of indigestion as indicative of biliary tract disease, and the presence of radiopaque gallstones in the lower abdomen causing a gallstone obstruction. Interpretation of the stones as either appendiceal or renal in origin will obviously lead to improper treatment.

Gallstone ileus is seen mainly in the elderly, and in those patients who have not had previous abdominal surgery obstructing gallstones account for a significant percentage of small intestinal obstructions. The stones gain access to the intestinal tract by forming fistulas, most commonly with the duodenum and less often with the colon, stomach, and jejunum.[30] Once the stone has entered the intestine, it will pass downwards and generally be passed per rectum. Nearly all stones less than 2.5 cm in diameter will pass spontaneously and cause no problems.[31] When the stones lodge, they will do so at the narrow portions of the GI tract, most commonly in the terminal ileum and less commonly in the sigmoid colon or duodenum.

The diagnosis of gallstone ileus is difficult only because it is uncommonly considered as a cause of intestinal obstruction. A number of radiologic signs have been described, including visualization of the radiopaque stones and documentation of their change in location within the abdomen on serial abdominal X rays, air in the biliary tree, and dilated loops of small intestine. In questionable cases, an upper GI tract X ray with a small bowel follow-through will accurately delineate the obturation.[32]

The treatment of such cases is operative, following adequate volume resuscitation. These patients are elderly and often have profound fluid and electrolyte derangements, and therefore a day or so of resuscitation may be required to prepare them for surgery. There is no danger of bowel perforation or gangrene in this condition, and so the added time is not detrimental to the patient. At operation, the entire intestinal tract should be examined, and when the point of obstruction is noted, the stone should be milked proximally into a dilated loop and an enterolithotomy performed. It is important to search for additional stones, as many cases have been reported in which two points of obstruction existed.[33] Following relief of the obstruction, the gallbladder and porta hepatis should be carefully examined, and if the patient is in good condition and the operation has proceeded well, the gallbladder should be removed and the fistulous tract excised. If, however, the patient is unstable or if there is an intense inflammatory response surrounding the gallbladder, this should be left undisturbed and the gallbladder removed electively at a later time.[33]

ANSWER: E.

5.9. A 46-year-old woman undergoes a radical total abdominal hysterectomy, followed by 5000 rads of radiotherapy to the pelvis and periaortic areas. Nine years later, she presents with a 6-hr history of crampy abdominal pain, gurgling intestinal sounds, and periodic diarrhea and flatus. She is afebrile; her abdomen is not distended. Bowel sounds are high-pitched and hyperactive. Her white blood cell count is 6800 cells/mm^3, and X rays of the abdomen disclose a few dilated small bowel loops with gas in the colon. Treatment at this time should consist of:

A. Celiotomy and lysis of adhesions.
B. Prolonged nasogastric suction.
C. Celiotomy and small bowel resection.
D. Celiotomy and small bowel bypass.
E. Prolonged nasogastric suction and corticosteroids.

This patient presents with typical signs and symptoms of a partial mechanical small bowel obstruction. Potential causes of this problem in this patient would be recurrent carcinoma, adhesions, and radiation enteritis. The partial nature of the bowel obstruction makes it probable that radiation enteritis is the cause, and in such a circumstance nonoperative therapy is indicated.

The incidence of small-bowel problems after abdominal radiotherapy is quite variable and dependent upon numerous host and technical factors. In a series of 1824 patients receiving abdominal radiotherapy, 5.1% of patients developed symptoms of small bowel enteritis, and of these one third required operation.[34] The incidence is surely dose related, being seen very infrequently when less than 4500 rads have been given and increasingly more frequently if between 5000 and 6000 rads have been given, a dose which yields approximately a 50% chance of some gut damage.[35] The incidence of radiation enteritis is increased by prior celiotomy and fixation of the bowel caused by adhesions, as freely movable small intestine is less likely to be damaged. However, innovations such as the use of megavoltage apparatus, a moderate daily dose fraction, a reasonable total dose, and careful computerized treatment planning of the ports can result in a decreased incidence of small bowel and colon complications. However, despite this, it is still recognized that even a patient who has undergone an easy course of radiotherapy in which few side effects were noted during the treatment is still subject to late complications.[35] The time from onset of radiotherapy to symptom presentation is very variable, ranging from several months to over 20 years.[35,36] In one series of 34 patients, the average time elapsed was 6.5 years.[37] In this series, 16 bowel resections were required, with 2 postoperative deaths. However, 7 patients suffered late perforations of the small intestine from 3 weeks to 6 months postoperatively, presumably owing to a progression of the radiation-induced intestinal vasculitis. Therefore, these authors advocated nonoperative therapy whenever possible. If operation is required, either a resection or a bypass will be needed. In one series of 40 patients, both resection and bypass were associated with a 30% anastomotic leak rate,[36] whereas other authors have found a much higher incidence of anastomotic breakdown with resection rather than intestinal bypass.[38]

ANSWER: B.

5.10. A 56-year-old woman underwent a total abdominal hysterectomy 16 years previously. Since that time, she was hospitalized on 14 occasions for bowel obstruction and required 9 celiotomies for lysis of adhesions. Two of these operations were followed by the formation of enterocutaneous fistulae, which closed with the support of total parenteral nutrition. She once again presents with a small bowel obstruction, and after 6 days of nasogastric suction has passed no gas nor stool. Celiotomy is carried out; dense adhesions are present throughout the abdomen, and multiple areas of small bowel are denuded of serosa. Following a complete release of all adhesions and kinks in the intestine, which of the following is not acceptable prior to closure?

A. Childs intestinal plication.
B. Nobel intestinal plication.
C. Stenting of the small bowel with a Baker tube inserted through the stomach and threaded to the cecum.
D. Stenting of the small bowel with a Baker tube inserted through the proximal jejunum and threaded to the cecum.
E. Arrangement of the small bowel loops in anatomical position and closure of the abdomen.

This case presents the difficult management problem of a patient who has undergone multiple celiotomies for recurrent bowel obstruction. Although a great deal is known concerning the etiology and pathogenesis of adhesion formation, little is known about the prevention of adhesions. Given such a patient, it is obvious that reobstruction will occur unless some additional means are utilized to prevent kinking and subsequent obstruction of bowel. All such recommendations recognize the reality that although adhesions cannot be prevented, at least the intestine can be laid down in an anatomic position so that recurrent obstruction is unlikely. Several methods have been utilized in this regard. Earliest of these was the Nobel plication, in which the loops of intestine were sutured to one another forming a gently curving pathway. Although this was successful in many cases of recurrent bowel obstruction, numerous complications arose, such as wound and intra-abdominal infection, fistulae, and recurrence of obstruction. In addition, the procedure tended to be an extremely long and difficult one, further reducing its appeal.[39] An improvement upon this was described by Childs, who recommended transfixing the mesentery with long sutures rather than suturing the intestine itself. This procedure had the advantage of speed and was associated with less infectious and fistulous complications.[40] More recently, internal stenting has been recommended, utilizing a large intraluminal tube that is passed throughout the length of the small intestine into the cecum. This Baker tube has been utilized successfully in many instances of recurrent obstruction. Insertion is accomplished through either the stomach or the proximal small intestine, and the tube is left in place for 8–10 days. It is then withdrawn, and the entrance site is allowed to seal over.[41]

On balance, it would appear that utilization of the Baker tube is presently the best technique for dealing with the patient with multiple recurrent bowel obstructions. It should be stressed that all of the preceding techniques are only uncommonly necessary and should be utilized only in those patients with multiple recurrent bowel obstructions and not in the patient with a simple uncomplicated bowel obstruction from adhesions.

ANSWER: E.

5.11. An 8-month-old female infant awakens crying from her sleep; after a few minutes, she vomits and falls asleep, only to reawaken two more times crying. She passes a loose bloody stool 5 hr after the onset of crying. She is brought to the emergency room. Her pulse is 140 and her temperature is 37.0°C. Her abdomen is mildly distended, with hyperactive bowel sounds present. No organs or masses are palpable. A rectal examination discloses only blood on the examining finger. The patient should next undergo:

A. Celiotomy.
B. Appendectomy.
C. Barium enema.
D. Insertion of a long intestinal tube.
E. Vagotomy and pyloroplasty.

This child presents with a classic history of intestinal intussusception. In most large series of cases, over one half of all intussusceptions are noted within the first year of life, with a predominance of cases during the summer months, a phenomenon that has never been adequately explained.[42] In a series of 344 children with intussusception reported from the Denver Children's Hospital, pain was present in 94%, vomiting in 91%, bloody diarrhea in 66%, and an abdominal mass was palpated in 59%. Ileocolic intussusceptions were found most commonly, followed by ileal-ileal and colocolic.[43]

The majority of intussusceptions in children, unlike those occurring in the adult, are idiopathic, with an anatomic lead point being noted in less than 10% of pediatric cases.[43,44] A Meckel's diverticulum is the most common lead point noted in children. Other causes, such as hypertrophied lymphoid patches, appendiceal stumps, and polyps, have also been described.

In any child presenting with a suspected intussusception who does not have evidence of ischemic bowel, a diagnostic and therapeutic barium enema should be carried out. The hydrostatic pressure of the barium enema will successfully reduce many intussusceptions, rendering an operation unnecessary. Barium enema reduction has been successful in 41% and 77% of two large series,[42,43] and recurrence after barium enema reduction is uncommon. Some patients will, however, require celiotomy. In general, there are three indications. One is the clinical suspicion of ischemic or dead bowel. Another is the failure of the barium enema to reduce the intussusception, and the other is the recurrence of the intussusception after barium enema reduction. If operation is necessary, the intussusception should be manually reduced by pushing the intussuscepted segment backward and proximally. If this is not successful, resection of the entire involved segment should be carried out, followed by primary anastomosis. Only if there is intestinal gangrene and marked peritoneal contamination should the ends of the resected intestine be brought out as stomas.

ANSWER: C.

References

1. Faulconer, H.T., Ferueson, J.A., VanZwalenburg, B.R.: The surgical significance of complete retrograde obstruction of the colon. *Dis. Colon Rectum* 14:428, 1971.
2. Welch, J.P., Donaldson, G.A.: Management of severe obstruction of the large bowel due to malignant disease. *Am. J. Surg.* 127:492, 1974.
3. Greenlee, H.B., Pienkos, E.J., Vanderbilt, P.C., Byrne, M.P., Mason, J.H., Banich, F.E., Freeark, R.J.: Acute large bowel obstruction: Comparison of County Veterans Administration and Community Hospital populations. *Arch. Surg.* 108:470, 1970.
4. Lowman, R.M., Davis, L.: An evaluation of cecal size in impending perforation of the cecum. *Surg. Gynecol. Obstet.* 103:711, 1956.
5. Ottinger, L.W., Austen, W.G.: A study of 136 patients with mesenteric infarction. *Surg. Gynecol. Obstet.* 124:251, 1967.
6. Bergan, J.J., Dean, R.H., Conn, J., Yao, J.S.T.: Revascularization in treatment of mesenteric infarction. *Ann. Surg.* 182:430, 1975.
7. Skinner, D.B., Zarins, C.K., Moossa, A.R.: Mesenteric vascular disease. *Am. J. Surg.* 128:835, 1974.
8. Singh, R.P., Shah, R.C., Lee, S.T.: Acute mesenteric vascular occlusion: A review of 32 patients. *Surgery* 78:613, 1975.
9. Van Way, C.W., Brockman, S.K., Rosenfeld, L.: Spontaneous thrombosis of the mesenteric veins. *Ann. Surg.* 173:561, 1971.
10. Boxer, M.A., Braun, J., Ellman, L.: Thromboembolic risk of postsplenectomy thrombocytosis. *Arch. Surg.* 113:808, 1978.
11. Coon, W.W., Penner, J., Clagett, G.P., Eos, N.: Deep venous thrombosis and postsplenectomy thrombocytosis. *Arch. Surg.* 113:429, 1978.
12. Butler, M.J., Britton, B.J., Hawkey, C., Smith, M., Irving, M.H.: The coagulation and fibrinolytic response to splenectomy. *Surg. Gynecol. Obstet.* 142:731, 1976.
13. Gordon, D.H., Schaffner, D., Bennett, J.M., Schwartz, S.I.: Postsplenectomy thrombocytosis. *Arch. Surg.* 113:713, 1978.
14. Balz, J., Minton, J.P.: Mesenteric thrombosis following splenectomy. *Ann. Surg.* 181:126, 1975.
15. Forward, A.D.: Hypokalemia associated with sigmoid volvulus. *Surg. Gynecol. Obstet.* 123:35, 1966.
16. Arnold, G.J., Nance, F.C.: Volvulus of the sigmoid colon. *Ann. Surg.* 177:527, 1973.
17. Drapans, T., Stuart, J.D.: Acute sigmoid volvulus: Concepts and surgical treatment. *Am. J. Surg.* 101:70, 1961.
18. Hines, J.R., Geurkink, R.E., Bass, R.T.: Recurrence and mortality rates in sigmoid volvulus. *Surg. Gynecol. Obstet.* 124:567, 1967.
19. String, S.T., Decosse, J.J.: Sigmoid volvulus: An examination of the mortality. *Am. J. Surg.* 121:293, 1971.
20. Smith, W.R., Goodwin, J.N.: Cecal volvulus. *Am. J. Surg.* 126:215, 1973.
21. Andersson, A., Bergdahl, L., VanDer Linden, W.: Volvulus of the cecum. *Ann. Surg.* 181:876, 1975.
22. Silen, W., Hein, M.F., Goldman, L.: Stangulation obstruction of the small intestine. *Arch. Surg.* 85:137, 1962.
23. Shatila, A.H., Chamberlain, B.E., Webb, W.R.: Current status of diagnosis and management of strangulation obstruction of the small bowel. *Am. J. Surg.* 132:299, 1976.
24. Leffall, L.D., Syphax, B.: Clinical aids in strangulation intestinal obstruction. *Am. J. Surg.* 120:756, 1970.
25. Stewardson, R.H., Bombeck, C.T., Nyhus, L.M.: Critical operative management of small bowel obstruction. *Ann. Surg.* 187:189, 1978.

26. Vasconez, L.O., Adams, J.T., Woodward, E.R.: Treatment of reluctant postvagotomy stoma with bethanechol. *Arch Surg*. 100:693, 1970.
27. McClelland, R.N., Horton, J.W.: Relief of acute, persistent, post-vagotomy atony by metroclopramide. *Ann. Surg*. 188:439, 1978.
28. Coletti, L., Bossart, P.A.: Intestinal obstruction during the early postoperative period. *Arch. Surg*. 88:774, 1964.
29. Sykes, P.A., Schofield, P.F.: Early postoperative small bowel obstruction. *Br. J. Surg*. 61:594, 1974.
30. Case 7-1979, Case records of the Massachusetts General Hospital: Weekly clinicopathologic exercises. *N. Engl. J. Med*. 300:355, 1979.
31. Day, E.A., Marks, C.: Gallstone ileus: Review of the literature and presentation of 34 new cases. *Am. J. Surg*. 129:552, 1975.
32. Cooperman, A.M., Dixon, F.R., ReMine, W.H.: Changing concepts in the surgical treatment of gallstone ileus. *Ann. Surg*. 167:377, 1968.
33. Warshaw, A.L., Bartlett, M.K.: Choice of operation for gallstone intestinal obstruction. *Ann. Surg*. 164:1051, 1966.
34. Cram, A.E., Pearlman, N.W., Jochimsen, P.R.: Surgical management of complications of radiation-injured gut. *Am. J. Surg*. 133:551, 1977.
35. Roswit, B.: Complications of radiation therapy: The alimentary tract. *Semin. Roentgenol*. 9:51, 1974.
36. Russell, J.C., Welch, J.P.: Operative management of radiation injuries of the intestinal tract. *Am. J. Surg*. 137:433, 1979.
37. DeCosse, J.J., Rhodes, R.S., Wentz, W.B., Reagan, J.W., Dworken, H.J., Holden, W.D.: The natural historv and management of radiation induced injury of the gastrointestinal tract. *Ann. Surg*. 170:369, 1969.
38. Swan, R.W., Fowler, W.C., Boronow, R.C.: Surgical management of radiation injury to the small intestine. *Surg. Gynecol. Obstet*. 142:325, 1976.
39. Wilson, N.D.: Complications of the Nobel procedure. *Am. J. Surg*. 108:264, 1964.
40. Childs, W.A., Phillips, R.B.: Experience with intestinal plication and a proposed modification. *Ann. Surg*. 152:258, 1960.
41. Baker, J.W.: Stitchless plication for recurring obstruction of the small bowel. *Am. J. Surg*. 116:316, 1968.
42. Larsen, E., Miller, R.C.: Clinical aspects of intussusception. *Am. J. Surg*. 124:69, 1972.
43. Wayne, E.R., Campbell, J.B., Burrington, J.D., Davis, W.S.: The management of 344 children with intussusception. *Radiology* 107:597, 1973.
44. Berman, E.J., Kimble, J.W.: Barium enema for intussusception in infants and children. *Arch. Surg*. 92:508, 1966.

6
INFLAMMATORY BOWEL DISEASE

6.1. A 73-year-old man presents to the emergency room with an 8-hr history of progressive lower abdominal pain. His temperature is 38.1°C, and his abdomen is diffusely tender, with peritoneal signs present in both lower quadrants. A white blood cell count is 9800 cells/mm^3, and four views of the abdomen disclose only ileus. After volume resuscitation and antibiotic treatment, he undergoes celiotomy. An inflammatory mass of the sigmoid colon is noted, with a small perforation partially sealed off by the omentum. Several hundred cc of turbid fluid are present in the pelvis. Treatment should consist of:

A. Sigmoid resection and primary anastomosis.
B. Sigmoid resection, end sigmoid colostomy, and oversewing of rectum.
C. Transverse colostomy.
D. Transverse colostomy and drainage of the mass.
E. Transverse colostomy, drainage of the mass, and postoperative peritoneal lavage.

This patient has a perforated inflammatory mass of the sigmoid colon with free-spreading peritonitis, presumably on the basis of perforated diverticulitis. For such a patient, it has often been noted that the performance of a colostomy alone has not led to clinical improvement, as the lower abdominal suppuration has continued to be fed by the contents of the defunctionalized transverse and descending colon.[1] Many of these patients have subsequently died of sepsis or complications resulting from it. Because of this, these patients should be operated upon immediately with primary resection of the involved area of the colon.[2–6] Although some authors have advocated primary anastomosis following left hemicolectomy in this instance,[7] this is generally not recommended because of the presumed increased risk of an anastomotic breakdown following the suture of inflamed tissues. The proximal end of the sigmoid colon is brought out as an end colostomy, and the distal end can either be brought out to the skin as a mucous fistula or oversewn and returned to the pelvis as a Hartmann procedure.

Following removal of the inflamed colon, the surgeon should open the resected specimen while still in the operating room to check for the presence of a perforating carcinoma, which can lead to a clinical picture indistinguishable from that of perforated diverticulitis. If a carcinoma is present, a more radical excision of the colon and its mesentery will be required, and this should be carried out at this time.

ANSWER: B.

6.2. A 62-year-old man gives a 4-week history of a dull, lower abdominal pain and urinary frequency and urgency, culminating in the passage of a large volume of gas with each urination. He is afebrile. Abdominal and rectal examinations are normal. Proctoscopy is normal to 14 cm, and the proctoscope cannot be inserted further because of pain. A barium enema shows narrowing and inflammation of the rectosigmoid colon with associated diverticuli. No extravasation of barium is noted. An intravenous pyelogram (IVP) and cystogram are normal. Cystoscopy reveals a localized area of inflammation in the bladder. The urinary sediment reveals numerous white blood cells, and *E. coli* is grown on culture. Treatment should consist of:

A. Long-term treatment with trimethoprim-sulfa (Septra).
B. Exploratory celiotomy and closure of fistula.
C. Transverse colostomy.
D. Exploratory celiotomy, sigmoid resection and anastomosis, and bladder repair.
E. Cystoscopy, biopsy, and fulguration of the bladder.

The diagnosis of pneumaturia in a male is obvious, and indicates that some portion of the GI tract must be in communication with the urinary tract. In women, the symptoms of pneumaturia can be overlooked, as females cannot directly visualize their urinary stream. The most common cause of fistulae between the GI tract and the bladder is diverticulitis, and males are affected far more frequently than females, probably because of the protection afforded to females by the presence of the uterus.[3]

In the evaluation of a patient presenting with pneumaturia, a urinalysis and culture should be performed. An IVP and cystogram will rarely disclose a fistula but should be carried out to ascertain the presence of two functioning kidneys if nothing else. Cytoscopy will demonstrate areas of inflammation in the bladder but will not usually visualize the fistula itself. However, if the fistula is the result of invasive carcinoma, this can be noted on cystoscopy. A barium enema will likewise uncommonly show the fistula, but in most cases it should be able to differentiate between diverticulitis and carcinoma of the colon.[8]

Traditionally, treatment of colovesical fistulae utilized a staged operative procedure. A transverse colostomy was first performed, and this decreased fistula drainage but usually did not eliminate the urinary tract infection. Following this, resection of the colon and repair of the fistula was carried out, with colostomy closure as a third step. However, it was noted that many fistulae were rather superficial on the bladder and unassociated with significant inflammatory reaction. For such fistulas, primary resection and anastomosis proved quite feasible, especially utilizing preoperative mechanical and antibiotic colon preparations. So basically, the decision of which operation to perform is based upon the results of the exploratory operation and, specifically, the appearance of the rectosigmoid colon and bladder. This will enable the surgeon to resect those fistulae that appear to be technically easy to resect, with diverting colostomy reserved for those patients who have a more intense inflammatory reaction, making resection and anastomosis more hazardous. Utilizing this approach, the majority of patients with colovesical fistulae can be resected safely in one stage.[3,8–10]

ANSWER: D.

6.3. A 67-year-old man has suffered from recurrent attacks of lower abdominal pain and constipation. He presents to the hospital with an 8-day history of persistent pain, which is now localized to the left lower quadrant. His temperature is 38.8°C. Abdominal examination discloses tenderness and guarding in the left lower quadrant coinciding with a palpable 8-cm mass. Rectal examination discloses pelvic tenderness, but no masses are appreciated. The white blood cell count is 15,800 cells/mm^3. A barium enema demonstrates diverticulitis of the rectosigmoid colon with narrowing and spasm. An abdominal ultrasound shows a 6-cm fluid-filled collection in the left lower quadrant. Treatment should consist of:

A. Exploratory celiotomy, transverse colostomy, and extraperitoneal drainage of the abscess.
B. Left hemicolectomy, end sigmoid colostomy, and oversewing of the rectum (Hartmann procedure).
C. Nasogastric tube and antibiotics.
D. Transverse colostomy.
E. Drainage of the intra-abdominal abscess.

This man has suffered from recurrent minor attacks of diverticulitis culminating in a perforation of the left colon with abscess formation. This question addresses the orderly diagnostic workup of a patient suspected to have diverticulitis, and stresses the early performance of an abdominal ultrasound and a barium enema. Although there has been hesitation in the past to perform proctoscopy and a barium enema in the presence of acute diverticulitis, these studies can be carefully performed with safety, and significant information may be gained.[3,11]

Many abscesses that form as a result of a perforated colonic diverticulum are enclosed within the mesentery of the colon, and often may be resected en bloc with no spillage of pus. Other abscesses form within the abdominal cavity itself and are walled off by the colon, omentum, small bowel, and parietal peritoneum. Obviously, an abscess in this location must be drained. It is generally impossible to determine preoperatively whether one is dealing with an abscess that can be resected or one that can only be drained. Therefore, an exploratory celiotomy is indicated. In the situation presented, the optimal approach would be an exploratory celiotomy along with a transverse colostomy and extraperitoneal drainage of the abscess if its anatomic location permits this. Performance of only a colostomy might lead to resolution of some inflammatory masses, but would not be expected to benefit an established abscess. Likewise, the performance of a colonic resection in the presence of an abscess should be attempted only for those collections of pus that are contained within the leaves of the mesentery. Drainage of the abscess alone would likely result in a fecal fistula, because proximal fecal diversion has not been established. Treatment with a nasogastric tube and antibiotics, although successful for localized phlegmons secondary to diverticulitis, are usually ineffectual in the treatment of established abscesses. One small series of patients with abscess formation secondary to diverticulitis demonstrated the superiority of colostomy and drainage of the abscess over colostomy alone. In this series, 5 out of 8 patients (62%) died when treated by colostomy alone, whereas only 5 of 19 patients (26%) died after colostomy and drainage of the abscess. Drainage was either trans- or extraperitoneal, depending upon anatomic considerations.[12]

ANSWER: A.

6.4. A 16-year-old boy presents to the emergency room with a 7-day history of right lower quadrant pain and difficulty with urination. His temperature is 38.8°C; his abdomen is distended and tender in the right lower quadrant, where a mass is palpated. A rectal examination discloses tenderness in the right lower quadrant. A white blood cell count is 14,600 cells/mm^3. Abdominal X rays are shown as Figures 6-1 and 6-2. An abdominal ultrasound shows a fluid-filled mass in the right lower quadrant. Treatment should consist of:

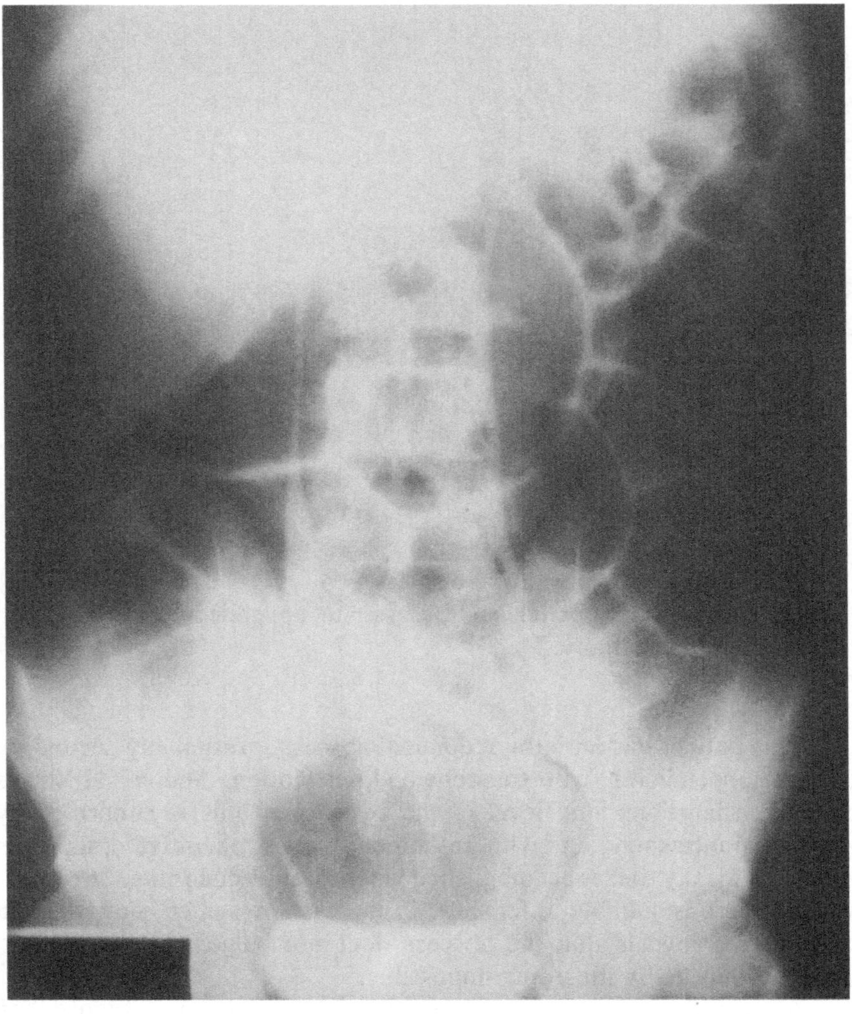

Figure 6-1

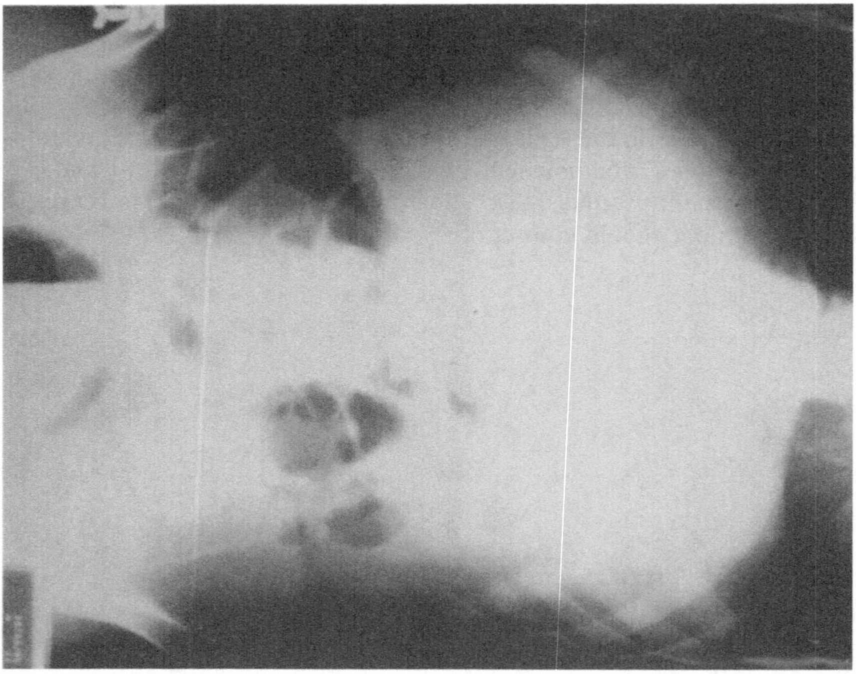

Figure 6-2

A. Antibiotics.
B. Appendectomy.
C. Drainage of appendiceal abscess.
D. Drainage of appendiceal abscess plus appendectomy.
E. Appendicostomy.

This patient has an intra-abdominal abscess, presumably secondary to acute appendicitis, with gangrene and perforation. Abdominal X rays disclose a large air fluid level in the pelvis, and this is confirmed by abdominal ultrasound. As with any other abscess, operative drainage is required. Ideally, this is accomplished via the transrectal route. The transvaginal route is suitable in females. In the case presented, however, an examination reveals that the abscess does not bulge into the rectum, making drainage by this route impossible.

At operation, technical problems are often encountered if more than simple abscess drainage is attempted. Usually, the tissues surrounding the abscess consists of omentum, coiled loops of small intestine, and the parietal peritoneum. Any effort to disturb this wall and perform appendectomy is fraught with complications of spreading intra-abdominal infection or fecal fistula and peritonitis. Indeed, the inflamed appendix is frequently not even identified at this time. In one series of 61 patients with appendiceal abscess, only 27% underwent drainage and appendectomy. The remainder underwent drainage alone, as either the appendix was not identified or appendectomy was felt to be too hazardous to perform.[13] Therefore, the operative plan in such a patient should be drainage of the appendiceal abscess, with appendectomy performed only if the appendix is easily identified and removable.

Whether or not patients who undergo only drainage should be readmitted to the hospital at a later time for interval appendectomy is an unclear issue. Although this recommendation has been made on the basis of a projected high incidence of recurrent appendicitis,[14] other studies have shown only 10%–20% risk of recurrent appendicitis and have recommended a more selective approach depending upon the patient's overall status.[13]

ANSWER: C.

6.5. A 16-year-old boy presents to the emergency room with a 7-day history of right lower quadrant pain and difficulty with urination. His temperature is 38.8°C; his abdomen is distended and tender in the right lower quadrant, where a mass is palpated. A rectal examination discloses tenderness in the right lower quadrant. A white blood cell count is 14,600 cells/mm^3, and four views of the abdomen are normal. A barium enema is shown as Figure 6-3. An abdominal ultrasound shows a solid mass in the right lower quadrant. Treatment should consist of:

A. Antibiotics.
B. Appendectomy.
C. Drainage of appendiceal abscess.
D. Drainage of appendiceal abscess plus appendectomy.
E. Appendicostomy.

Although the clinical presentation of this patient is similar to the previous one, the pathologic process is presumably different. In the former case, an air fluid level was demonstrated, indicating a collection of pus. In the present case, a solid mass compressing the cecum is noted. Traditionally, all patients with appendicitis were operated upon when the diagnosis was made. In patients presenting many days after the onset of symptoms, often a phlegmonous mass was encountered at operation and attempts to dissect this led to significant bleeding or bowel injury with subsequent peritonitis, abscess formation, or fistula. Because of this, recommendations have evolved for treatment of such patients with antibiotics alone, in the expectation that the majority will resolve their inflammatory process and can be subjected to interval appendectomy weeks later. This type of treatment will be satisfactory in the majority of patients in whom it is attempted. Those patients who harbor an abscess that was not detected or whose inflammatory process progresses to an abscess will require drainage of that abscess. The rest will resolve during 5–10 days of broad-spectrum antibiotic therapy.[13,15,16] Interval appendectomy should be carried out 6–8 weeks after the acute attack; this allows sufficient time for the inflammatory process to subside and for the technical aspects of appendectomy to improve, and also limits the amount of time the patient is at risk for recurrent appendicitis.

ANSWER: A.

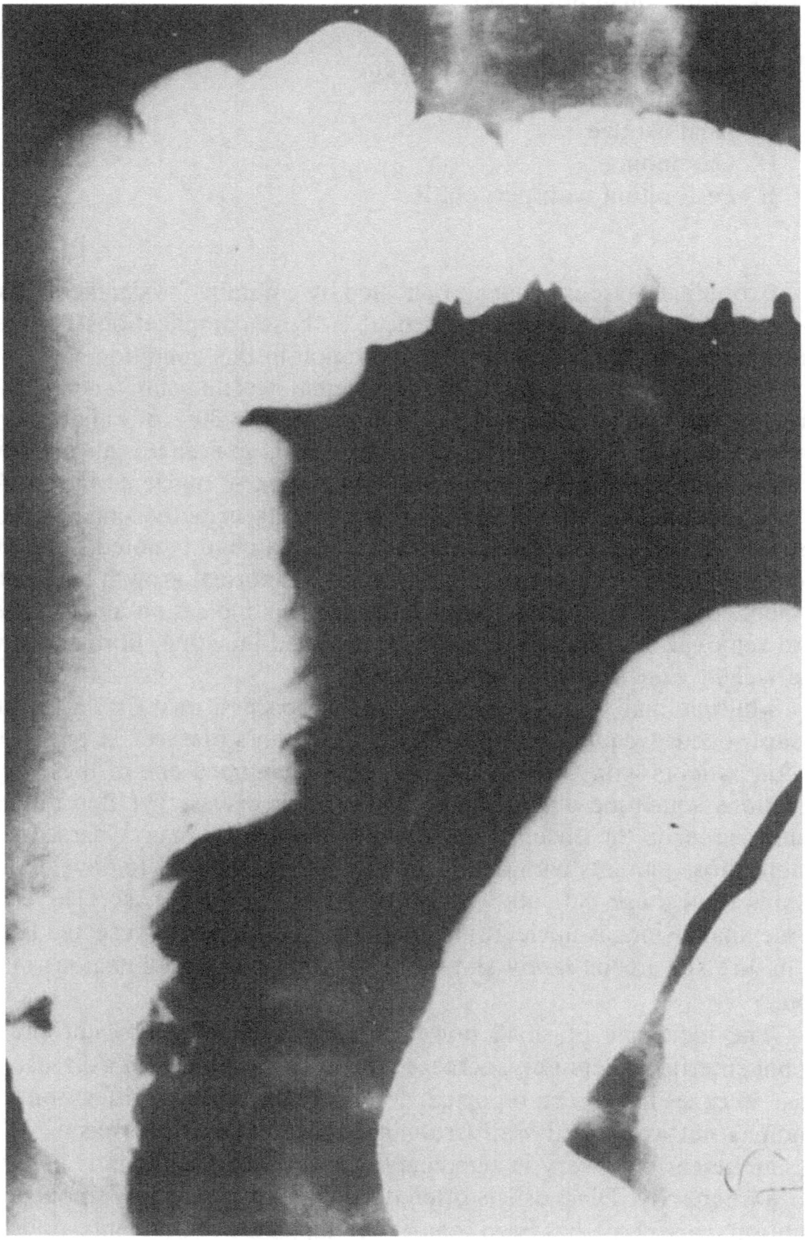

Figure 6-3

6.6. Which of the following is not a recognized complication of Crohn's disease of the small intestine?

A. Growth retardation in children.
B. Intussusception.
C. Anal fistulae.
D. Carcinoma.
E. Perforation with peritonitis.

Crohn's disease is often complicated by a number of significant local and systemic complications. Indeed, it is these complications that generally represent the indications for operation in this condition.[17]

Decreased linear growth, below-normal weight gain, and delayed onset of sexual maturation occur in from 18% to 30% of children with Crohn's disease. The underlying mechanism is multifactorial, including decreased nutrient intake, decreased absorption of nutrients by the diseased intestine, increased energy requirements of active inflammatory disease, and the use of corticosteroids. Once a child is noted to be progressively falling behind his peers in terms of normal growth and development, operation must be considered for this indication alone. Often, with removal of a limited segment of diseased intestine, normal growth and weight gains can be accomplished.[18,19]

Multiple anal lesions, including rectal abscess, anal fistula, or anal fissure, occur frequently in patients with Crohn's disease. In one series of 503 patients with Crohn's disease, 28% developed one of these complications sometime during the course of their disease.[20] Often the anal lesions precede the onset of intestinal symptoms by many years. In addition, those patients with Crohn's colitis are more likely to develop anal lesions than those patients with purely small bowel disease. The cause of the anal lesions is unclear, and histologic evaluation of resected fistula or fissure specimens rarely shows any evidence of granulomatous infection.

The incidence of small bowel carcinoma complicating chronic regional enteritis is definitely increased in patients with Crohn's disease. At least 50 cases have been reported.[17,21] These carcinomas differ from carcinomas not associated with Crohn's disease in several respects. Mean age at cancer discovery is significantly lower, and the ileum is involved more frequently. Diagnosis is often delayed, and cure is less frequent. In addition, carcinoma has been reported in segments of small intestine containing regional enteritis that had been previously bypassed, providing yet another reason for avoidance of bypass procedures in preference to resectional procedures in this condition.[22]

Free perforation of Crohn's disease is uncommon, as the inflammatory process tends to be a chronic one with the tendency towards abscess and fistula formation rather than frank perforation. About 100 cases have been reported in the literature, and the clinical manifestations are those one would expect from an acute perforation of the small intestine with a rapidly spreading fecal peritonitis.[23] The treatment of this condition will be governed by the general condition of the patient and local findings at operation. In the patient with a relatively early peritonitis, primary resection and anastomosis can be carried out. Mere oversewing of the involved area or bypass of the involved area should not be attempted, as these procedures will invariably be unsuccessful. In the situation where either the patient is critically ill or severe fecal peritonitis exists, the segment of bowel can be resected, with the formation of an ileostomy and a mucous fistula. Intestinal reconstitution can be carried out at a later time.

ANSWER: B.

6.7. A 24-year-old man has had Crohn's disease documented radiologically for 2 years. He is taking sulfa drugs and 20 mg of prednisone a day. He gives a 2-month history of increasing lower abdominal cramping pain, postprandial gurgling, and abdominal distention; all symptoms are increased by eating and relieved by the passage of gas and stool. Hematocrit is 33%; albumin level is 3.2 g. A barium enema is shown as Figure 6-4. Treatment at this time should consist of:

A. Increase in prednisone to 40 mg q.d.
B. Addition of azathioprine.
C. Addition of ACTH and azathioprine.
D. Ileo-ascending colostomy with bypass of the diseased segment.
E. Ileocolic resection and anastomosis.

This patient presents with a classic picture of increasing small-bowel obstruction. The barium enema discloses a severe narrowing of the terminal ileum with dilated proximal small intestine. Further indication of the severity of the chronic disorder is the anemia and the hypoalbuminemia. In the presence of such a high-grade small-bowel obstruction, operation will be necessary. In two large series of patients with Crohn's disease encompassing experience with over 1000 patients, approximately 75% of patients with ileocolic Crohn's disease ultimately required operation for complications such as obstruction, fistula, and medical intractability.[24,25] Operation has been objected to in Crohn's disease because of the "inevitable" chances of recurrence. However, this has been quite overstated in the literature. In one series of 64 patients with terminal-ileal disease who were treated by ileocolectomy and primary anastomosis, 55% had no recurrent disease, with all patients being followed for at least 10 years and having a mean duration of follow-up of over 17 years.[26]

In the present situation, with a fixed cicatrix of small intestine being present, any form of medical management is unlikely to bring about lasting relief from obstructive symptoms. Increases in corticosteroids, induced by administration of either cortisone or ACTH, will benefit some patients with an acute edematous obstruction but rarely a patient with a fixed fibrotic narrowing.[24] Likewise, azathioprine (Imuran) has been extensively studied, but the results of its effectiveness are quite contradictory.[27,28]

Once operation is decided upon, resection of the diseased bowel is indicated. The results of bypass of the diseased segment have been very disappointing, with active disease manifested by persistent symptoms, fistulae, or the development of carcinoma in the bypassed segments in at least 75% of such patients.[29]

ANSWER: E.

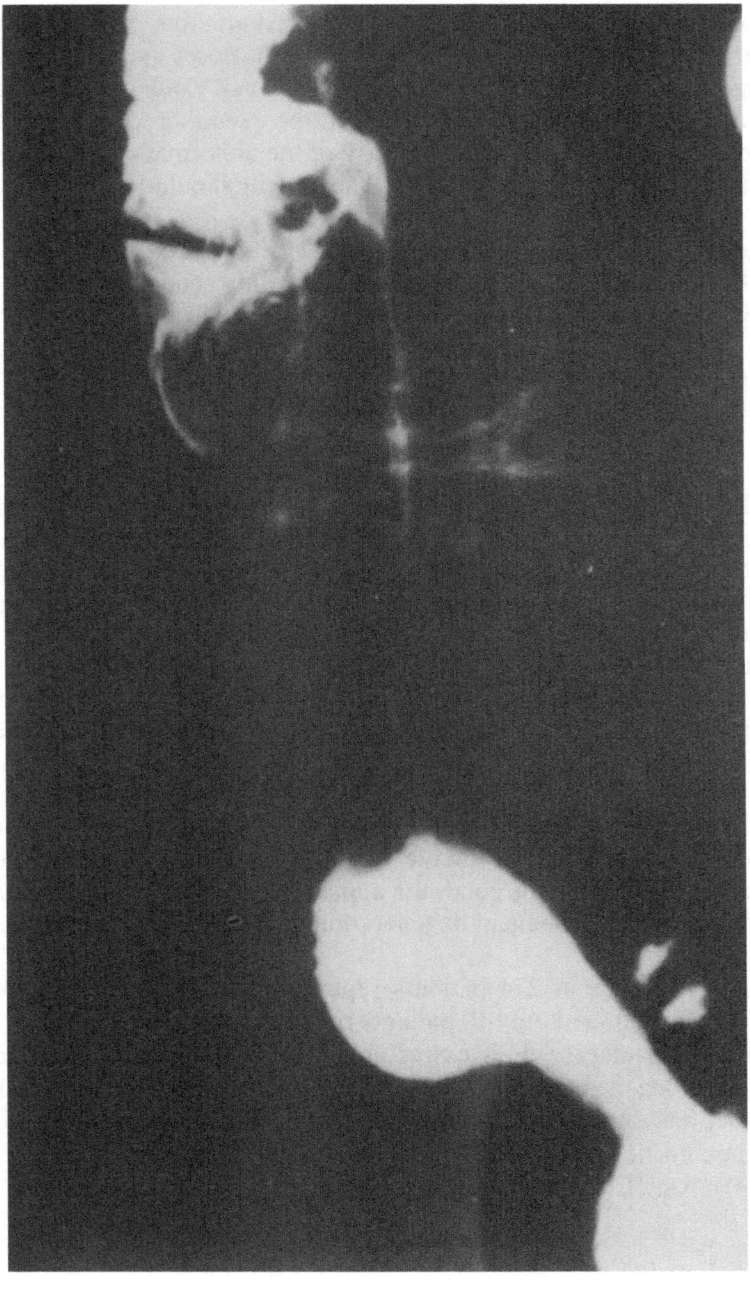

Figure 6-4

6.8. A 28-year-old man gives a 6-month history of intermittent diarrhea that is sometimes bloody. He has no other symptoms. A barium enema is performed and is normal. Proctoscopy discloses mild inflammatory changes with focal hemorrhagic areas up to 20 cm. Colonoscopy is carried out, and the entire colonic mucosa with the exception of the previously noted distal 20 cm is normal. A biopsy of the abnormal area is taken and interpreted as "ulcerative colitis." The patient should be advised that:

A. Malignant degeneration is likely with the passage of years.
B. Treatment with systemic corticosteroids should be begun.
C. Symptomatic treatment, utilizing antidiarrheal medications, sulfa drugs, or cortisone enemas, should prove beneficial.
D. Diffuse involvement of the colon is likely to occur.
E. An ileostomy will prove beneficial at this time.

Physicians are generally more aware of the manifestations of diffuse ulcerative colitis than they are with the entity designated as ulcerative proctitis. This condition generally follows a benign clinical course with few of the complications of ulcerative colitis. Although gross and microscopic appearances of the rectum in this condition are identical with those noted in diffuse ulcerative colitis, the entity is distinguished by its sparing of the abdominal colon. The condition tends to appear in the younger age groups, as does idiopathic ulcerative colitis. It is generally manifested by diarrhea and moderate rectal bleeding. The course of the condition is punctuated by frequent exacerbations and remissions, and it may be treated symptomatically with antidiarrheal medications and sometimes corticosteroid enemas. Systemic complications are only uncommonly noted. In a few cases, the condition appears to be the forerunner of diffuse ulcerative colitis. Malignant degeneration in the affected rectum does not occur.[30]

In one series of 234 patients reported from the Lahey Clinic, no deaths occurred, and only 10 patients required operation on the colon for control of the disease. Few extracolonic manifestations occurred and no malignant degeneration was noted. The authors of this series concluded that diet and supportive therapy along with oral sulfa drugs and local or systemic corticosteroids were beneficial.[31]

ANSWER: C.

6.9. A 23-year-old woman has had ulcerative colitis for 5 years. She has taken Azulfidine and 20 mg of prednisone daily for 1½ years. When she enters the hospital, she has had six to eight bloody bowel movements per day for 1 week and abdominal distention associated with crampy pain. Her temperature is 38.2°C. Her abdomen is diffusely tender, distended, and tympanitic, with hypoactive bowel sounds present. No peritoneal signs are present. Proctoscopy reveals a markedly hemorrhagic rectal mucosa. Laboratory studies disclose the following values: hematocrit, 24%; white blood cell count, 16,200 cells/mm^3; serum potassium, 3.1 mEq/liter; serum albumin, 2.9 g%. A supine abdominal X ray is shown as Figure 6-5. Treatment should consist of:

A. Proctocolectomy.
B. An increase in the corticosteroid dosage.
C. Administration of ACTH intravenously.
D. Ileostomy and transverse colostomy.
E. Abdominal colectomy and ileostomy with oversewing of the rectal stump.

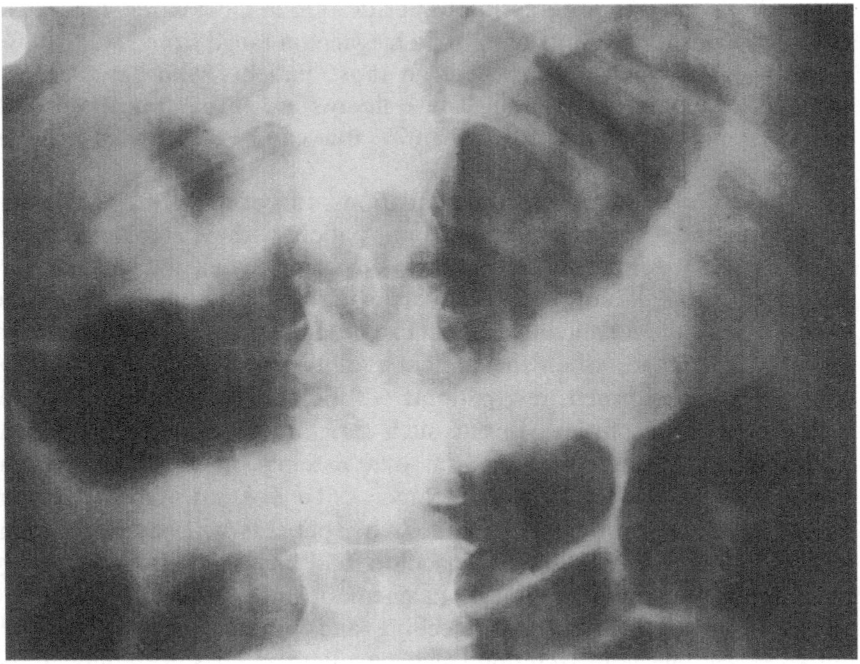

Figure 6-5

This patient is presenting with toxic megacolon, one of the grave consequences of uncontrolled ulcerative colitis. The occurrence of this condition implies extensive involvement of all layers of the colonic wall, with the real possibility of perforation. The complication is related to the severity, not the duration, of the patient's disease, and many patients will contract a toxic megacolon during their first attack of ulcerative colitis.[32] Toxic megacolon is also noted in granulomatous colitis and other less-common forms of colitis, such as amebic colitis. It is important to recognize that a contributing factor in the development of toxic megacolon may be excessive use of antidiarrheal medications. In a patient who has been ingesting large quantities of these drugs, cessation of the medication alone will often lead to a resolution of the condition.

For the majority of patients, however, the onset of toxic megacolon will signify that the disease is no longer controlable medically. Even if the condition is brought under control by medical management, the vast majority of these patients will still require removal of the colon in the future because of the uncontrolable symptoms.[33] Therefore, the prudent management of most patients with toxic megacolon will entail early operation as soon as the patient is volume resuscitated, transfused, given vitamin K supplements, and begun on a regimen of systemic antibiotics. This will obviate the progression to perforation in most cases. Operative mortality rates for patients with toxic megacolon range from 25% to 50%, with the higher figures being seen in those patients who have already suffered a colonic perforation. These figures are to be contrasted with operative mortality rates of less than 2% that can be anticipated from an elective proctocolectomy.[34]

There are numerous recommendations concerning the specific operative treatment of this condition. In the patient without significant rectal hemorrhage, abdominal colectomy can be performed easily, with the formation of an ileostomy and the oversewing of the rectal stump or the creation of a sigmoid mucous fistula. The proctectomy can then be carried out at a later time, when the patient is not critically ill. If abdominal colectomy is performed, few patients will be able to undergo ileorectal anastomosis in the future. In one such series of 43 patients, no patient ever had a functioning rectum.[35] In some patients, however, the rectum may remain in place until reanastomosis is carried out, and the patient will have minimal problems from it. Other patients will have significant bleeding along with the toxic megacolon, and for these, protocolectomy remains the treatment of choice. In one series of 28 patients with toxic megacolon, 8 had significant bleeding and proctocolectomy was required.[36] Another approach that has been advocated has been dubbed the "blow-hole" operation.[37] The rationale behind this operation was the authors' frequent finding at the time of operation for toxic megacolon of sealed-off perforations, which were then reopened with mobilization of the colon causing fecal spillage. By performing merely an ileostomy and transverse and sigmoid colostomy, the authors felt that this problem was obviated. It is recognized that this approach will cure the toxic megacolon, but many patients will have continued activity of their inflammatory disease, with toxicity or hemorrhage, and require proctocolectomy shortly thereafter.

ANSWER: A.

6.10. A 32-year-old man has suffered from granulomatous colitis for 11 years, requiring long-term treatment with large doses of prednisone and multiple hospitalizations for uncontrolled disease. He has undergone drainage of four perirectal abscesses and two incisions of anal fistulae. He enters the hospital with profuse bloody diarrhea. He is afebrile, and his abdomen is nontender. Proctoscopy reveals severe inflammation and ulceration throughout the rectum. Rectal examination shows a markedly decreased anal sphincter tone. Hematocrit is 24%; albumin concentration is 2.8 g%. A barium enema is shown as Figure 6-6. Treatment should consist of:

A. Proctocolectomy and ileostomy.
B. Abdominal colectomy and ileoproctostomy.
C. Ileostomy alone.
D. Abdominal colectomy, ileostomy, and oversewing of the rectal stump.
E. Ileostomy, and transverse and sigmoid colostomies.

This patient obviously has severe diffuse granulomatous colitis as manifested by the chronicity of the disease, the proctoscopic and barium enema findings, and the hematologic values showing anemia and hypoalbuminemia. Few would argue that some form of operation is indicated. In this situation, with an extensively involved rectum, it is unlikely that any procedure that spares the rectum will be successful in bringing the patient's symptoms under control. At the very least, abdominal colectomy must be carried out along with an ileostomy. Whether the rectum is left in place as a defunctionalized pouch or is removed is more debatable, but in the situation presented, the rectal disease is sufficiently severe to warrant removal.

Many authorities have reported series of patients in whom abdominal colectomy was carried out with either primary ileoproctostomy or an ileostomy alone, with subsequent reanastomosis. With few exceptions, these patients have suffered recurrence of the disease in the rectal segment necessitating removal of the rectum. In one series, only 2 out of 49 patients retained a functioning rectal segment, when patients with both ulcerative and granulomatous colitis were considered.[38] Another series of 111 patients disclosed that only 15% of patients were left with a functioning rectum, with little difference noted between those patients with ulcerative and granulomatous colitis. However, in this study, a long duration of the disease had a more unfavorable outlook.[39] In the patient presented, the presence of significant rectal disease, with perianal suppuration and di-

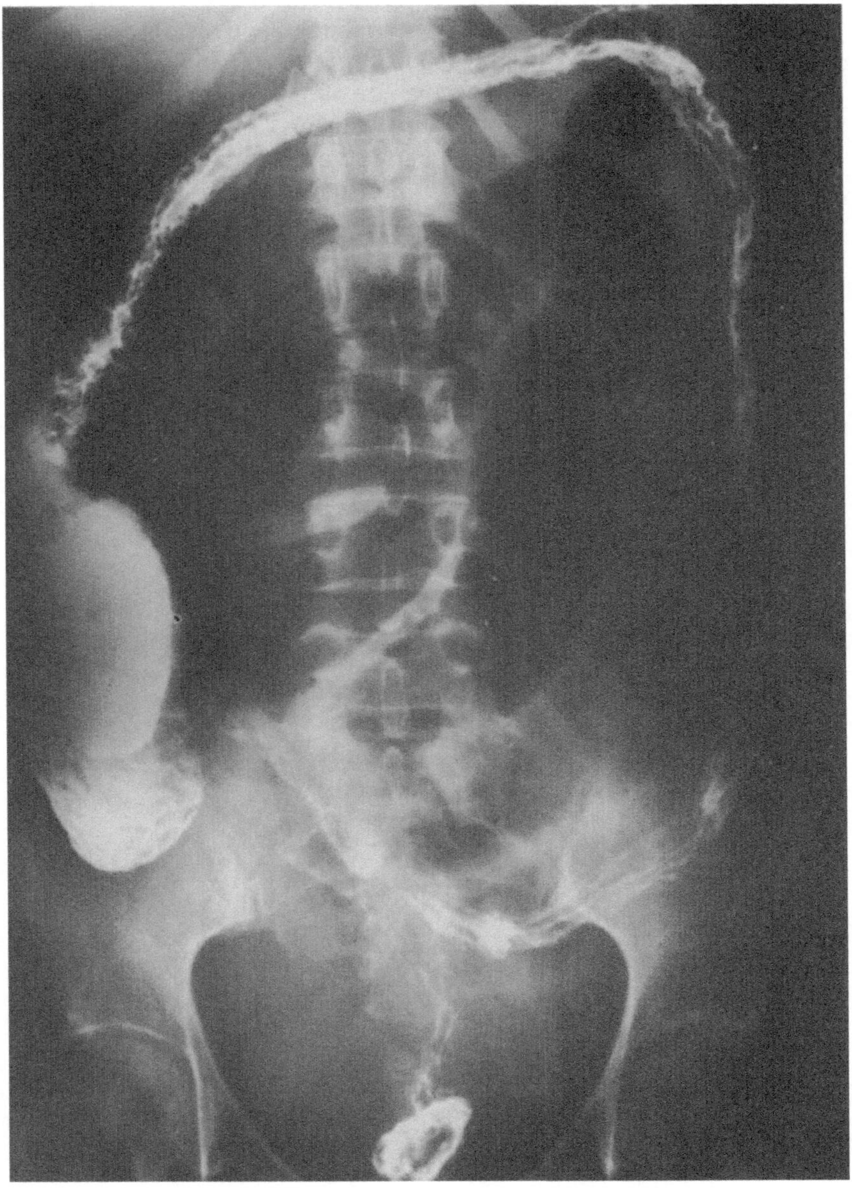

Figure 6-6

minished sphincter tone, further precludes any attempt at anastomosis.

If an ileostomy is performed in a patient with Crohn's disease, there is a risk of the inflammatory process affecting the ileostomy or proximal small intestine. This risk has ranged from 7% to 46% in three well-studied series of patients.[40,41] In addition, the rate of recurrence seems to increase with the length of patient follow-up, with one series showing an 18% recurrence rate in those patients followed up for a minimum of 5 years, but a 43% recurrence rate for those patients followed up for a minimum of 15 years.[41]

ANSWER: A.

6.11. A 32-year-old previously well patient presents to the hospital with a 3-day history of severe bloody diarrhea, refractory to large doses of nonprescription antidiarrheal medications. Proctoscopy discloses ulcerations and a severely hemorrhagic rectal mucosa. A biopsy is interpreted as ulcerative colitis; a fresh swab is taken, and trophozoites of *Entamoeba histolytica* are identified. The hematocrit is 26%. Treatment should consist of:

A. Metronidazole (Flagyl).
B. Intravenous corticosteroids.
C. Proctocolectomy.
D. Abdominal colectomy and ileostomy with sigmoid mucous fistula.
E. Intravenous corticosteroids, cortisone enemas, and broad-spectrum antibiotics.

The management of a patient with fulminant acute colitis may be thwarted by the failure of the physician to consider varieties of colitis other than ulcerative or granulomatous. Specifically, amebic colitis is rarely considered in these emergency situations. In the case presented, the demonstration of the trophozoite form of *E. histolytica* should provide sufficient evidence that this is the cause in this instance.

In this country, it is estimated that the incidence of the asymptomatic carrier state of intestinal cysts and trophozoites of *E. histolytica* is 5%, with higher figures noted in rural or low socioeconomic areas.[43] Because of its rarity in this country, amebic colitis is often not considered in the differential diagnosis of a patient with acute colitis. Clinical features of amebic or ulcerative colitis may be indistinguishable, and proctoscopic findings and barium enema changes may be similar in both conditions.[44] Physicians from Latin American countries have had extensive experience with invasive intestinal amebiasis and attest to the fact that the entity that clinicians in the United States call ulcerative colitis would pass for amebic colitis in their countries and frequently would be successfully treated with amebicidal drugs. The usual course in the United States is one in which the diagnosis of amebic colitis is rapidly discarded if it is considered at all, once a stool specimen for ova and parasites is found to be negative. This overlooks the marked difficulty in demonstrating the trophozoites of *E. histolytica*. A wide variety of substances can interfere with the detection of these organisms.[45] Most of the common antidiarrheal medications and broad spectrum antibiotics, cleansing enemas, or barium enemas can lead to failure to isolate the organism for several weeks afterwards. The indirect hemagglutination test is quite specific for amebiasis but takes considerable time to perform. Therefore, the careful obtaining of wet fresh rectal swabs and their prompt evaluation under the microscope is essential. Several reports have been published in this country of patients harboring amebic colitis in whom the original assumption of ulcerative colitis proved incorrect, with subsequent catastrophic results when therapy with corticosteroids was attempted.[45,46]

ANSWER: A.

6.12. A 67-year-old man is hospitalized following 3 days of left lower quadrant abdominal pain and bloody diarrhea. His temperature is 38.0°C; an abdominal exam discloses tenderness in the left lower quadrant with guarding and local peritoneal signs. A proctoscopy discloses normal mucosa up to 16 cm, where severe hemorrhagic changes and ulcerations are noted. A biopsy is interpreted as ulcerative colitis. The white blood cell count is 12,600 cells/mm^3. A barium enema is performed and is shown as Figure 6-7. Four days later the patient's fever is 38.9°C, his abdominal findings are unchanged, and the white blood cell count is 16,200 cells/mm^3. A repeat barium enema is performed, and the rectosigmoid area is shown in Figure 6-8. Treatment at this time should consist of:

A. Intravenous corticosteroids, antibiotics, and steroid enemas.
B. Proctocolectomy.
C. Left hemicolectomy, end sigmoid colostomy, and Hartmann procedure.
D. Abdominal colectomy and ileoproctostomy.
E. Metronidazole (Flagyl) orally.

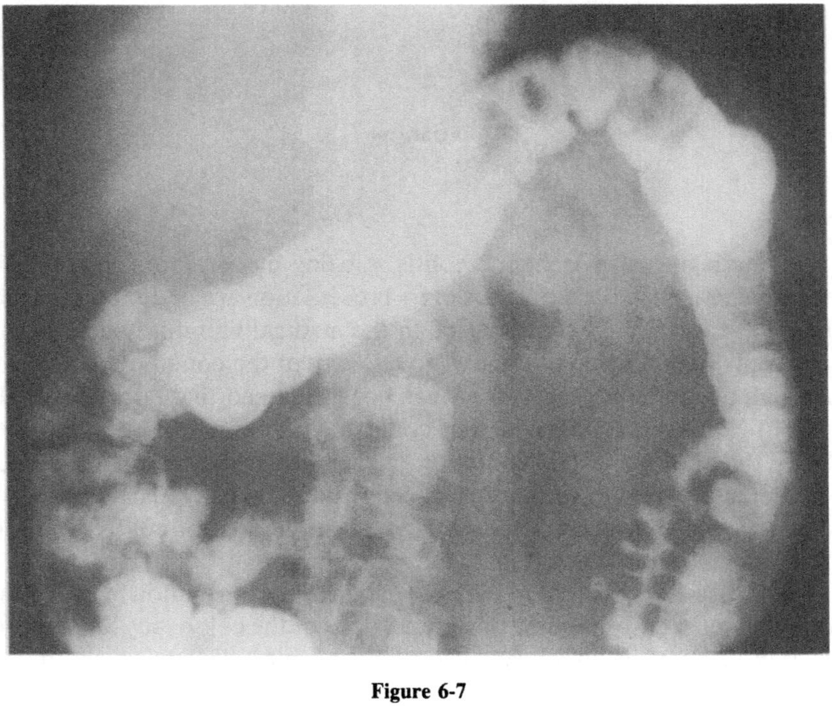

Figure 6-7

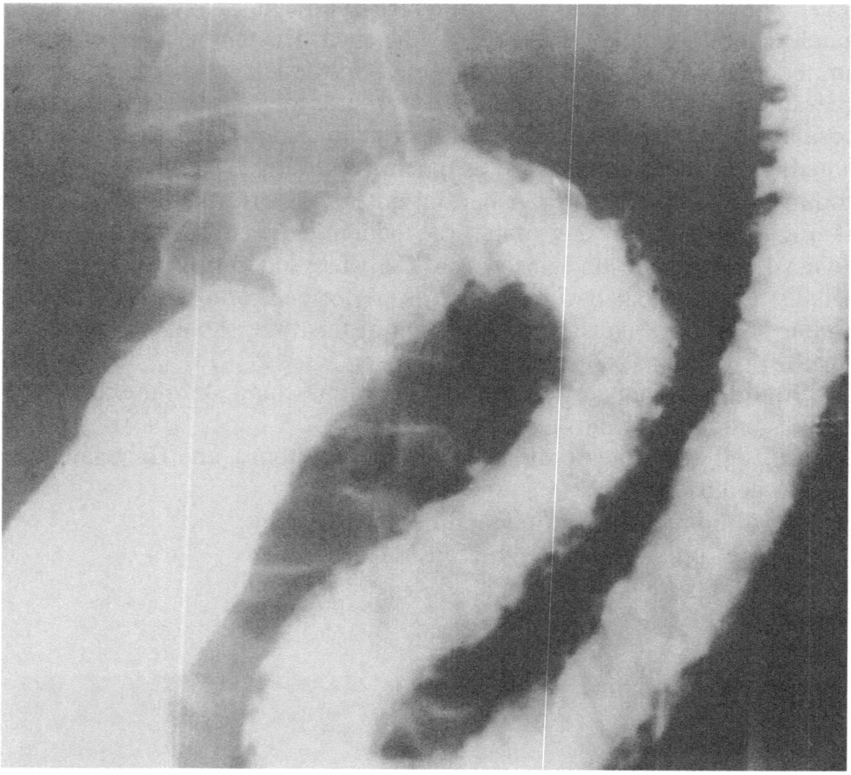

Figure 6-8

The diagnosis of ischemic colitis is being made more frequently in recent years, since the subtleties of its presentation are better recognized. Over 300 cases have been reported in the medical literature and all were in patients over 45 years of age. The etiology of the condition is unclear, although as the name suggests, it has been assumed that large- or small-vessel occlusion accounts for the clinical syndrome.[47] In an attempt to clarify the etiology of this condition, mesenteric arteriograms have been performed, frequently with rather mixed results. In many instances, major visceral segmental occlusions were noted in the area of colitis, while in other instances the angiograms have proven normal.[47,48]

The disease is characterized by its segmental distribution in the colon. Although most cases involve the left portions of the colon, any area except the rectum may be involved. The clinical course is one of abdominal distention, pain, and bloody diarrhea. The course of the illness can take many forms. In its most extreme forms, the condition may progress to full thickness colonic slough, with evidence of spreading peritonitis. Far more usual, however, is a variable period of time in which the patient manifests local evidence of inflammation that gradually subsides on supportive treatment only. Approximately 75% of all patients fall into this self-limited category. Some of these patients will go on to develop a later stricture, which can closely resemble an obstructing neoplasm of the colon.[47-49]

The indications for operation in this condition will be either signs of colonic perforation during the acute phase or a late stricture. In over 300 cases presented in the literature, no patient has had to be operated on for a persistence of bleeding.[47] Obviously, the proper treatment demands differentiation of this entity from other forms of colitis, such as ulcerative or amebic. This is usually easy because of lack of prior symptoms, the age group of the patients involved, and the sharply segmental nature of the ischemic lesions. If, as in the patient presented, operation is indicated for impending colon perforation, a limited colon resection should be carried out, with an end colostomy and oversewing of the rectal stump. Removal of the entire colon is unnecessary in this condition, and primary anastomosis would carry an additional hazard in these critically ill patients.

ANSWER: C.

6.13. Three years following a total abdominal hysterectomy for cervical carcinoma that was followed by intracavitary and external beam radiotherapy, a 54-year-old woman notes a feculent vaginal discharge. Multiple biopsies of the vaginal cuff disclose only inflammatory tissue. A barium enema is shown as Figure 6-9. Treatment should consist of:

A. Steroid enemas and vaginal antibiotic suppositories.
B. Temporary end sigmoid colostomy with closure 6–12 months later.
C. Permanent end sigmoid colostomy.
D. Excision of rectovaginal fistula.
E. Excision of rectovaginal fistula plus sigmoid colostomy.

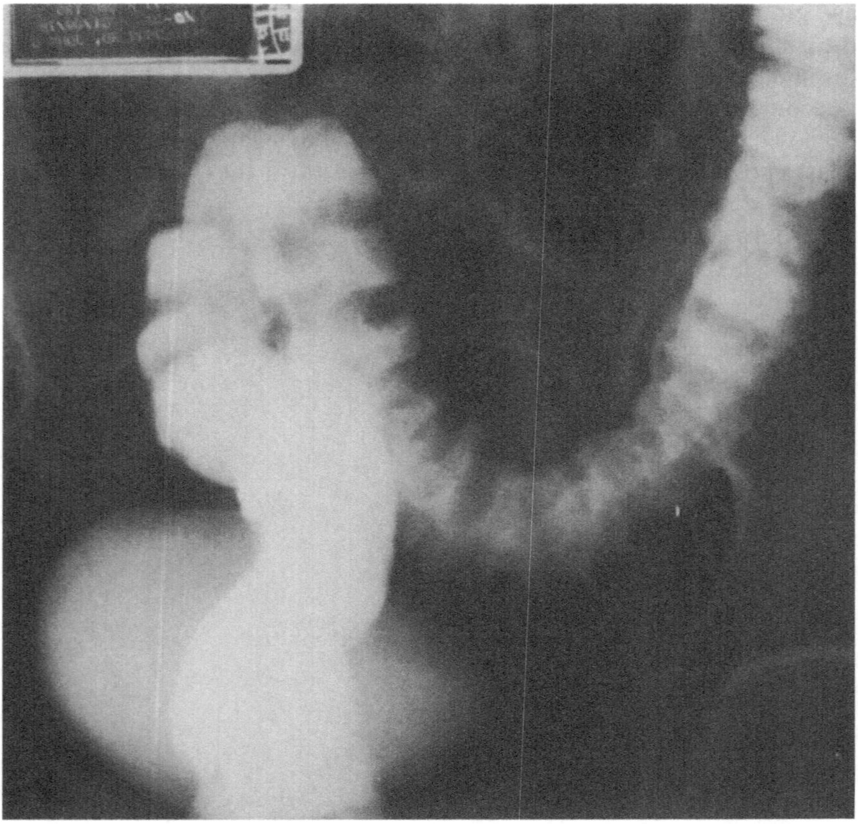

Figure 6-9

This patient has a presumably nonmalignant rectovaginal fistula secondary to severe radiation proctitis and colitis. The barium enema discloses marked inflammatory changes in the rectosigmoid colon. Although the rectum is alleged to be the most tolerant portion of the intestinal tract, generally requiring the administration of over 6000 rads to obtain a significant effect,[50] many instances of permanent damage to the colon and the rectum have occurred with dosages less than this. Radiation damage to the intestinal tract can take many forms, with radiation proctitis, rectovaginal fistula, and radiation enteritis being the most common.[51] Other forms include rectal ulceration and stricture, radiation colitis, and the late development of rectal neoplasms.[51,52] Some form of symptomatic intestinal injury is noted in over 11% of cases following radiotherapy for cervical carcinoma,[51] a figure which, however, is disputed by many radiotherapists.

The onset of symptoms of radiation-induced intestinal damage is quite variable. Mild or severe symptoms may begin as early as two months or as late as 30 years following treatment. Approximately three quarters of all cases, however, are manifest within four years.[53] Various factors have been said to be associated with an increased incidence of radiation-induced bowel damage. Among these are prior laparotomy, which can lead to adhesion formation and therefore fixation of the small intestine in one location, chemotherapy, hypertension, and diabetes mellitus.[51,53]

Many treatments have been attempted for those unfortunate patients with rectovaginal fistulas. Local nonoperative treatments are always unsuccessful, and any operative treatment that attempts excision or closure of the fistula that does not include proximal fecal diversion as well is doomed to failure. However, the general experience has been that even when fecal diversion is employed and the fistula is excised, when intestinal continuity is restored by closure of the colostomy the vast majority of fistulas recur. Therefore, it is felt that in this situation a permanent diverting colostomy is the most effective and realistic treatment.[53,54]

ANSWER: C.

References

1. Smiley, D.F.: Perforated sigmoid diverticulitis with spreading peritonitis. *Am. J. Surg.* 111:431, 1966.
2. Asch, M.J., Markowitz, A.M.: Diverticulitis coli: A surgical appraisal. *Surgery* 62:239, 1967.
3. Colcock, B.P.: Diverticular disease: Proven surgical management. *Clin. Gastroenterol.* 4:99, 1975.
4. Miller, D.W., Wichern, W.A.: Perforated sigmoid diverticulitis: Appriasal of primary versus delayed resection. *Am. J. Surg.* 121:536, 1971.
5. Rodkey, G.V., Welch, C.E.: Surgical management of colonic diverticulitis with free perforation or abscess formation. *Am. J. Surg.* 117:265, 1969.
6. Byrne, J.J., Garick, E.I.: Surgical treatment of diverticulitis. *Am. J. Surg.* 121:379, 1971.
7. Madden, J.L.: Primary resection and anastomosis in the treatment of perforated lesions of the colon. *Am. Surg.* 31:781, 1965.
8. Small, W.P., Smith, A.N.: Fistula and conditions associated with diverticular disease of the colon. *Clin. Gastroenterol.* 4:171, 1975.
9. Colcock, B.P., Stahmann, F.D.: Fistulas complicating diverticular disease of the sigmoid colon. *Ann. Surg.* 175:838, 1972.
10. Carpenter, W.S., Allaben, R.D., Kambouris, A.A.: Fistulas complicating diverticulitis of the colon. *Surg. Gynecol. Obstet.* 134:625, 1972.
11. Patient Management Problem #4, SESAP III. American College of Surgeons Surgical Education and Self Assessment Program III Syllabus. Chicago, Illinois, 1979, pp 28–37, 163–166.
12. Byrne, J.J., Garick, E.I.: Surgical treatment of diverticulitis. *Am. J. Surg.* 121:379, 1971.
13. Bradley, E.L., Isaacs, J.: Appendiceal abscess revisited. *Arch. Surg.* 113:130, 1978.
14. Stone, H.H., Sanders, S.L., Martin, J.D.: Perforated appendicitis in children. *Surgery* 69:673, 1971.
15. McPherson, A.G., Kinmonth, J.B.: Acute appendicitis and the appendix mass. *Br. J. Surg.* 32:365, 1945.
16. Thomas, D.R.: Conservative management of the appendix mass. *Surgery* 73:677, 1973.
17. Kirsner, J.B.: The local and systemic complications of inflammatory bowel disease. *J.A.M.A.* 242:1177, 1979.
18. Beeken, W.L.: Absorptive defects in young children with regional enteritis. *Pediatrics* 52:69, 1973.
19. Block, G.E., Moossa, A.R., Simonowitz, D.: The operative treatment of Crohn's disease in childhood. *Surg. Gynecol. Obstet.* 144:713, 1977.
20. Homan, W.P., Tang, C., Thorbjarnarson, B.: Anal lesions complicating Crohn disease. *Arch. Surg.* 111:1333, 1976.
21. Hoffman, J.P., Taft, D.A., Wheelis, R.F., Walker, J.H.: Adenocarcinoma and regional enteritis of the small intestine. *Arch. Surg.* 112:606, 1977.
22. Greenstein, A.J., Sachar, D., Pucillo, A., Kreel, I., Geller, S., Janowitz, H.D., Aufses, A.: Cancer in Crohn's disease after diversionary surgery. *Am. J. Surg.* 135:86, 1978.
23. Menguy, R.: Surgical Management of free perforation of the samll intestine complicating regional enteritis. *Ann. Surg.* 175:178, 1972.
24. Wall, A.J.: The use of glucocorticoids in intestinal disease. *Med. Clin. North Am.* 57:1241, 1973.
25. Farmer, R.G.: The protean manifestations of Crohn's disease. *Postgrad. Med.* 57:129, 1975.

26. Gump, F.E., Sakellariadis, P., Wolff, M., Broell, J.R.: Clinical pathological investigation of regional enteritis as a guide to prognosis. *Ann. Surg.* 176:233, 1972.
27. Rosenberg, J.L., Levin, B., Wall, A.J., Kirsner, J.B.: A controlled trial of azathioprine in Crohn's disease. *Am. J. Dig. Dis.* 20:721, 1975.
28. Klein, M., Binder, H.J., Mitchell, M., Aaronson, R., Spiro, H.: Treatment of Crohn's disease with azathioprine: A controlled evaluation. *Gastroenterology* 66:916, 1974.
29. Homan, W.P., Dineen, P. Comparison of the results of resection, bypass, and bypass with exclusion for ileocecal Crohn's disease. *Ann.. Surg.* 187:530, 1978.
30. Folley, J.H.: Ulcerative proctitis. *N. Engl. J. Med.* 282:1362, 1970.
31. Nugent, F.W., Veidenheimer, M.C., Zuberi, S., Garabedian, M.M., Parikh, N.K.: Clinical course of ulcerative proctosigmoiditis. *Digestive Diseases* 15:321, 1970.
32. Scott, H.W., Sawyers, J.L., Gobbel, W.G., Graves, H.A., Shull, H.J.: Surgical management of toxic dilitation of the colon inulculerative colitis. *Ann. Surg.* 179:647, 1974.
33. Neschis, M., Siegelman, S.S., Parker, J.G.: Diagnosis and management of megacolon of ulcerative colitis. *Gastroenterology* 55:251, 1968.
34. VanHeerden, J.A., McIlrath, D.C., Adson, M.A.: The surgical aspects of chronic mucosal inflammatory bowel disease (chronic ulcerative colitis). *Ann. Surg.* 187:536, 1978.
35. Binder, S.C., Miller, H.H., Deterling, R.A.: Emergency and urgent operations for ulcerative colitis. *Arch. Surg.* 110:284, 1975.
36. Foley, W.J., Coon, W.W., Bonfield, R.E.: Toxic megacolon in acute fulminate ulcerative colitis. *Am. J. Surg.* 120:769, 1970.
37. Turnball, R.B., Hawk, W.A., Weakley, F.L.: Surgical treatment of toxic megacolon: Ileostomy and colostomy to prepare patients for colectomy. *Am. J. Surg.* 122:325, 1971.
38. Binder, S.C., Miller, H.H., Deterling, R.A.: Fate of the retained rectum after subtotal colectomy for inflammatory disease of the colon. *Am. J. Surg.* 131:201, 1976.
39. Tompkins, R.K., Weinstein, M.H., Foroozan, P., Marx, F.W., Barker, W.F.: Reappraisal of rectum-retaining operations for ulcerative and granulomatous colitis. *Am. J.Surg.* 125:159, 1973.
40. Korelitz, B.I., Present, D.H., Alpert, L.I., Marshak, R.H., and Janowitz, H.D.: Recurrent regional ileitis after ileostomy and colectomy for granulomatous colitis. *N. Engl. J. Med.* 287:110, 1972.
41. Goligher, J.C.: The outcome of excisional operations for primary and recurrent Crohn's disease of the large intestine. *Surg. Gynecol. Obstet.* 148:1, 1979.
42. Lockhart-Mummery, H.E.: Crohn's disease of the large bowel. *Br. J. Surg.* 59:823, 1972.
43. Brooke, M.M.: Epidemiology of amebiasis in the U.S. *J.A.M.A.* 188:519, 1964.
44. Ittman, F.E., El-Hashimi, W.K., Pittman, J.C.: Studies of human amebiasis. *Gastroenterology* 65:581, 1975.
45. Tucker, P.C., Webster, P.D., Kilpatrick, Z.M.: Amebic colitis mistaken for inflammatory bowel disease. *Arch. Intern. Med.* 135:681, 1975.
46. Giacchino, J.L., Pickleman, J.R., Bartizal, J.F., Banich, F.E.: The therapeutic dilemma of acute amebic and ulcerative colitis. *Surg. Gynecol. Obstet.* 146:599, 1978.
47. Williams, L.F., Wittenberg, J.: Ischemic colitis: A useful clinical diagnosis, but is it ischemic? *Ann. Surg.* 182:439, 1975.
48. Hagihara, P.F., Parker, J.C., Griffen, W.O.: Spontaneous ischemic colitis. *Dis. Colon Rectum* 20:236, 1977.
49. Davis, J.E.: Reversible vascular occlusion of the colon. *Ann. Surg.* 171:789, 1970.
50. Roswit, B.: Complications of radiation therapy: The alimentary tract. *Semin. Roentgenol.* 9:51, 1974.
51. DeCosse, J.J., Rhodes, R.S., Wentz, W.B., Reagan, J.W., Dworken, H.J. Holden, W.D.: The natural history and management of radiation induced injury of the gastrointestinal tract. *Ann. Surg.* 170:369, 1969.

52. MacMahon, C.E., Rowe, J.W.: Rectal reaction following radiation therapy of cervical carcinoma: Particular reference to subsequent occurrence of rectal carcinoma. *Ann. Surg.* 173:264, 1971.
53. Russell, J.C., Welch, J.P.: Operative management of radiation injuries of the intestinal tract. *Am. J. Surg.* 137:433, 1979.
54. Smith, J.S., Milford, H.E.: Management of colitis caused by irradiation. *Surg. Gynecol. Obstet.* 142:569, 1976.

7
GASTROINTESTINAL CANCER

7.1. A 66-year-old man with no prior history of illness gives a 7-month history of progressive dysphagia so that he now can swallow only liquids. An esophagogram is shown as Figure 7-1. An esophagoscopy reveals a

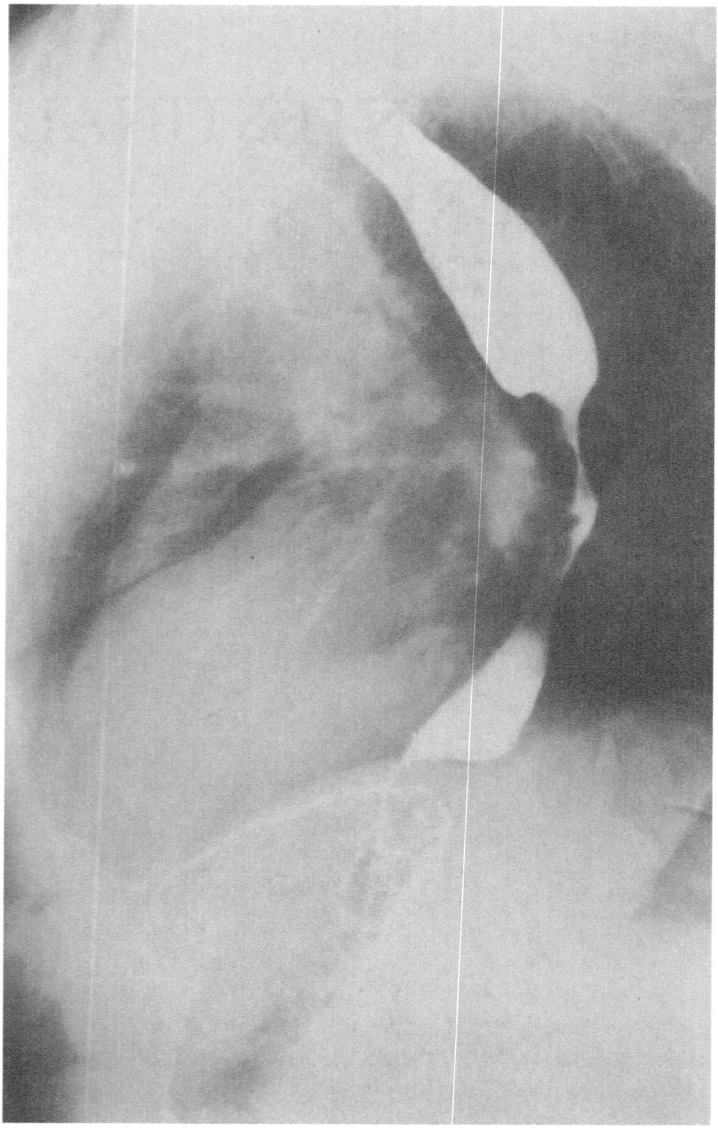

Figure 7-1

midesophageal friable tumor, and a biopsy revealing squamous cell carcinoma is obtained. A chest X ray and a liver scan are normal. Treatment of this patient should consist of:

A. Radiotherapy.
B. Insertion of an internal stent.
C. Esophagectomy with colon interposition.
D. Esophagectomy with jejunal interposition.
E. Esophagectomy with gastric interposition.

In previous years, the results of treatment of esophageal carcinoma were so poor that many surgeons developed a nihilistic attitude when confronted with a patient with this condition. Large series of patients were published with 5-year survival figures of less than 1%, regardless of the method of treatment.[1] Because of the high operative mortality rates attending esophagectomy, the trend in treatment of midesophageal lesions favored curative radiotherapy. However, this was tempered by the frequent complications that often resulted, such as aspiration pneumonia, tracheoesophageal fistula, mediastinal perforation, esophageal stricture, and radiation-induced spinal cord myelitis. Additionally, it was found that in those cases receiving preoperative radiotherapy residual carcinoma was often found in the esophageal specimen.[2] Because of these factors, surgery once again became favored, with various reconstruction techniques recommended since, in general, removal of the lesion tended to give better long-term palliation and relieve the obstruction more reliably than did radiation.[3]

Although there are still proponents of jejunal and colon interposition, it would appear that the best results currently obtainable for midesophageal cancer resections are obtained when the stomach is mobilized and swung up into an intrathoracic position, with the formation of a high esophagogastrostomy. This eliminates reliance upon the more tenuous blood supply of the colon, the resultant need for three anastomoses, and the problems of obtaining adequate length of either colon or jejunum. Operative mortality rates utilizing these two procedures have ranged between 15% and 25%. Utilizing separate right thoracotomy and celiotomy incisions with mobilization of the stomach upwards into the chest, operative mortality rates ranging from 3% to 12% have been obtained.[4,5] These series have noted an average survival of 21 months in 82 patients who were suitable for resection[4] and a 5-year survival rate of 9%.[5]

ANSWER: E.

7.2. A 54-year-old man complains of 3 months of indigestion, epigastric pain, and anorexia associated with a 15-lb weight loss. An upper GI tract study is performed and is shown as Figure 7-2. Gastroscopy discloses a 7-cm ulcerated lesion at the gastric cardia, and biopsies disclose adenocarcinoma. A chest X ray and a liver scan are normal. The patient should receive:

A. Celiotomy plus right thoracotomy, with distal esophagectomy and total gastrectomy.
B. Celiotomy plus left thoracotomy, with distal esophagectomy and total gastrectomy.
C. Celiotomy and total gastrectomy.
D. Celiotomy and proximal gastrectomy.
E. Chemotherapy and radiotherapy only.

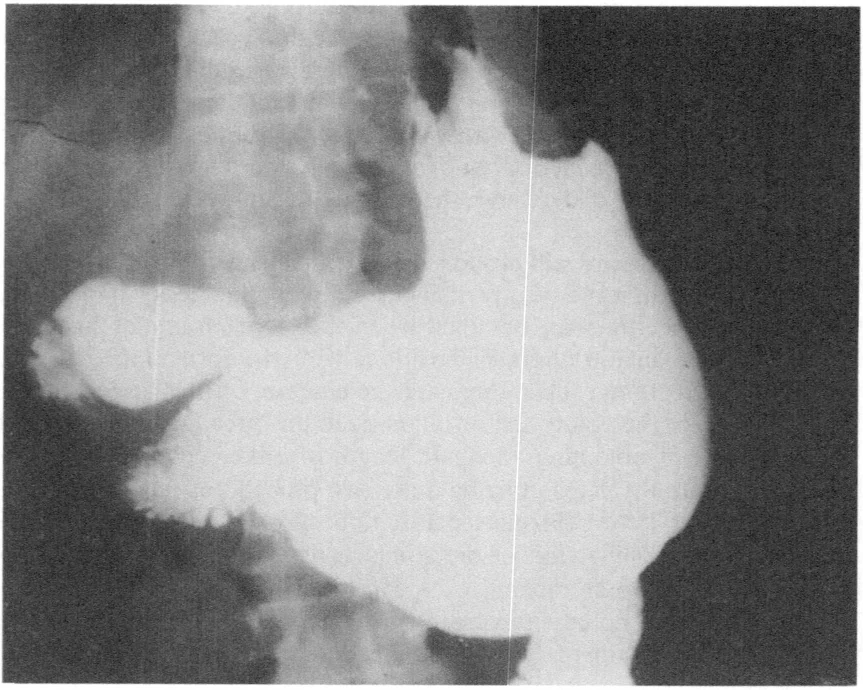

Figure 7-2

The problems in management of a patient with a proximal gastric carcinoma are complicated by the poor prognosis of such lesions and the extensive operations that are required to attempt cure. These operations are dictated by the characteristic spread of these tumors. In one series of 101 patients, 64% had positive splenic nodes, 80% had positive lesser omental nodes, 40% had positive greater omental nodes, and 12% had supra- or subpyloric nodes.[6] In addition to nodal spread, extensive submucosal spread occurs within the stomach and proximally into the esophagus. In one series of 100 patients, 35% had residual carcinoma at the proximal esophageal margin. It was found that this number could be significantly decreased by using frozen-section analysis of the transected margin at the time of operation and also by going further proximally on the esophagus, up to 12 cm proximal to the gross lesion. Interestingly, in this series the presence of positive margins did not seem to predispose to anastomotic breakdown.[7]

Because of these factors, adenocarcinoma of the cardia is best treated by total gastrectomy. Proximal gastrectomy enables the antrum of the stomach to be spared, but the resultant operative mortality rates are equal to if not greater than those noted with total gastrectomy, and the patient's alimentation is often not as satisfactory. Utilizing a left thoraco-abdominal approach, sufficient margins of proximal esophagus can be obtained for most gastric adenocarcinomas. Reconstruction by an end-to-side Roux-en-Y esophagojejunostomy completes the procedure. Utilizing total gastrectomy along with a radical nodal excision, including the splenic and distal pancreatic nodes, one series noted that 83% of patients with either localized gastric cancers or those involving only adjacent nodes survived for 5 years.[6]

ANSWER: B.

7.3. A 76-year-old woman undergoes a cholecystectomy for symptomatic gallstones. Four days postoperatively, she is making a normal recovery, and the pathologist informs you that the gallbladder contains carcinoma. Microscopically, it invades the muscularis mucosa of the gallbladder. You should advise your patient that she should undergo:

A. No further treatment at this time.
B. Right hepatic lobectomy.
C. Radiotherapy to the liver bed.
D. Wedge excision of the liver underlying the gallbladder bed.
E. Portal node dissection.

Carcinoma of the gallbladder is an extremely uncommon GI tract neoplasm and usually either presents as advanced metastatic disease with jaundice or is fortuitously noted in gallbladders removed for acute cholecystitis or recurrent biliary colic. Two factors appear to predispose to gallbladder carcinoma. The first is a calcified gallbladder; approximately 20% of these will harbor carcinoma.[8] Calcified gallbladders should, therefore, be removed when first diagnosed. The other association is cholelithiasis. In one large review of the literature, gallstones were noted in 72% of all cases of carcinoma of the gallbladder.[9] However, as many as 88% of some series of carcinomas of the gallbladder have been associated with gallstones.[10] In general, the vast majority of the long-term survivors of this disease are those patients in whom the gallbladder was removed for gallstone disease and harbored occult noninvasive carcinoma. In one series of such patients, 21 patients with full thickness invasion of the gallbladder wall all succumbed with cancer within 2½ years of their operation. Eleven other patients, however, had carcinoma confined to the submucosa; none underwent any further treatment and 7 of 11 survived 5 years.[10] In another series of 115 patients, only 2 patients survived 5 years, and these were likewise superficially situated carcinomas in gallbladders removed for gallstones.[11] This was confirmed in another series of 82 patients in whom the 10 1-year survivors were analyzed. In 4 patients, carcinoma was suspected at laparotomy and all patients subsequently died of their disease. However, 5 of 6 patients whose diagnosis was unsuspected at the time of laparotomy survived for 5 years with no evidence of disease.[12]

Because of the poor results noted in most patients with this disease, many authorities have advocated further surgery, with recommendations ranging from portal node dissection or hepatic wedge excision to formal right hepatic lobectomy.[11,13] However, careful analysis of the results of most of these operations fails to indicate any significant advantage in terms of long-term survival. Recently, local radiotherapy has been utilized with increasing success.[14,15] In the patient presented, because of her age and the fact that further radical surgery would be unlikely to benefit her, it would be reasonable to recommend a course of local radiotherapy.

ANSWER: C.

7.4. A 56-year-old man presents with a 2-week history of increasing, painless jaundice. Physical examination is normal; no abdominal masses are palpated. The serum bilirubin level is 11.6 mg%, the alkaline phosphatase content is 560 IU and the SGOT level is 120 U/ml. A liver scan and an abdominal ultrasound are normal. A percutaneous transhepatic cholangiogram and an endoscopic retrograde cholangiopancreatogram (ERCP) are performed and are shown as Figures 7-3 and 7-4. Celiotomy is carried out, and a 4-cm mass is palpated at the junction of the hepatic

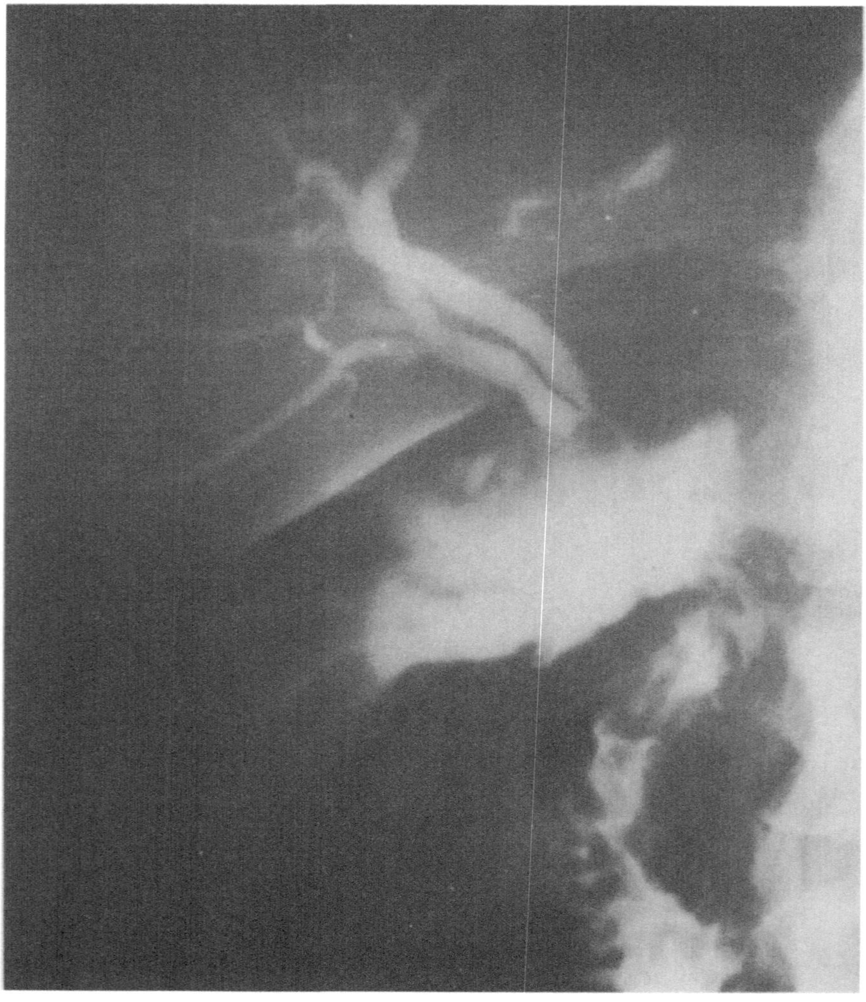

Figure 7-3

ducts. Needle biopsy of the mass discloses carcinoma. The surgeon should now attempt:

A. Intubation of the tumor with subsequent radiotherapy.
B. Extended right hepatic lobectomy.
C. Extended left hepatic lobectomy.
D. Closure of the patient and referral for hepatic transplantation.
E. Resection of the tumor and Roux-en-Y hepaticojejunostomy.

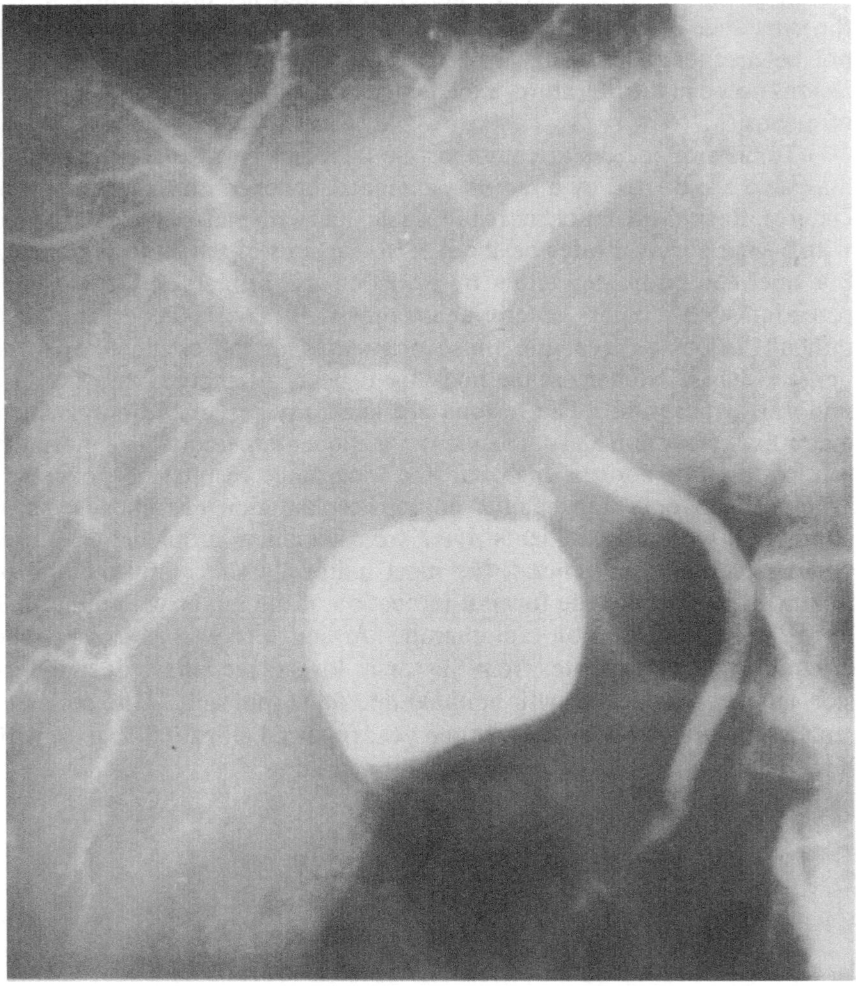

Figure 7-4

In this patient presenting with the biochemical picture of obstructive jaundice and a nonpalpable gallbladder, the chances are increased that he harbors gallstones with resultant common duct obstruction or an obstruction in the proximal hepatic ducts, as opposed to the more typical distal bile duct obstruction caused by cancer. The percutaneous cholangiogram and the ERCP clearly demonstrate an obstruction at the junction of the hepatic ducts. In general, malignant tumors of the extrahepatic bile ducts are slow growing and only infrequently metastasize. However, they are often lethal because of the technical problems that they impose in achieving decompression of the biliary tree. Tumors at the hepatic duct bifurcation can be easily missed at celiotomy, as they are often nearly within the substance of the liver, and even biopsies of suspicious areas will often not be diagnosed as malignant. Although there are few cures of these lesions noted in the literature, excellent palliation is possible with a variety of means.

Tumors of the distal common bile duct present as a periampullary mass and are treated by a radical pancreatoduodenectomy (Whipple procedure). Results are much more favorable than with pancreatic carcinoma, with 5-year survival rates of about 30%. Lesions of the central common bile duct can be treated either by resection and primary anastomosis or resection with a biliary-enteric anastomosis. By far, however, the most difficult lesions to treat are those originating at the confluence of the hepatic ducts. Numerous methods have been attempted, and few are uniformly successful. The lesions are generally resectable only with a major liver resection and subsequent hepaticoenterostomy. The mortality rate of this operation is high and the long-range results are poor.[16–18] Total hepatectomy and hepatic homotransplantation has likewise been attempted, with most patients dying from technical problems or subsequent rejection.[17] In general, the most uniformly successful method of treatment has been some form of intubation of the tumor with either a T or a Y tube, followed by radiotherapy. Although the tubes cause some discomfort at the exit sites from the torso, long-range biliary decompression has been achieved with minimal operative mortality. One series of ten patients followed for at least one year reported all patients alive, with three patients alive 2–3 years following operation.[19]

ANSWER: A.

7.5. A 62-year-old nonalcoholic man presents with painless jaundice, anorexia, and a 14-lb weight loss. On examination, an enlarged gallbladder is palpated. Total bilirubin concentration is 12.4 mg%, alkaline phosphatase content is 460 IU, and SGOT level is 118 U/ml. A liver scan is normal, and ultrasound discloses a 4-cm mass in the head of the pancreas. A percutaneous transhepatic cholangiogram is shown as Figure 7-5. At the time of celiotomy, the liver is normal and no abnormal lymph nodes are noted. The mass does not appear to be firmly fixed to the retroperitoneum. Two biopsies of the mass disclose only chronic pancreatitis on frozen section. The surgeons should perform:

A. Radical pancreatoduodenectomy (Whipple procedure).
B. A radical pancreatoduodenectomy with a total pancreatectomy.
C. A cholecystoenterostomy.
D. A choledochoduodenostomy.
E. Insertion of a T tube into the common duct.

This patient presents many of the problems one encounters in the management of a patient with an obstructing periampullary lesion. The clinical and laboratory picture are highly suggestive of an obstructive etiology for the jaundice, and therefore tests are undertaken immediately that will delineate this. Once ultrasound discloses a definite mass in the pancreas, a percutaneous transhepatic cholangiogram is performed and shows the characteristic distal common bile duct narrowing of carcinoma. Alternatively, an endoscopic retrograde cholangiopancreatogram could have been performed. The advantage of the percutaneous cholangiogram, however, is that if extremely high levels of bilirubin are present, an indwelling tube can be left in the liver to afford preoperative decompression of the bilary tree, with a resultant drop in the serum bilirubin. This has been shown to decrease postoperative morbidity significantly.[20]

In the presence of a negative history for alcohol abuse, and in the presence of a dilated gallbladder without stones, nearly all patients with a mass in the head of the pancreas will harbor a malignancy. Because of this, it is not necessary to insist upon a tissue diagnosis of carcinoma before embarking upon radical surgery. Often the carcinoma is surrounded by an area of pancreatitis, and positive biopsies cannot be obtained by either direct or needle biopsy. The surgeon, therefore, must be willing to act on the basis of the clinical information.

In recent years, significant dissatisfaction has surfaced regarding the classical radical pancreatoduodenectomy or Whipple procedure. Operative mortality has been high, and long-term survivors of this procedure

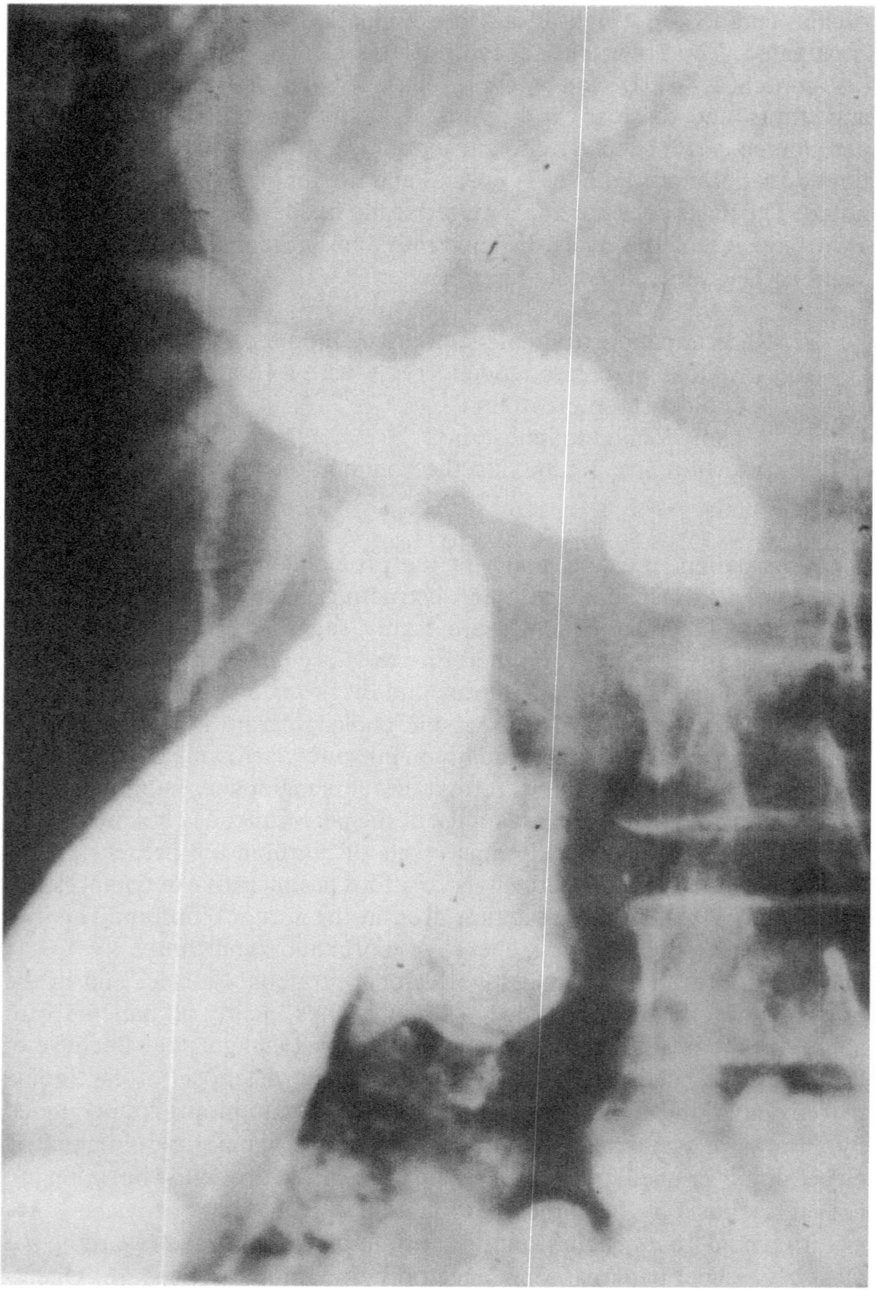

Figure 7-5

in patients harboring pancreatic carcinoma are rare. In analyzing these failures, two points became apparent. First, many patients died with locally recurrent carcinoma and not widespread metastatic disease, and second, a large percentage of patients who died in the postoperative period suffered local complications, of which the most common was leakage of the pancreaticoenteric anastomosis. Because of this, radical pancreatoduodenectomy with total pancreatectomy has been recently advised. This stand is further supported by the findings of multicentric pancreatic carcinoma in approximately one third of such patients, who presumably could not have been cured with a classical Whipple resection, as tumor would have been left behind in the pancreatic remnant.[21,22] With experience, these authors were able to perform the operation with a 30-day operative mortality of 12%–14%, and on long-term follow-up, several 5-year survivors were obtained. Besides the factors of multicentricity and the avoidance of a hazardous pancreatic anastomosis, total pancreatectomy also eliminates the possibility of postoperative pancreatitis. That subsequent exocrine and endocrine pancreatic function is superior when the Whipple procedure is employed is doubtful.[23] Preoperative diabetes mellitus in patients with pancreatic carcinoma and significant numbers of patients with postoperative diabetes are seen after Whipple resection, so the argument that all patients are made diabetic with a total pancreatectomy loses some of its force.[24] In addition, exocrine function is usually found to be minimal on long-term follow-up after Whipple procedures. In the largest series of total pancreatectomies, the subsequent diabetic management was considered easy in 76% of patients, with an average daily insulin requirement of 20–25 units.[21] Others have noted, however, a more brittle diabetic state and have experienced more difficulty in dealing with it. Regardless of which operation is chosen, a vagotomy and partial gastrectomy should probably be included. In one series, 6% of patients following a Whipple procedure and 18% of patients following a total pancreatectomy suffered from anastomotic ulceration if no vagotomy was carried out.[25]

ANSWER: B.

7.6. A 58-year-old woman gives a 1-year history of intermittent low abdominal cramps, aggravated by eating. For 3 months she has noted periodic warmth and flushing of the face and neck and episodic diarrhea. A small bowel series reveals kinking of the terminal ileum and proximal distention of bowel. A liver scan discloses a 6-cm defect in the left lateral lobe. Urinary 5-HIAA levels are elevated. Treatment should consist of:

A. Small bowel resection and biopsy of the liver tumor.
B. Small bowel resection and wedge excision of the liver tumor.
C. Small bowel resection and left hepatic lobectomy.
D. Small bowel bypass and wedge excision of the liver tumor.
E. Small bowel bypass and left hepatic lobectomy.

This patient presents with the classical signs and symptoms of a small-bowel carcinoid metastatic to the liver. Carcinoid tumors may arise from any level of the GI tract, but origins in the appendix and ileum are most frequent. Ileal carcinoids rarely spread unless the primary tumor is greater than 1 cm in diameter, and characteristically these tumors elicit a desmoplastic fibrotic reaction in the small bowel, leading to kinking and symptoms of small-bowel obstruction.[26] In addition, the patient with a small-bowel carcinoid is likely to harbor a carcinoid in another location. In one series, 40% of such patients harbored multiple carcinoids.[27] In a significant percentage of cases they are also associated with carcinomas.[27,28]

The carcinoid syndrome generally occurs only in the presence of metastatic carcinoid to the liver, usually originating from the small intestine. If no liver metastases are present, the elevated levels of serotonin and other hormonally active substances are degraded in the liver. Rare exceptions to this occur in the presence of bronchial or ovarian carcinoids, in which the peptides are released directly into the systemic circulation.[29]

As with many endocrine tumors, carcinoids often exhibit slow rates of growth, and therefore prolonged survival is possible. This justifies a radical operative approach for the primary lesions. In the case of symptomatic hepatic lesions, they should be removed with the least damaging resection possible, providing this can be done safely. This will often control the symptoms of the carcinoid syndrome and significantly improve the quality and duration of survival.[28,30] In recent years, the use of systemic chemotherapy also has been quite successful in patients with metastatic carcinoid.

In the patient presented, an aggressive surgical approach is indicated, as the small bowel disease appears limited to one area. A formal left hepatic lobectomy would obviously encompass all of the visible tumor, but a wedge excision of the liver can be carried out more safely.

ANSWER: B.

7.7. A 56-year-old man undergoes sigmoidoscopy because of several episodes of rectal bleeding. A 3-cm polyp on a 0.5-cm stalk is removed piecemeal. A portion of the polyp is shown in Figure 7-6. A few areas from the stalk are sectioned and show no evidence of carcinoma. The patient should be advised that he requires:

A. No further treatment at this time.
B. Repeat sigmoidoscopy and biopsy in 3 months.
C. Exploratory celiotomy, colotomy, and wedge excision of the remaining stalk.
D. Exploratory celiotomy and segmental left colon resection.
E. Exploratory celiotomy and radical left hemicolectomy.

This patient points out some of the many problems encountered in the management of a patient with colonic polyps. With the advent of colonoscopy, more and more polyps are being removed, and a certain percentage of these show evidence of carcinoma, ranging from carcinoma in situ to frankly invasive lesions. The management of these patients can be difficult.

Although there has been considerable debate over the years, most authorities today agree that there is a relationship between benign adenomatous polyps and colon carcinomas. Indeed, most people feel that a certain percentage of adenomatous polyps, if left in place, will become carcinomatous.[31-33] Recent data based on large numbers of colonoscopic polypectomies have substantiated the impressions that the incidence of carcinoma rises with the size of the polyp, is increased in polyps with villous features, and increases with the presence of multiple polyps.[31]

There is uniform agreement that snare removal of a pedunculated adenomatous polyp is sufficient treatment. This is true even if there is a focus of carcinoma in situ within that polyp. When, however, there is invasive carcinoma through the muscularis mucosa, as in the case presented, there is a potential for lymphatic dissemination of tumor, as there are lymphatics in the submucosal areas within the polyp. Although some authorities have attempted to argue that such a situation can be regarded as a carcinoma in situ if the stalk is sectioned and found to be free of tumor, routine sectioning may fail to note the presence of tumor within the stalk, and metastases are quite possible in the absence of such stalk invasion. Therefore, some form of additional treatment is required in the presence of a polyp containing invasive carcinoma. The operative mortality and morbidity following exploratory celiotomy and colotomy are similar to those following celiotomy and colonic resection. Therefore, this patient should be advised to undergo a left hemicolectomy with a wide nodal excision to try to remove all potential lymphatic drainage sites.

ANSWER: E.

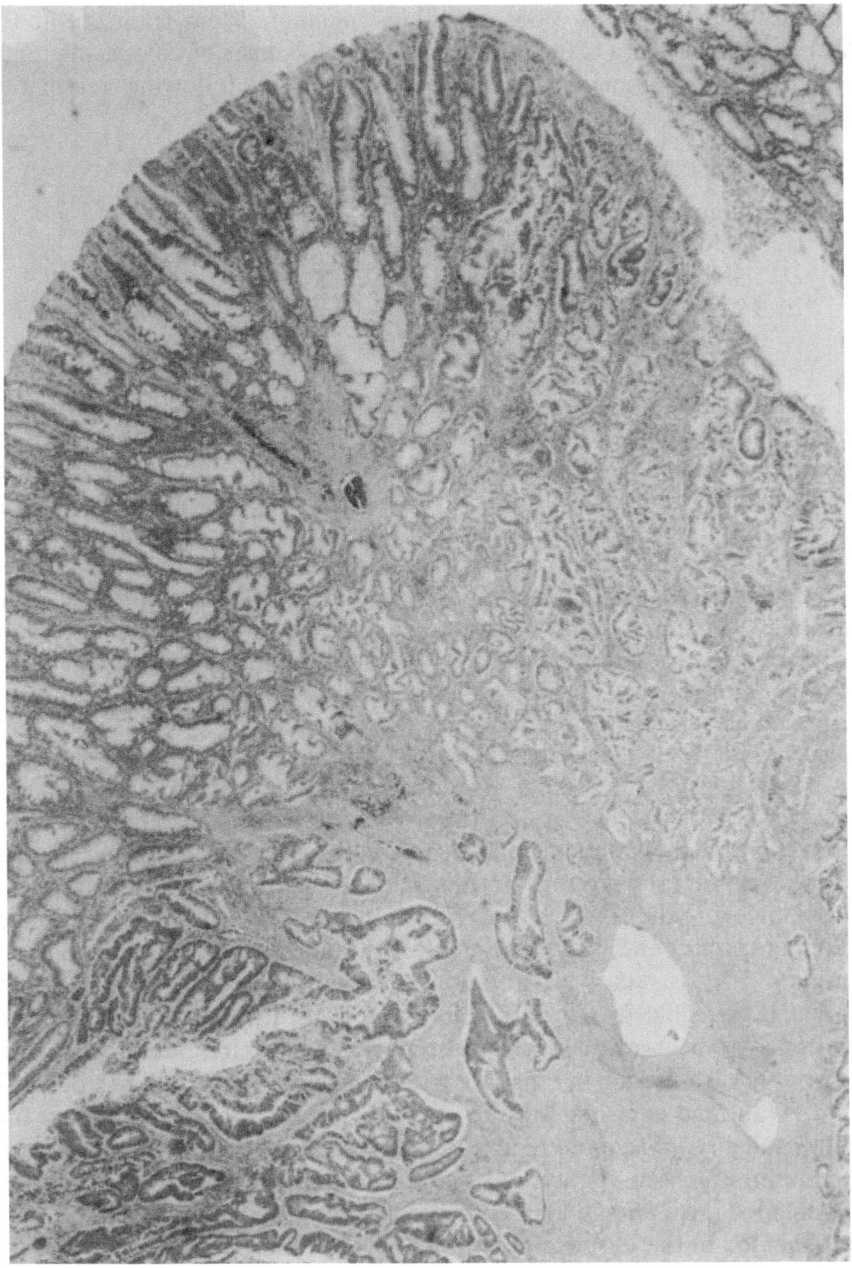

Figure 7-6

7.8. A 48-year-old woman presents with rectal bleeding and is found to have a 4-cm posteriorly located villous adenoma 9 cm from the anus. Multiple biopsies are taken, and a histologic diagnosis of villous adenoma with foci of carcinoma in situ is made. Which of the following treatments is not suitable for this patient?

A. Transanal excision of the tumor.
B. Fulguration.
C. Abdomino-perineal resection.
D. Abdomino-transsacral excision.
E. Low anterior resection.

Villous tumors of the colon, although found far less commonly than adenomatous polyps, are more important clinically, as the incidence of carcinoma in such polyps is high. Approximately 70% of these lesions are found in the rectum or rectosigmoid colon, further compounding the therapeutic problems.[34] Although it is recognized that the incidence of malignancy increases with the size of these tumors,[35,36] biopsy of such lesions can be misleading, as areas of invasive carcinoma can be missed.[34,35] The incidence of carcinoma in villous adenomas ranges from 35% to 48% in several large series of patients.[34,36–38] In addition, these tumors can recur after incomplete excision, and it is frequently noted that tumors previously regarded as benign may recur as invasive carcinoma, a circumstance that occurred in 17% of local recurrences in one series.[35]

Therefore, the treatment of villous adenomas must take these factors into consideration. Tumors arising above the peritoneal reflection pose no real problem, as they may be treated with a standard colon carcinoma operation with primary anastomosis. Tumors below the peritoneal reflection, however, should be extensively biopsied, and if no foci of invasive carcinoma are found, should be treated by some form of sphincter-saving surgery. In this regard, fulguration has been successfully utilized and would be feasible in the patient presented, as the lesion is below the peritoneal reflection and located posteriorly. With a circumferential lesion or one that is anterior in a female patient, fulguration would not be suitable. Transanal excision is quite possible, even for fairly high-lying tumors, and any subsequent recurrences can be either snared or reresected. Abdomino-transsacral excisions and low anterior resections are likewise suitable for this patient.[39] An abdomino-perineal resection would be contraindicated in the absence of definite proof of invasive malignancy.

ANSWER: C.

7.9. A 60-year-old man is admitted to the hospital because of weakness. Physical examination is normal, but his hemoglobin level is 5.8 g% and his stools are strongly positive for occult blood. A barium enema reveals a large fungating tumor in the sigmoid colon. The carcinoembryonic antigen level is 240 ng/ml and a liver scan discloses multiple bilateral filling defects. He should be advised that he should receive:

A. Iron therapy.
B. Systemic chemotherapy.
C. Radiotherapy to the colon tumor.
D. Transverse colostomy.
E. Resection of the colon tumor with primary anastomosis.

The management of patients with incurable colon carcinoma presents difficult problems, owing to the high risks involved with most forms of treatment and the limited life expectancy that these patients have. Survival of patients with colon carcinoma metastatic to the liver generally averages between 9 and 12 months from the time of diagnosis. However, many of these do not succumb to the effects of widespread cancer but rather to local effects of the tumor itself, such as hemorrhage, either acute or chronic, obstruction, or perforation. For these reasons, palliative colon resections may be indicated in certain people with colon carcinoma. In one series of 78 patients undergoing palliative colon resection, the operative mortality rate was 6.4%, and 20% of patients had major postoperative complications.[40] Those who survived operation had a mean survival of 12.4 months. These authors concluded that palliative resection was indicated for those patients with incurable colon carcinoma manifesting chronic GI tract bleeding or presenting with a large-bowel obstruction. Another series investigated the usefulness of palliative resections for all types of GI tract carcinomas. Overall, an operative mortality of 26% was noted; this figure however was only 13% for those patients with colon carcinoma.[41] Survival of patients with stomach or pancreatic cancer averaged less than 5 months. However, those patients with colon carcinoma enjoyed longer survival: 10 months in this series. These authors noted that the best results were obtained in those patients who presented with GI tract blood loss; the next most favorable group were the patients presenting with colon obstruction. No patient who presented with a perforated cancer and peritonitis survived the operation.

In view of these factors, an attempt at palliation is indicated in this patient. Any treatment that does not remove the primary tumor is likely to be negated by local complications. Local radiotherapy might precipitate an acute obstruction or perforation. Therefore, in a good-risk patient, a limited colon resection and anastomosis is warranted.

ANSWER: E.

7.10. Which of the following statements regarding carcinoembryonic antigen (CEA) is false?

A. CEA may be elevated in benign GI tract disorders.
B. CEA may be elevated in non-GI-tract cancers.
C. The highest CEA levels are noted in patients with liver metastases.
D. CEA levels may be elevated in patients who smoke cigarettes.
E. CEA is a relatively low-cost screening test for colon cancer.

Since its first use in 1965, the measurement of CEA levels has become extremely useful in the monitoring of patients with a variety of malignancies. CEA is an antigen shared by many carcinomas and fetal tissues; it is measured by a relatively simple radioimmunoassay. Although it is most widely used in the care of patients with colon cancer, CEA levels are also elevated in many GI tract cancers as well as in non-GI-tract cancers such as those of the lung, ovary, and breast. Additionally, a wide variety of benign disorders may be associated with elevations in the serum CEA level. Among these are hepatitis, cirrhosis, pancreatitis, inflammatory bowel disease, and diverticulitis. Persons who smoke may also have modest elevations in their CEA level. Because of the test's lack of specificity for colon carcinoma, it cannot be used as a screening test for this disorder.

Basically, the level of CEA correlates with the stage of the colon cancer, with the higher levels being noted in the more advanced cancers.[42,43] The levels tend to decrease postoperatively and increase at the time of tumor recurrence. The highest levels detected are generally in those patients with metastatic disease to the liver. Because of these factors, the major usefulness of serum CEA determinations lies in the postoperative follow-up of these patients. A patient who has had an elevated level that returns to normal postoperatively undergoes sequential determinations of CEA. Any sustained rise in the level of CEA nearly always connotes recurrent disease, and this information may then be used as a guide to second-look operations, at which time removal of obvious recurrent disease can be carried out with the hope of cure.[44,45]

ANSWER: E.

7.11. A 56-year-old man undergoes a radical left hemicolectomy for a colon carcinoma. Three out of 14 lymph nodes are involved by tumor. Fourteen months later, he is noted to have an elevated carcinoembryonic antigen level, and a liver scan shows a 4-cm solitary defect in the right lobe that was not previously present. The patient should undergo:

A. Systemic chemotherapy.
B. Hepatic artery infusion chemotherapy.
C. Excision of the metastasis.
D. Liver irradiation.
E. Hepatic artery ligation.

Patients with malignancies metastatic to the liver have a poor prognosis. In one large series of patients with hepatic metastases who were untreated, the median survival of patients with colon carcinoma was 5 months. However, 21% of patients survived over 10 months. In this series, the survival was equal for carcinomas of the colon and rectum but was strikingly superior to the survivals in other patients with metastatic gastric or pancreatic carcinomas. No statistically different survivals were noted between those patients with solitary metastases, multiple metastases in one lobe, or bilateral metastases.[46] Since then, several large series have demonstrated that patients with colorectal carcinoma metastatic to the liver can be afforded long-term survival by removal of the liver metastases. In a multi-institutional review of this problem, patients with hepatic metastases who were not treated rarely survived for 5 years. With appropriate hepatic resection, a 22% 5-year survival rate was noted. In these combined series, no difference in ultimate survival time was noted whether the liver metastasis was removed at the same time as the colectomy or was done at a later time, and wedge resections of the liver provided survival rates equal to those after major hepatic resections.[47] In this series, patients with solitary metastases and those with multiple metastases in one lobe enjoyed similar survivals. However, another study showed clearly that patients with solitary metastases fared better. In that series, 15 out of 36 patients with solitary lesions survived for 5 years, whereas no patient with multiple metastases did so.[48] Subsequently, the same group undated their experience with patients with metastatic colorectal cancer who had sufficiently large metastatic deposits in the liver that a major hepatic resection was required. In this group also prolonged survival was obtained, with 41% of patients being alive more than 3 years postoperatively and three patients surviving over 10 years postoperatively.[49]

In comparison to these relatively good results, the results of chemotherapy in patients with metastatic colorectal carcinoma have been disappointing. In one multi-institution series, no differences in survival were noted between intravenous and regional hepatic chemotherapy, although survival was definitely prolonged in those patients who did respond. Likewise, liver irradiation has not proven to yield meaningful long-term survival. So, at the present time, the best opportunity to achieve long-term survival in patients with metastatic colorectal carcinoma lies in resection of the localized disease.

ANSWER: C.

7.12. A 66-year-old man has been unsuccessfully treated by his local physician for hemorrhoids for 6 months. He is referred for surgery. On examination, he has a 1.5-cm ulcerated area at the anal verge that prolapses with straining. The remainder of the rectal examination is normal. There is no abnormal lymphadenopathy. Biopsy of the area reveals squamous cell carcinoma. A sigmoidoscopy, a liver scan, and the carcinoembryonic antigen level are normal. The patient should be advised to undergo:

A. Abdomino-perineal resection.
B. Local radiotherapy.
C. Local excision.
D. Local excision and radiotherapy.
E. Radiotherapy followed by abdomino-perineal resection.

Patients with squamous cell carcinoma of the anus or anal canal are often treated for inordinately long periods of time for benign disease. Studies of large series of patients have disclosed that as many as one third of these patients saw doctors previously for benign anorectal disorders and the true diagnosis was unsuspected.[50,51] Certain authorities have attempted to make a prognostic distinction between anal canal carcinomas (those originating at or just below the pectinate line) and anal carcinomas (those originating from the anal verge or perianal skin). However, while this may pathologically be a valid concept, the management and prognosis of these patients does not differ, and they can therefore be considered together.[51]

The major importance in differentiating squamous carcinomas of the anus and anal canal from the more common adenocarcinomas of the rectum lies in the propensity of the former to metastasize to the inguinal lymph nodes. Several studies have shown that approximately one third of all patients will have positive mesenteric lymph node metastases and another third will have positive inguinal metastases. It has generally been noted that if the metastases to the inguinal lymph nodes are detected at the time of initial presentation of the anal cancer, cure of the patient is unlikely, even though an inguinal node dissection is carried out. Two series of patients have disclosed only a 20% 5-year salvage of such patients, but most of these patients subsequently died from their disease.[51,52] If, however, the inguinal lymph node metastases appeared after 3 months following treatment of the primary lesion, 60%–70% of such patients could be alive and free of disease 5 years following treatment of the primary lesion and subsequent radical groin dissection.[51,52] Approximately one third of patients will also have metastases to the obturator and hypogastric lymph nodes.[51]

On the basis of this data, treatment guidelines have been formulated. For lesions less than 2 cm in diameter, wide local excision can be satisfactory treatment.[51–53] This treatment may be curative in as many as two thirds of patients.[51] For those patients with larger or histologically invasive lesions, abdomino-perineal resection should be carried out, and the obturator and hypogastric nodes should be removed as part of this operation.[51] Prophylactic bilateral inguinal lymph node dissection is not recommended, as the majority of patients with carcinoma of the anus do not develop inguinal metastases. If abnormal groin nodes are palpable at the time of presentation, a groin dissection should be carried out along with treatment of the primary lesion, but in such cases the outlook is poor. If groin metastases develop after treatment of the primary lesion, a therapeutic groin dissection should be carried out.[51] Although radiotherapy has been used successfully for some small anal carcinomas, the present experience is too limited to make conclusions.

ANSWER: C.

References

1. Lowe, W.C.: Survival with carcinoma of the esophagus. *Ann. Intern. Med.* 77:915, 1972.
2. Parker, E.F., Gregorie, H.B.: Carcinoma of the esophagus. *J.A.M.A.* 235:1018, 1976.
3. Piccone, V.A., LeVeen, H.H., Ahmed, N., Grosberg, S.: Reappraisal of esophagogastrectomy for esophageal malignancy. *Am. J. Surg.* 137:32, 1979.
4. Ellis, F.H., Gibb, S.P.: Esophagogastrectomy for carcinoma. *Ann. Surg.* 190:699, 1979.
5. Gunnlaugsson, G.H., Wychulis, A.R., Roland, C., Ellis, F.H.: Analysis of the records of 1,657 patients with carcinoma of the esophagus and cardia of the stomach. *Surg. Gynecol. Obstet.* 130:997, 1979.
6. Papachristou, D.N., Fortner, J.G.: Adenocarcinoma of the gastric cardia: The choice of gastrectomy. *Ann. Surg.* 192:58, 1980.
7. Papachristou, D.N., Agnanti, N., D'Agostino, H., Fortner, J.G.: Histologically positive esophageal margin in the surgical treatment of gastric cancer. *Am. J. Surg.* 139:711, 1980.
8. Polk, H.C.: Carcinoma and the calcified gallbladder. *Gastroenterology* 50:582, 1966.
9. Strauch, G.O.: Primary carcinoma of the gallbladder. *Surgery* 47:368, 1960.
10. Bergdahl, L.: Gallbladder carcinoma first diagnosed at microscopic examination of gallbladders removed for presumed benign disease. *Ann. Surg.* 191:19, 1980.
11. Beltz, W.R., Codon, R.E.: Primary carcinoma of the gallbladder. *Ann. Surg.* 180:180, 1974.
12. Moossa, A.R., Anagnost, M., Hall, A.W., Moraldi, A., Skinner, D.B.: The continuing challenge of gallbladder cancer. *Am. J. Surg.* 130:57, 1975.
13. Piehler, J.M., Crichlow, R.W.: Primary carcinoma of the gallbladder. *Surg. Gynecol. Obstet.* 147:929, 1978.
14. Smoron, G.L.: Radiation therapy of carcinoma of gallbladder and biliary tract. *Cancer* 40:1422, 1977.
15. Treadwell, T.A., Hardin, W.J.: Primary carcinoma of the gallbladder. *Am. J. Surg.* 132:703, 1976.
16. Longmire, W.P., McArthur, M.S., Bastounis, E.A., Hiatt, J.: Carcinoma of the extrahepatic biliary tract. *Ann Surg.* 178:333, 1973.
17. Fortner, J.G., Kallum, B.O., Kim, D.K.: Surgical management of carcinoma of the junction of the main hepatic ducts. *Ann. Surg.* 184:68, 1976.
18. McDermott, W.V., Peinert, R.A.: Carcinoma in the supra-ampullary portion of the bile ducts. *Surg. Gynecol. Obstet.* 149:681, 1979.
19. Terblanche, J., Saunders, S.J., Louw, J.H.: Prolonged palliation in carcinoma of the main hepatic duct junction. *Surgery* 71:720, 1972.
20. Nakayama, T., Ikeda, A., Okuda, K.: Percutaneous transhepatic drainage of the biliary tract: Technique and results in 104 cases. *Gastroenterology* 74:554, 1978.
21. Pliam, M.B., ReMine, W.H.: Further evaluation of total pancreatectomy. *Arch. Surg.* 110:506, 1975.
22. Tryka, A.F., Brooks, J.R.: Histopathology in the evaluation of total pancreatectomy for ductal carcinoma. *Ann. Surg.* 190:373, 1979.
23. Forrest, J.F., Longmire, W.P.: Carcinoma of the pancreas and periampullary region: A study of 279 patients. *Ann. Surg.* 189:129, 1979.
24. Ihse, I., Lilja, P., Arnesjo, B., Bengmark, S.: Total pancreatectomy for cancer. *Ann. Surg.* 186:675, 1977.
25. Grant, C.S., VanHeerden, J.A.: Anastomotical ulceration following subtotal and total pancreatectomy. *Ann. Surg.* 190:1, 1979.

26. Case 16-1979, Case records of the Massachusetts General Hospital: Weekly clinicopathologic exercises. *N. Engl. J. Med.* 300:909, 1979.
27. Morgan, J.G., Marks, C., Hearn, D.: Carcinoid tumors of the gastrointestinal tract. *Ann. Surg.* 180:720, 1974.
28. Peskin, G.W., Kaplan, E.L.: The surgery of carcinoid tumors. *Surg. Clin. North Am.* 49:137, 1969.
29. Teitelbaum, S.L.: The carcinoid. *Am. J. Surg.* 123:564, 1972.
30. Davis, Z., Moertel, C.G., McIlrath, D.C.: The malignant carcinoid syndrome. *Surg. Gynecol. Obstet.* 137:637, 1973.
31. Shinya, H., Wolff, W.I.: Morphology, Anatomic distribution, and cancer potential of colonic polyps. *Ann. Surg.* 190:679, 1979.
32. Welch, C.E.: Polyps and cancer of the colon. *Am. J. Surg.* 138:625, 1979.
33. Buntain, W.L., ReMine, W.H., Farrow, G.M.: Premalignancy of polyps of the colon. *Surg. Gynecol. Obstet.* 134:499, 1972.
34. McCabe, J.C., McSherry, C.K., Sussman, E.B., Gray, G.F.: Villous tumors of the large bowel. *Am. J. Surg.* 126:336, 1973.
35. Jahadi, M.R., Baldwin, A.: Villous adenomas of the colon and rectum. *Am. J. Surg.* 130:729, 1975.
36. Olson, R.O., Davis, W.C.: Villous adenomas of the colon, benign or malignant? *Arch. Surg.* 98:487, 1969.
37. Orringer, M.B., Eggleston, J.C.: Papillary (villous) adenomas of the colon and rectum. *Surgery* 72:378, 1972.
38. Bacon, H.E., Eisenberg, S.W.: Papillary adenoma of villous tumor of the rectum and colon. *Ann. Surg.* 174:1002, 1971.
39. Localio, S.A., Baron, B.: Abdomino-transsacral resection and anastomosis for midrectal cancer. *Ann. Surg.* 178:540, 1973.
40. Takaki, H.S., Ujiki, G.T., Shields, T.S.: Palliative resections in the treatment of primary colorectal cancer. *Am. J. Surg.* 133:548, 1977.
41. Borwn, P.W., Terz, J.J., Lawrence, W., Blievernicht, S.W.: Survival after palliative surgery for advanced intraabdominal cancer. *Am. J. Surg.* 134:575, 1977.
42. Slater, G., Papatestas, A.E., Aufses, A.H.: Preoperative carcinoembryonic antigen levels in colorectal carcinoma. *Arch. Surg.* 114:52, 1979.
43. Livingstone, A.S., Hampson, L.G., Schuster, J., Gold, P., Hinchey, E.J.: Carcinoembryonic antigen in the diagnosis and management of colorectal carcinoma. *Arch. Surg.* 109:259, 1974.
44. Cohen, A.M., Wood, W.C.: Carcinoembryonic antigen levels as an indicator for reoperation in patients with carcinoma of the colon and rectum. *Surg. Gynecol. Obstet.* 149:22, 1979.
45. Wanebo, H.J., Stearns, M., Schwartz, M.K.: Use of CEA as an indicator of early recurrence and as a guide to a selected second-look procedure in patients with colorectal cancer. *Ann. Surg.* 188:481, 1978.
46. Jaffi, B.M., Donegan, W.L., Watson, F., Spratt, J.S.: Factors influencing survival in patients with untreated hepatic metastases. *Surg. Gynecol. Obstet.* 127:1, 1968.
47. Foster, J.H.: Survival after liver resection for secondary tumors. *Am. J. Surg.* 135:389, 1978.
48. Wilson, S.M., Adson, M.A.: Surgical treatment of hepatic metastases from colorectal cancers. *Arch. Surg.* 111:330, 1976.
49. Adson, M.A., VanHeerden, J.A.: Major hepatic resections for metastatic colorectal cancer. *Ann. Surg.* 191:576, 1980.
50. Brennan, J.T., Stewart, C.F.: Epidermoid carcinoma of the anus. *Ann. Surg.* 176:787, 1972.

51. Stearns, M.W., Quan, S.H.Q.: Epidermoid carcinoma of the anorectum. *Surg. Gynecol. Obstet.* 131:953, 1970.
52. Golden, G.T., Horsley, J.S.: Surgical management of epidermoid carcinoma of the anus. *Am. J. Surg.* 131:275, 1976.
53. Al-Jurf, A.S., Turnbull, R.B., Fazio, V.W.: Local treatment of squamous cell carcinoma of the anus. *Surg. Gynecol. Obstet.* 148:576, 1979.

8
ENDOCRINE SURGERY

8.1. Which of the following is not currently considered to be an acceptable treatment for Cushing's disease?

A. Subtotal adrenalectomy.
B. Transphenoidal hypophysectomy.
C. Total adrenalectomy.
D. Pituitary irradiation.
E. Adrenocorticolytic drugs (*o,p*-DDD).

Chronic circulating excesses of adrenal corticosteroids bring about devastating physical sequelae. Central obesity, marked weakness, and easy bruiseability are all noted commonly, as are severe osteoporosis, hypertension, and diabetes. Although it has been classically thought that Cushing's disease results from a pituitary adenoma secreting excessive amounts of ACTH with resultant adrenal hyperplasia, more recent evidence suggests a neurohypothalamic origin of Cushing's disease. In addition, Cushing's syndrome may also be caused by benign or malignant adrenal tumors or by carcinomas that secrete excessive amounts of ACTH.

The diagnosis of Cushing's disease depends upon the biochemical demonstration of adrenocorticoid excess. Elevated levels of urinary 17-hydroxycorticosteroids are noted, along with elevated rates of cortisol secretion and elevated urinary cortisol levels. Plasma cortisol and ACTH levels are elevated, and the normal circadian rhythm of cortisol and ACTH levels in plasma are altered. In addition, the hyperplastic adrenal glands may be suppressed by the oral administration of dexamethasone.

At this time, there are several competing treatments that are effective against Cushing's disease. Bilateral total adrenalectomy has proven to be quite effective, immediately bringing the excess cortisol secretion under control. This approach, of course, does not directly attack the cause of the problem, namely the pituitary adenoma, but long-term follow-ups have demonstrated excellent sustained results.[1] Disadvantages of this method include the need for lifelong corticosteroid support and the possibility that a rarely occurring ACTH-secreting pituitary lesion that can cause local compressive symptoms and hyperpigmentation (Nelson's syndrome) will arise. Alternatively, with the advent of transphenoidal pituitary microsurgery, microadenomas of the pituitary gland can be carefully dissected out, preserving the remainder of the anterior pituitary gland. In several series of cases, this has ameliorated the symptoms of Cushing's disease, but thus far, follow-up of these patients has not been carried out long enough to say that this procedure has definite long-term merit.[2,3] Advocates of this approach stress the normal adrenal function that can be maintained after the procedure without exogenous steroid supplements. Pituitary irradiation has also been employed in an attempt to destroy the pituitary lesion. This has proven successful in many cases, but disadvantages are the permanent hypopituitary state and the long time elapsed before the treatment takes effect, up to one year in some instances.[4] More recently, the adrenocorticolytic drug *o,p*-DDD has been successfully used. Once again, an excessive time is required for the drug effect to occur, and many patients relapse following treatment.[5]

Subtotal adrenalectomy, either intentional or accidental owing to technical reasons, is an inadequate operation, as the adrenal remnant often hyperfunctions, leading to a recurrence of clinical symptoms.

ANSWER: A.

8.2. A 46-year-old woman gives a 3-year history of progressive obesity, easy bruiseability, and cutaneous striae. Her blood pressure is 160/100, and a fasting blood glucose level is 140 mg%. Cushing's disease is suspected, and biochemical tests of adrenocortical function are carried out. Urinary 17-hydroxycorticosteroids are elevated, as are plasma and urinary cortisol levels. Following administration of 8 mg of dexamethasone, urinary 17-hydroxycorticosteroid secretion is unchanged. A chest X ray and intravenous pyelogram are normal, and an abdominal CAT scan is shown as Figure 8-1. Treatment should consist of:

A. Transphenoidal hypophysectomy.
B. Pituitary irradiation.
C. Left adrenalectomy.
D. Right adrenalectomy.
E. Total adrenalectomy.

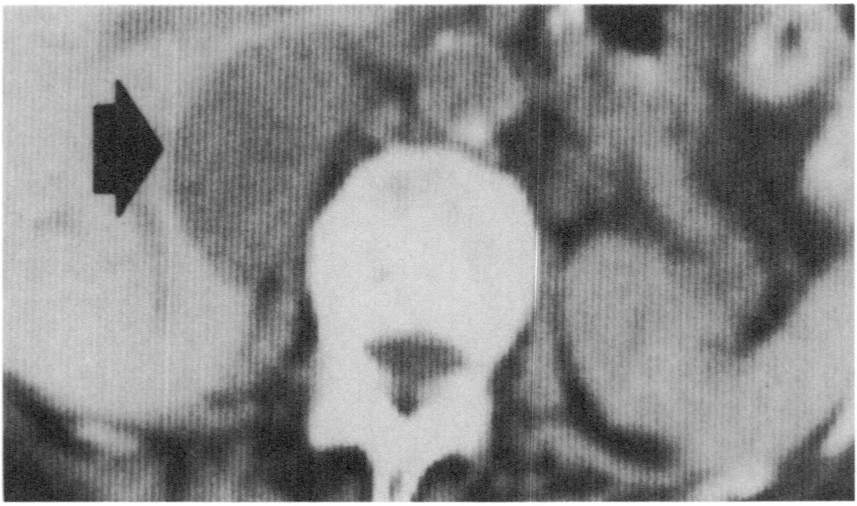

Figure 8-1

This patient has the classic clinical and biochemical evidence of cortisol excess. The problem, at this point, is to differentiate between a pituitary adenoma secreting excessive amounts of ACTH associated with adrenal hyperplasia, an ACTH-producing tumor associated with adrenal hyperplasia, and a primary adrenal tumor such as an adenoma or carcinoma. The failure of high levels of dexamethasone to suppress the urinary 17-hydroxycorticosteroid excretion eleminates the possibility of a pituitary lesion. The normal chest X ray helps to rule out an ACTH-producing tumor, because most of these tumors originate in the lung. When the abdominal CAT scan discloses an enlarged adrenal gland on the right side, the diagnosis of adrenal adenoma or carcinoma is secure, and unilateral adrenalectomy should be carried out.[6]

Once operation has been decided upon, the surgeon must choose between a transabdominal approach, a flank approach, or a combined thoracoabdominal incision. As only a unilateral adrenalectomy is required in this instance, a flank approach is preferred by many, as it gives adequate access to the area and is associated with minimal postoperative morbidity.

ANSWER: D.

8.3. A 42-year-woman with blood pressure levels up to 180/120 is referred for investigation of hypertension. An intravenous pyelogram is normal. Vanillylmandelic acid levels are normal, as are urinary metanephrine and normetanephrine levels. Plasma renin activity is low, and urinary aldosterone levels are elevated. Urinary 17-hydroxycorticosteroid levels are normal. Serum electrolytes are: sodium, 146 mEq/liter; potassium, 2.6 mEq/liter; and chloride, 101 mEq/liter. An abdominal CAT scan discloses a 2-cm mass in the left adrenal gland. The most likely diagnosis is:

A. Pheochromocytoma.
B. Cushing's syndrome secondary to adrenal adenoma.
C. Right renal artery stenosis.
D. Left renal artery stenosis.
E. Aldosteronoma.

Primary aldosteronism is an uncommon disorder, but an important one, as it represents a potentially curable form of hypertension. The hallmarks of this condition—hypokalemia, increased secretion of aldosterone, and low plasma renin activity—are often seen but do not necessarily indicate that the patient has a form of aldosteronism that will respond to adrenalectomy. It has become apparent that a number of patients harbor bilateral adrenal cortical hyperplasia without a single autonomous tumor, and in this group of patients, the results of surgical excision are variable.[7–10]

In view of the 60%–90% cure rate that can be anticipated when an adrenal adenoma is present, the diagnostic work-up of these patients assumes great importance. The biochemical determinations that suggest the diagnosis will be hypokalemia and a high aldosterone secretion that cannot be suppressed by high sodium intake. In addition, plasma renin activities, both supine after overnight bedrest and again after three hours of walking or standing, are low. Following these biochemical determinations suggestive of the diagnosis, differentiation between adrenal hyperplasia and adenoma must be made. Adrenal venography and adrenal vein blood analysis have been used with success,[8] as have iodocholesterol adrenal scans.[8,9] With the advent of highly accurate abdominal CAT scanning, this modality may well prove to be the simplest method to detect an adrenal tumor, however.[10] As nearly all of the potentially surgically curable forms of this disorder are unilateral, a posterior flank approach gives easy access to the affected adrenal gland and allows for minimal postoperative morbidity.[8–10]

ANSWER: E.

8.4. A 52-year-old man has a 3-year history of gradually increasing hypertension. He complains of frequent attacks of facial flushing, nausea, pounding headaches, and palpitations. Conventional antihypertensive drugs poorly control the hypertension, and he is hospitalized for diagnostic evaluation. Vanillylmandelic acid (VMA) levels are elevated, as are urinary metanephrine and normetanephrine levels. An intravenous pyelogram (IVP) is normal, and an abdominal CAT scan is shown as Figure 8-2. Which of the following drugs would not be useful in the perioperative period in this patient?

A. Isoproterenol (Isuprel).
B. Propranolol (Inderal).
C. Phenoxybenzamine (Dibenzyline).
D. Phentolamine (Regitine).
E. Lidocaine (Xylocaine).

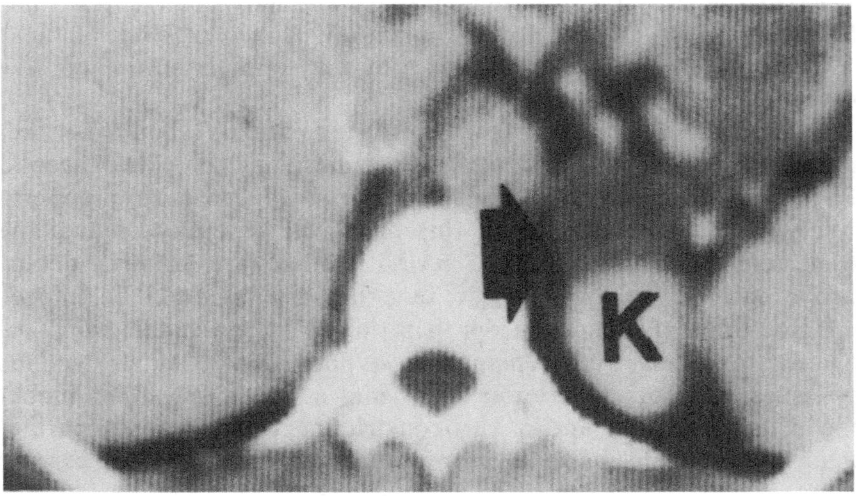

Figure 8-2

This patient manifests a classical presentation of a pheochromocytoma, with episodic hypertension, flushing, pounding headaches, and palpitations. Patients with pheochromocytomas may have either episodic or sustained hypertension, and therefore do not necessarily have to suffer from attacks of high blood pressure. In a series of 138 cases reported from the Mayo Clinic, 5% of tumors were bilateral, 10% were found in extra-adrenal sites originating from sympathetic nervous tissue, and 13% were malignant.[11]

Adrenal pheochromocytomas normally secrete both epinephrine and norepinephrine, and the metabolites of these hormones can be recovered in the urine as increased levels of metanephrine and normetanephrine. VMA is also an end product of catecholamine metabolism and can be measured in the urine. It is important to remember that numerous substances can interfere with these determinations, including food substances such as vanilla, tea, coffee, and bananas, antibiotics such as tetracycline and ampicillin, and commonly used antihypertensive drugs such as methyldopa (Aldomet). Once the diagnosis is suspected, a chest X ray is indicated to rule out the presence of the rare intrathoracic tumors. An IVP with tomograms will give accurate localizing information concerning the adrenal tumors in at least two thirds of patients.[11] Abdominal CAT scanning will give additional information concerning the localization of the tumor. In this case, a large left adrenal tumor is noted. Other tests that have been used in the past include angiography, and provocative tests utilizing histamine and Regitine stimulation. However, each of these tests is potentially dangerous, as they may stimulate an excessive catecholamine release.

Once the diagnosis has been made, patients should be prepared for operation utilizing alpha-adrenergic blocking agents. Phenoxybenzamine is given orally for 1 to 2 weeks preoperatively, and administration of this drug will generally control the hypertension. If during this period cardiac arrhythmias occur, propranolol, a beta-adrenergic blocking drug, should be added. At the time of operation, preparation must be made to guard against extreme hypertension or hypotension. Central venous pressure monitoring, arterial lines, and a fast-acting alpha-blocking drug (Regitine) and a vasoconstricting drug (norepinephrine) must be available, as must propranolol and Xylocaine for cardiac arrhythmias.[11–14] Utilizing this perioperative management, operative mortality rates of less than 3% can be anticipated.[11,12]

ANSWER: A.

8.5. A 31-year-old woman has suffered from recurrent ulcerative colitis for 10 years, being treated with Sulfasalazine and 30 mg prednisone daily for the previous year. Because of increasing bloody diarrhea, proctocolectomy is performed. The anesthetic utilized is halothane, and the operation lasts 5 hr; 6 units of blood are transfused. Twenty-four hours postoperatively in the intensive care unit, the patient's pulse is 140, blood pressure is 90/40, and temperature is 39.2°C. The patient complains of profound weakness. At this time, she should be treated with:

A. Dopamine.
B. Broad-spectrum antibiotics.
C. Corticosteroids.
D. Hypertonic glucose solution.
E. Prompt reoperation.

This patient is suffering from an acute adrenal crisis. It is presumed that during her year's treatment with prednisone, the long-term suppression of ACTH and resultant adrenal cortical atrophy rendered the patient hypoadrenal. Therefore, at a time of stress such as a lengthy operation necessitating multiple transfusions for bleeding, the suppressed adrenal glands could not respond to the demand for increased corticosteroid output. The patient's symptoms of tachycardia, hypotension, weakness, fever, nausea, and abdominal pain are all typical.

Although there are many case reports in the literature concerning patients whose adrenal glands have allegedly been suppressed over long periods of time by exogenous administration of corticosteroids, definite proof of adrenal nonresponsiveness has been much more difficult to document. Surely, there are many patients documented who have been treated with corticosteroids and have then undergone a stressful situation who did not respond with symptoms of adrenal crisis. In these situations, the adrenal glands were presumably able to increase their corticosteroid output.[15,16] In view of the fact that no one particular test of adrenal function can definitely screen those patients who have clinically significant adrenal suppression, it would seem prudent to recommend additional steroid coverage during periods of stress for any patient who has undergone systemic steroid therapy within the previous year. There is no evidence that a short course of corticosteroids, rapidly tapered down postoperatively, increases morbidity following abdominal surgery.

One other instance in which a hypoadrenal state may occur is in the patient who is suffering from severe sepsis. In much the same way that various organs can dysfunction in this setting, such as the lungs, kidneys, heart, liver, and pancreas, the adrenal glands can likewise malfunction, giving rise to an acute hypoadrenal state. Therefore, in any patient who is septic and does not promptly respond to proper treatment, including eradication of the septic focus, appropriate antibiotics, and fluid therapy, corticosteroid supplementation should be considered.[17,18]

ANSWER: C.

8.6. A 42-year-old man is admitted to the hospital with an upper GI tract hemorrhage. He gives a history of ulcerlike symptoms on and off for years, and has one sister who has undergone an operation for a duodenal ulcer. Endoscopy reveals a duodenal ulcer, and after a transfusion of 5 units of blood, bleeding ceases. Subsequent gastric analysis reveals a basal acid output (BAO) of 22 mEq/hr and a maximal acid output (MAO) of 30 mEq/hr. The serum gastrin level is 600 pg/ml, the serum calcium level is 11.6 mg%, and a serum parathormone level is 700 pg/ml. Treatment at this time should consist of:

A. Parathyroidectomy and cimetidine.
B. Total gastrectomy.
C. Vagotomy and antrectomy.
D. Exploratory celiotomy and excision of pancreatic tumor.
E. Cimetidine.

The Zollinger–Ellison syndrome was first described in 1955, when two patients with a fulminant ulcer diathesis associated with pancreatic islet cell tumors were described. Since that time, the syndrome has been commonly recognized as occurring either sporadically or in a familial fashion as part of the multiple endocrine neoplasia (MEN-I) syndrome, along with endocrinopathies involving the pituitary and parathyroid glands.[19] These patients present with severe peptic ulceration, often recurrent after "definitive" ulcer surgery. Upper GI tract X rays often disclose typical duodenal ulcers, sometimes along with ulcers in the stomach and other portions of the duodenum. Giant rugal folds of the stomach are also noted. Approximately 60% of these tumors are malignant, often with lymph node and liver metastases, while a smaller number are solitary pancreatic tumors. Perhaps 10% of patients will harbor hyperplasia or microadenomatosis of the pancreatic islets, accounting for the syndrome. In addition to their occurrence in the pancreas, these tumors can also originate in the duodenal wall.

The diagnosis of gastrinoma is important, as the operations usually employed for duodenal ulcer are generally unsuccessful in this condition. Gastric analysis will demonstrate a hypersecretion of acid and an increased volume of gastric juice. BAOs can be strikingly elevated, and characteristically respond only moderately to administration of pentagastrin. In most cases, the BAO/MAO ratio will be greater than 0.6 in the presence of a gastrinoma.[20] In recent years, the use of abdominal CAT scanning has allowed identification of pancreatic tumors, and this can aid in their excision. Some patients with Zollinger–Ellison syndrome will not have strikingly elevated serum gastrin levels, and several stimulation tests have been devised. The most useful of these are the calcium and secretin infusion tests, both of which cause a marked rise in the serum gastrin level in the presence of a gastrinoma.[21] It must be remembered, however, that other entities may cause hypergastrinemia. Among these are antral G-cell hyperplasia, which can be diagnosed by an increase in hypergastrinemia secondary to a protein meal and is treated by antrectomy[22]; gastric outlet obstruction; atrophic gastritis and achlorhydria; hyperparathyroidism; and isolated antrum secondary to a Billroth II gastrectomy.

A great deal of attention has centered around the very occasional reports of "spontaneous regression" following total gastrectomy in this condition, but this phenomenon remains a very uncommon exception.[23] Most patients with this syndrome die from their disease, as a result either of inadequately treated peptic ulceration or of metastatic tumor. The former complication, of course, can be completely prevented by the performance of total gastrectomy.[24] For those patients with documented metastatic disease, the use of streptozotocin has recently shown promise.[25]

An alternative to total gastrectomy has recently become available with the advent of cimetidine, a histamine receptor antagonist that profoundly lowers gastric acid. Initial results with the use of this drug have shown great promise in controlling the effects of uncontrolled acid output, with most but not all patients gaining temporary relief.[26] However, as this condition represents a lifelong disease, it is not known at this time whether patients should remain on cimetidine for many years or if they would be better served by the performance of total gastrectomy. Also, the effects of cimetidine on the growth rate of the malignant tumor are as yet unknown.

In the patient presented, evidence for both hyperparathyroidism and hypergastrinemia is present. It has been found that in such a patient a parathyroidectomy should be performed first, as in some cases this will bring about a reduction in the serum gastrin levels and the gastric acid hypersecretion. Although some of these patients subsequently will have a recurrence of their gastric hypersecretion, some appear to be very well controlled by the parathyroidectomy alone, and this should always be carried out initially.[27]

ANSWER: A.

8.7. A 40-year-old man seeks medical attention because of a generalized skin rash manifested by crops of papules that gradually fade and crust over. His blood glucose level is 196 mg%. A liver–spleen scan is shown as Figure 8-3. An arteriogram shows a hypervascular mass in the body of the pancreas. The most likely diagnosis is:

A. Benign insulinoma.
B. Malignant insulinoma.
C. Gastrinoma.
D. WDHA pancreatic tumor.
E. Glucagonoma.

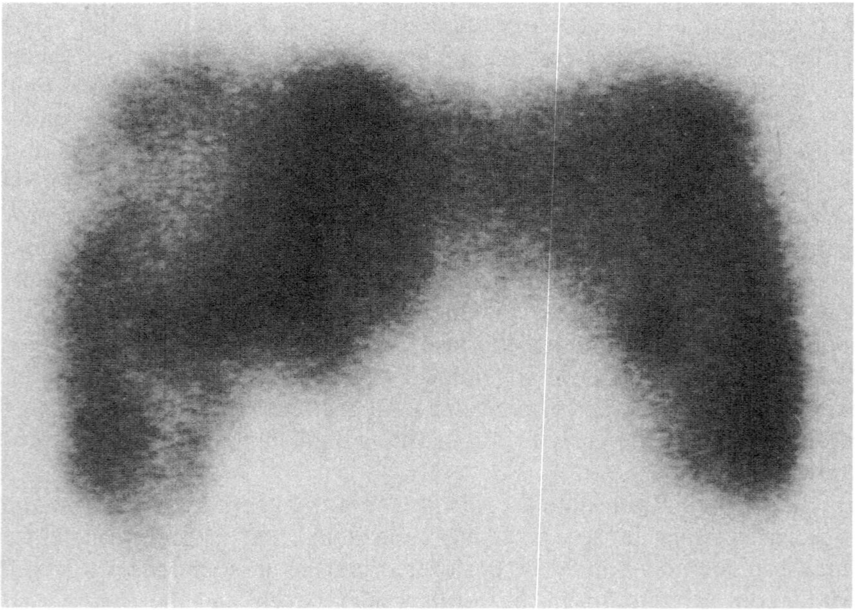

Figure 8-3

This patient harbors a glucagonoma associated with liver metastases. The syndrome has been only recently described, and there are approximately 50 cases in the English literature. Adults of both sexes are affected, and the condition may be either sporadic or familial. This alpha-cell disorder of the pancreas may appear in the form of a generalized islet hyperplasia or as either discrete single or multiple tumors. The hypersecretion of glucagon may exist as one component of the polyglandular APUD (amine precursor uptake and decarboxylation)-cell system. These cells are widely distributed in the body and derive their name from the initial letters of their first three and most important properties, namely (1) a high uptake of amine; (2) the capacity for amine precursor uptake; and (3) the presence of amino acid decarboxylase for the conversion of the amino acid precursors into amines.[28] It is thought that all of these cells arise from the primitive neural crest, and the system includes cells of the pituitary, thyroid, and adrenal glands; the stomach; the duodenum; the small and large intestines; and the pancreatic islets. At least six varieties of islet cell hyperfunction have been described, resulting in excesses of insulin, glucagon, gastrin, somatostatin, pancreatic polypeptide, and vasoactive intestinal polypeptide.

The glucagonoma syndrome is important in that it represents a potentially surgically curable form of diabetes. Most of these patients have overt diabetes or at least an altered glucose tolerance, and some manifest symptoms of a widespread malignancy. The characteristic skin lesion is a necrolytic migratory erythema. Individual lesions evolve over 7–14 days, beginning as macules or papules that become pale, then blister, and then crust. The pancreatic tumors can be located utilizing abdominal CAT scanning or arteriography.[29,30] Further tumor localization can be accomplished by percutaneous transhepatic catheterization of the portal vein with subsequent pancreatic vein sampling for glucagon immunoassay.[31] Treatment consists of local tumor excision, if this is feasible, or subtotal pancreatectomy if hyperplasia of the islets exists. For those patients presenting with metastatic disease, streptozotocin has been proven to be beneficial, bringing about tumor regression and improvement in the diabetic state in some patients.[32]

ANSWER: E.

8.8. A 42-year-old woman gives a 2-year history of intermittent watery diarrhea, with up to 14 liquid bowel movements daily. In the 2 weeks prior to admission, her symptoms have worsened, and she appears weak and dehydrated. Following intravenous hydration and insertion of a nasogastric tube, the diarrhea decreases in amount and frequency. A proctoscopic examination and a barium enema are normal. Excess secretion of which of the following hormones would not be associated with this syndrome?

A. Vasoactive intestinal polypeptide (VIP).
B. Prostaglandin E (PGE).
C. Human pancreatic polypeptide (HPP).
D. Gastrointestinal inhibitory polypeptide (GIP).
E. Parathormone (PTH).

The watery diarrhea syndrome associated with a nonbeta islet-cell tumor of the pancreas was originally thought to be a variant of the Zollinger–Ellison syndrome, in which patients had a gastrin-producing tumor associated with excessive gastric acid secretion. As more became known about both syndromes, however, they soon became separated, with the diarrheagenic syndrome achieving its own individual identity. Other names, such as pancreatic cholera and WDHA (watery diarrhea, hypokalemia, achlorhydria) tumor have also been used to describe this syndrome. Significant disagreement, however, exists regarding the hormone responsible for the syndrome. Although it was originally felt to be secretin, recent reports have implicated VIP,[33,34] prostaglandins,[35,36] GIP,[37] and HPP.[38] However, despite the fact that serum and tissue determinations of each of these hormones have been described in patients with this syndrome, not all patients with pancreatic cholera have elevated hormone levels, and those that do tend to have any of the various hormones secreted in excess.

It would thus appear likely that many hormones produced by islet cell tumors of the pancreas can mediate this syndrome, and that primary treatment should be directed toward excision of the pancreatic tumor if it can be located. For metastatic or unresectable tumors, streptozotocin chemotherapy may provide significant symptomatic relief.[39]

ANSWER: E.

8.9. A 46-year-old woman gives a history of 4 months of periodic sweating and palpitations. Her husband describes her behavior as strange during these periods and discloses that her memory has recently become impaired. An insulinoma is suspected because of a single fasting blood glucose level of 54 mg%. Which of the following tests would *not* prove useful in confirming the diagnosis?

A. Abdominal CAT scan.
B. Arteriography.
C. Prolonged fasting.
D. Abdominal ultrasound.
E. Tolbutamide test.

This patient presents with many of the classical signs and symptoms of insulin overdose. In addition, convulsions and coma are seen in some patients, and the total duration of symptoms may range up to several years owing to a delay in seeking medical help or a delayed diagnosis. Often the patients will note that the symptoms are aggravated by food deprivation and relieved by eating. This may lead to a significant weight gain in some patients. Because of the bizarre nature of these symptoms, many patients will be initially diagnosed as having some form of mental disturbance.

The diagnosis of insulinoma depends upon the demonstration of increased levels of circulating insulin at the same time the blood glucose concentration is less than 45 mg%.[40] Factitious hyperinsulinemia can be excluded by the absence of circulating insulin antibodies. In some patients, however, symptoms will be so infrequent that provocative testing will be necessary. The most reliable test is a prolonged fast. In the Mayo Clinic Series, typical symptoms occurred within 12 hr of fasting in 33% of patients, within 24 hr in 80% of patients, within 48 hr in 90%, and within 72 hr of fasting in 100%.[40] In addition, the intravenous tolbutamide test will often be positive, with insulinoma patients showing a greater than normal drop in serum glucose levels and a delayed recovery of normal glucose levels. Recently, a new provocative test for insulinoma has been described, employing a calcium infusion. This test resulted in significant hypoglycemia and hyperinsulinemia in nine of ten patients.[41]

Insulinomas are evenly distributed throughout the pancreas, being found in roughly equal numbers in the head, body, and tail regions. The majority of patients will have a solitary islet-cell adenoma, but multiple adenomas or islet-cell hyperplasia can also occur.[40,42] Because of this, preoperative localization of the insulinoma is crucial, as the operative demonstration of these nodules can be extremely difficult owing to their small size. In one large series, nearly three quarters of all adenomas were less than 1.5 cm in diameter.[40] Recently, abdominal CAT scanning has been utilized with success in localizing these tumors, as has arteriography. In the Mayo Clinic Series of 58 patients who have undergone angiography, 92% had positive findings, making this test the most useful study in the preoperative diagnostic workup of a patient suspected of harboring an insulinoma.[40] Another recently described test depends upon percutaneous transhepatic catheterization of a portal venous branch within the liver with subsequent sampling of the portal, mesenteric, and splenic veins, looking for regional increases in insulin levels.[43]

At the time of operation, a thorough mobilization and exploration of the entire pancreas is necessary. If any lymph nodes are palpable these should be biopsied, as up to 10% of islet cell tumors are malignant. After systemic palpation of the entire pancreas, most adenomas will be located, and these can be simply enucleated. If no tumor is found, a subtotal pancreatectomy should be performed. This will sometimes disclose either islet-cell hyperplasia or microadenomatosis, and the patient's symptoms will be relieved. The operative management of these patients has been simplified by the recent introduction of the so-called artificial beta cell. This is a machine that continuously monitors plasma glucose and, using a computer, administers to the patient through an infusion pump the precise amount of insulin required to maintain blood glucose at a normal level.[44]

ANSWER: D.

8.10. A male infant who was born after a normal gestation is well until his fourth month, when he begins to suffer from generalized tonic–clonic seizures. The serum glucose level is found to be less than 30 mg% on several occasions, and the serum insulin level is inappropriately elevated. At celiotomy, the pancreas is normal to palpation and the remainder of the abdominal exploration is normal. The surgeon should now:

A. Close the abdomen and treat the patient medically.
B. Perform a distal pancreatectomy.
C. Perform a distal pancreatectomy and splenectomy.
D. Perform a subtotal pancreatectomy.
E. Perform a subtotal pancreatectomy and splenectomy.

This child has definite evidence of hyperinsulinism, and most such infants will harbor abnormal pancreatic islets. There are several varieties of islet-cell hyperfunction found in infants, but of these nesidioblastosis is probably the most common. In one review of the world literature since nesidioblastosis was first described in 1970, this entity occurred in 34% of patients, with hyperplasia and islet-cell adenomas each seen in 29%. Eight percent of patients had a normal pancreas.[45] The three major entities can usually be differentiated histologically. Islet-cell adenomas will consist of an isolated nodule or multiple nodules in clumps. Islet-cell hyperplasia represents an increased number of islets with normal intralobular distribution. Nesidioblastosis is recognized by a diffuse increase in differentiated endocrine cells within the ductal epithelium, and these islet cells are thought to arise from pancreatic ductal epithelium.[46,47]

Because of the devastating effects of recurrent hypoglycemia in infants, any infant who suffers hypoglycemic attacks that cannot be controlled by medical means must be operated upon promptly. Failure to do so will lead to a significant incidence of brain damage and mental retardation. At the time of operation, if a single nodule is noted in the pancreas, this should be excised. However, as is usually the case, the pancreas will be grossly normal to palpation, and in this instance, a subtotal pancreatectomy, removing 85%–90% of the pancreas, should be employed. This will bring about a cure of the hypoglycemic attacks in most infants.[45,46] If at all possible, the spleen should be preserved because of the markedly increased risk of overwhelming sepsis in the splenectomized child.

ANSWER: D.

8.11. A 42-year-old woman is found to be hypercalcemic. She has had renal stones on three separate occasions in the past and has taken antacids for a "nervous stomach." Her blood pressure is 160/105, and her neck examination is normal. Laboratory studies disclose the following values: serum BUN, 12 mg%; calcium, 12.6 mg%; phosphorus, 2.1 mg%; sodium, 146 mEq/liter; potassium, 4.8 mEq/liter; chloride, 109 mEq/liter; serum parathormone, normal. A diagnosis of primary hyperparathyroidism is suspected, and a neck exploration is carried out; a 2.5-g parathyroid gland is found in the right superior position. The surgeon should now:

A. Remove the tumor and close the neck.
B. Remove the tumor and biopsy at least one other parathyroid gland.
C. Remove the tumor and transplant a portion of it into a forearm muscle.
D. Perform a subtotal parathyroidectomy (3½-gland excision).
E. Remove the tumor after identifying the other three glands.

The differential diagnosis of hypercalcemia must include other conditions besides primary hyperparathyroidism. Myeloma, sarcoidosis, and hyperthyroidism can all cause hypercalcemia but are usually readily apparent. Likewise, any malignancy metastatic to bone or any malignancy producing parathyroid hormone can cause hypercalcemia. In addition, the thiazide diuretics may cause an elevation of the serum calcium.

The patient presented clearly has primary hyperparathyroidism. She has no renal failure that could account for secondary hyperparathyroidism. Her calcium level is significantly elevated, with a marked depression in her serum phosphorus level and associated hyperchloremia. Depending upon the parathormone immunoassay utilized and the serum calcium level at the time the blood is drawn, the parathormone level may be normal or elevated, making it important not to rely on an elevated parathormone level alone for the diagnosis. In addition, her history of recurrent renal stones, upper GI tract complaints, and hypertension are all suggestive of the diagnosis.

The operative treatment of the patient with primary hyperparathyroidism has remained controversial, with suggestions ranging from removal of the adenoma alone[48] to subtotal parathyroidectomy.[49] This has partly resulted from a failure of pathologists to agree on a strict definition of single-gland involvement (adenoma) versus multiple-gland involvement (hyperplasia). It has become apparent that size of the gland or histological appearance cannot accurately differentiate single from multiple gland involvement. It is also recognized that there is a significant incidence of persistent or recurrent hyperparathyroidism following parathyroid surgery, but this occurs mainly in those patients who have multiple-gland disease or hyperplasia, often in the presence of the multiple endocrine neoplasia syndrome or a positive family history for hyperparathyroidism.[50–52] On the other hand, in the vast majority of patients with single-gland enlargement and grossly normal remaining parathyroid glands, excision of the single gland will prove curative.[48] Today, most endocrine surgeons would agree that excision of the dominant enlarged gland is essential, with an attempt to identify all other glands. Double parathyroid adenomas will be found in 3%–5% of cases, and in these instances both glands should be removed. Whether or not the remaining grossly normal glands should be biopsied is controversial, but many surgeons feel that at least one gland should be biopsied to verify the normal parathyroid histology.

ANSWER: B.

8.12. Which of the following treatments is not useful in the definitive management of a patient with diffuse toxic goiter (Graves disease)?

A. Subtotal thyroidectomy.
B. Propylthiouracil.
C. Propranalol.
D. Radioiodine (^{131}I).
E. Total thyroidectomy.

As in most instances in which there are several competing forms of therapy for a given disease, it will usually be determined that no one form of therapy is clearly superior to the others. This is nowhere more true than in the definitive management of the patient with diffuse toxic goiter or Graves disease. Fortunately, today there are at least three effective means of treating the patient with Graves disease that offer a hope of permanent remission of the condition. Each, however, has significant advantages and disadvantages, and everyone would recognize the need for individualizing treatment. Subtotal removal of the thyroid gland is a time-tested method of achieving permanent control of the symptoms of Graves disease. Ideally, several grams of functioning thyroid tissue are left bilaterally. This renders the patient euthyroid and minimizes the chance of recurrent laryngeal nerve damage and hypoparathyroidism. In experienced hands, this operation will lead to a persistence of the hyperthyroidism in less than 5% of patients, but hypothyroidism may manifest itself in the future in 5%–25% of patients. Because of the possibility of persistent or recurrence of the disease, some have advocated total thyroidectomy and have shown that this can be carried out safely with minimal morbidity.[53]

In this country, the use of radioiodine has gained prominence. Originally, large doses were utilized, and this led to a virtual 100% incidence of hypothyroidism. Because of this, progressively lower doses have been utilized, and although it is expected that the ultimate rates of hypothyroidism in the future will be very great, initial short-term studies have shown a lower rate of permanent hypofunction.[54] Several problems, however, exist with the use of radioiodine. Ionizing radiation has been implicated as a cause of thyroid carcinoma, usually after a lag period of 20 or more years.[55–57] Because of this, it has been hypothesized that some patients treated with low dosages of ^{131}I might develop thyroid carcinomas in the future. Although there has been no statistically valid study showing that a higher incidence of thyroid carcinoma will result from this treatment, there are numerous cases in the medical literature of thyroid carcinoma following ^{131}I therapy for Graves disease. At the least, the question still remains open, with some authorities withholding ^{131}I treatment because of the potential carcinogenic or teratogenic effect it may have.[58] Antithyroid drugs such as propylthiouracil have been shown to lead to permanent remission rates in from 15% to 80% of patients depending upon the series quoted.[59] However, problems of patient compliance, the unpredictability of response, and potential side effects of the drugs have limited their widespread usefulness.

In recent years, propranalol (Inderal) has been used to bring the thyrotoxic symptoms of Graves disease quickly under control, usually in preparation for operation. Although thyrotoxicosis is associated with increased levels of circulating thyroid hormone, many of the physiologic effects appear to be caused by circulating catecholamines. Therefore, it appeared logical to treat these symptoms with catecholamine blocking agents, such as propranolol, a beta adrenergic blocking drug. Many patients who cannot be brought under control with antithyroid drugs will readily respond to propranalol, making this a useful drug for routine preoperative preparation and also for the treatment of thyroid storm. However, owing to the side effects and potential complications of long-term propranalol therapy, the drug has generally been restricted to short-term use, and is not recommended for the permanent treatment and control of thyrotoxicosis.[60–62]

ANSWER: C.

8.13. A 32-year-old man presents with a lump in his neck. A 2-cm mass in the right thyroid lobe is noted by palpation and confirmed as a cold nodule on a thyroid scan. No lymph nodes are palpable. Thyroid function tests are normal. The patient should be advised that:

A. The nodule should be observed for growth.
B. A subtotal thyroidectomy should be performed.
C. He should be treated with suppressive doses of thyroid extract.
D. A right thyroid lobectomy should be performed.
E. Therapeutic doses of radioiodine should be administered.

The managment of thyroid nodules remains an extremely controversial area. Obviously, the primary concern about thyroid nodules is that they might harbor malignancy. Unfortunately, no absolute set of clinical or laboratory criteria are available that clearly differentiate between benign and malignant lesions. Depending upon how these clinical and laboratory criteria are weighed, various reported series of patients with thyroid nodules will indicate rates of malignancy in 5% to 40% of patients.

The age and sex of the patient are important considerations. In patients under the age of 20, most thyroid nodules will be found to be malignant, and a higher percentage of thyroid nodules in males are malignant when compared with those in females.[63,64] A history of irradiation of the head and neck area during childhood should be sought, as this definitely predisposes patients to the development of thyroid malignancies later in life.[55–57] Carcinoma is more likely to be present in a solitary thyroid nodule than in a diffusely nodular gland, but widely varying frequencies are noted in both of these groups depending upon patient selection. Obviously, if there are palpable lymph nodes present or if the nodule is very hard or fixed to surrounding structures, the nodule is more likely to be a carcinoma. Laboratory tests usually do not prove helpful. Most patients with thyroid nodules are euthyroid, and so thyroid function tests do not aid in the differentiation. Likewise, thyroid antibodies can be found in patients with either benign or malignant thyroid lesions. Radioactive thyroid scans can confirm the solitary nature of the thyroid lesion, and most benign or malignant thyroid nodules will appear as a cold area on the scan. A hot nodule, which concentrates iodine on a scan, will usually but not always prove benign.

Because of all of these uncertainties, most patients who have solitary thyroid nodules should undergo operation. In addition, most male patients at any age must be highly suspect of harboring carcinoma. The operation of choice is a thyroid lobectomy on the side of the lesion, with subtotal or total removal of the other side if the frozen section report discloses carcinoma.[64] A subtotal thyroidectomy without prior substantiation of malignancy is not indicated. Suppressive doses of thyroid extract would not be suitable treatment for malignant growths, although some will appear to decrease in size with treatment. Likewise, therapeutic doses of radioiodine are not indicated prior to thyroidectomy.

ANSWER: D.

8.14. A 35-year-old woman presents with a lump in the neck. At age 5, she had undergone "X-ray treatments" for enlarged tonsils. Examination discloses a 2.5-cm mass in the lower pole of the right lobe of the thyroid with some questionable nodularity in the left lobe. No lymph nodes are palpable. A thyroid scan confirms the location of the right thyroid nodule and it is interpreted as a cold nodule. Treatment should consist of:

A. Subtotal thyroidectomy.
B. Total thyroidectomy.
C. Right thyroid lobectomy.
D. Right thyroid lobectomy and right radical neck dissection.
E. Total thyroidectomy and right radical neck dissection.

This patient must be highly suspect of harboring a differentiated papillary–follicular carcinoma of the thyroid secondary to her childhood irradiation. Large series of patients who underwent prior irradiation to the head and neck for enlarged thymus as infants, tonsillar hypertrophy as young children, or acne during adolescence point out the increased risk of thyroid carcinoma in these individuals. In the original Chicago series, 7% of unselected patients with prior irradiation harbored carcinoma.[65] This incidence has gradually become higher since publication of the article in 1975, as extensive patient recall and surveillance programs have been organized. Of those patients with palpable abnormalities of the thyroid gland along with scan defects, 30%–60% have been shown to harbor carcinoma, while the others harbor benign and hyperplastic changes within their thyroids.[55,66]

Total thyroidectomy is currently advocated for these patients for a variety of reasons. First of all, the carcinoma tends to be multicentric and bilateral in 30%–80% of patients who are carefully studied.[57,67,68] In addition, approximately half of these patients harbor lymph node metastases, which may be on either side of the neck.[57] Total thyroidectomy prevents the occurrence of transformation into the highly virulent anaplastic thyroid carcinoma in the future.[67] Also, it facilitates the utilization of radioactive iodine in the follow-up evaluation and treatment of patients with metastatic papillary or follicular carcinoma. Only if all normal functioning thyroid tissue is removed from the neck can this be effectively accomplished, for any normal thyroid remnant will selectively take up radioiodine preferentially over thyroid metastases.[67] Several series of patients have domonstrated that the prognosis for thyroid carcinoma patients with lymph node metastases is poorer than in those without nodal metastases, but if total thyroidectomy and selective nodal excision is carried out, patient survival can be improved.[69] In addition, it has been shown that the subsequent use of therapeutic ^{131}I can lead to improved patient survival.[70,71]

While most would agree with the foregoing statements, many authorities still feel that the morbidity of total thyroidectomy for such a slow-growing tumor outweighs the potential advantage. One series of 184 cases demonstrated a 5% incidence of permanent recurrent laryngeal nerve damage and a 5% incidence of permanent hypoparathyroidism.[67,70] Other larger series, however, have not demonstrated this high percentage of complications, reflecting the increased surgical expertise that is possible with experience.[72] Others have found a useful means of virtually eliminating permanent postoperative hypoparathyroidism in the autotransplantation of any parathyroid tissue that is identified and devascularized. By merely mincing the normal parathyroid up into small pieces and implanting it into a pocket of muscle, normal parathyroid function will be assured within several months.[57] Because of these factors, it would appear that total thyroidectomy is the treatment of choice in all patients with thyroid carcinomas larger than 2 cm, regardless of whether they are associated with a prior history of irradiation. Although radical neck dissection may be indicated for those patients with extensive cervical nodal metastases, selective removal of nodes for those with minimal metastases can be quite effective in some patients.

ANSWER: B.

8.15. A 20-year-old woman undergoes a right thyroid lobectomy for a mixed papillary–follicular carcinoma of the thyroid. Several positive lymph nodes are removed, but no formal neck dissection is carried out. She is well until 26 years later, when she begins to have symptoms of dysphagia, dyspnea, and hoarseness, and notices enlargement of her neck. A markedly enlarged multinodular thyroid is palpated bilaterally. Which of the following treatments might be expected to benefit this patient at this time?

A. Radioiodine (^{131}I).
B. Thyroid suppression.
C. Chemotherapy.
D. Thyroidectomy.
E. External irradiation.

The sudden change of a pre-existing goiter or any sudden growth in a patient known to have thyroid disease often indicates that an undifferentiated or anaplastic carcinoma of the thyroid is present. The symptoms of hoarseness are often due to recurrent laryngeal nerve paralysis, and dyspnea, dysphagia, and a sensation of neck pressure are common complaints. The case presented points out the progression of differentiated thyroid neoplasms to the anaplastic variety. This has been substantiated in many instances of surgically treated anaplastic thyroid carcinomas, in which differentiated papillary–follicular elements were noted in the excised thyroid.[73–76] This transformation is another reason to consider total thyroidectomy as the initial treatment in patients with differentiated thyroid carcinomas.

The outlook for patients with anaplastic thyroid carcinoma is extremely poor. Early mortality is the rule, with average survivals of 6 months noted in many series.[74,77] There is a certain amount of confusion regarding these tumors because of the well-known difficulty in differentiating small-cell neoplasms of the thyroid gland from primary thyroid lymphomas, which have a much better overall prognosis.[77,78] Because of this, several series of patients with alleged anaplastic carcinomas of the thyroid have reported quite favorable 5-year survival statistics. It is likely that the more favorable cases represented patients with thyroid lymphomas rather than carcinomas.

Treatment is directed at symptomatic relief only. When possible, excision of the gland should be carried out, as this will minimize compressive symptoms by the tumor.[77] However, in most instances, owing to direct invasion of surrounding structures, excision will be impossible, and operation can only lead to a markedly increased complication rate from infection and hemorrhage.[75] Once unresectability has been determined, external irradiation may give temporary respite from symptoms, but this is usually brief, and the disease grows locally at a rapid rate and causes strangulation. ^{131}I and chemotherapy have proven disappointing in the vast majority of cases in which they were attempted.

ANSWER: E.

8.16. A 46-year-old man presents with a neck mass. On examination, his blood pressure is 170/110, and he has a 4-cm right thyroid mass with several 1-cm anterior cervical nodes on the right. The remainder of his examination is normal. A thyroid scan confirms the cold area on the right lobe. The serum calcium level is 12.2 mg%, and urinary catecholamines are elevated. An abdominal CAT scan shows an enlarged left adrenal gland. The operative procedure of choice at this time is:

A. Right thyroid lobectomy.
B. Total thyroidectomy.
C. Right thyroid lobectomy and subtotal parathyroidectomy.
D. Bilateral adrenalectomy.
E. Left adrenalectomy.

Any patient with a thyroid nodule who is also hypertensive must be carefully screened to rule out the presence of an associated pheochromocytoma. In the patient presented, the thyroid nodule, the elevated urine catecholamines, and the hypercalcemia all indicate that this patient has Sipple's syndrome (MEN-IIA syndrome). This syndrome may occur sporadically or it may be familial. In the multiple endocrine neoplasia IIA syndrome, the parathyroids are often hyperactive and histologically usually show diffuse hyperplasia, whether or not they are enlarged. Hypercalcemia may or may not be present. In the other variant of this syndrome, MEN-IIB, parathyroid abnormalities are not commonly noted, but the patients manifest a marfanoid habitus, have broad lips, low-set ears, and mucosal neuromas. This variant tends to be much more highly lethal than the MEN-IIA variety, with rapid spread of the medullary cancer.[79]

Medullary thyroid cancer is distinct from the other differentiated thyroid carcinomas and histologically contains large areas of amyloidlike stroma. The tumor is usually multicentric and involves lymph nodes in over half of the cases. These tumors secrete thyrocalcitonin, and this substance can be measured by immunoassay preoperatively to confirm the diagnosis.[80] In some patients, provocative tests using a calcium or pentagastrin infusion or both must be utilized in order to obtain elevated calcitonin levels, and these have been shown to be highly accurate.[81,82] Since the widespread application of these stimulation tests, many patients have been operated upon who had elevated levels of thyrocalcitonin but harbored no carcinoma. These patients have demonstrated C-cell hyperplasia of the thyroid glands, and this is now recognized to be the precursor of medullary carcinoma of the thyroid.[81]

Similarly, it is now well-recognized that adrenal medullary hyperplasia often antedates the development of actual pheochromocytomas and that both conditions can be associated with elevated catecholamine production. It would appear that this adrenal defect is bilateral in most cases, even if the glands appear normal grossly. This has led many authorities to advocate total adrenalectomy as the treatment of choice.[83–85] As always, treatment of the adrenal medullary disease should be preceded by alpha-adrenergic blockade to control the hypertension and beta adrenergic blockade in those patients suffering from tachycardia or cardiac arrhythmias. Following recovery from adrenalectomy, a total thyroidectomy and excision of any positive lymph nodes in the neck should be carried out for the medullary thyroid cancer. At that time, in those patients who are hypercalcemic or have grossly enlarged parathyroid glands, the enlarged glands should be removed.[83] If all four parathyroid glands must be removed, a portion of one should be taken for an autotransplantation into the forearm musculature.[86] In any patient thought to have medullary carcinoma of the thyroid with or without associated pheochromocytomas, all close family members should be screened by serum calcitonin and urinary catecholamine determinations, as both conditions may be clinically silent for a period of time.[87] It has been recently noted that some patients who have undergone total thyroidectomy and lymph node excision have had persistent elevations of calcitonin levels even though all gross disease in the neck was removed. These calcitonin levels have remained stable for many years, and their clinical significance is, therefore, unknown. It is suggested that microscopic metastases from medullary thyroid carcinoma may remain dormant for years causing this abnormality. This further points out the need for lifelong calcitonin screening of these patients.[88]

ANSWER: D.

8.17. A 54-year-old man with no familial history of hypertension is found to have a blood pressure of 180/100. Serum BUN and creatinine levels are normal. An intravenous pyelogram demonstrates somewhat delayed excretion bilaterally. A renal arteriogram discloses bilateral renal artery stenosis, worse on the left side. Peripheral renin levels are normal. Differential renal vein renin levels disclose elevated values bilaterally, worse on the left side. Treatment should consist of:

A. Right aorto-renal bypass.
B. Left aorto-renal bypass.
C. Right nephrectomy.
D. Left nephrectomy.
E. Bilateral aorto-renal bypass.

Renin is an enzyme produced by the juxtaglomerular cells of the kidney; it acts on a protein substrate in plasma globulins to produce a peptide, angiotensin I. This peptide, after passage through the pulmonary circulation, is converted to another peptide, angiotensin II, which is a very potent vasopressor substance. In addition to this vasopressor action, angiotensin II also acts on the adrenal cortex causing the release of the sodium-retaining hormone aldosterone. When blood flow to the juxtaglomerular apparatus of the kidneys is decreased by a proximal renal artery lesion, renin is produced in excess, thus accounting for renovascular hypertension.[89,90]

Clinically, renovascular hypertension occurs in two major groups of patients. One consists of those patients with stenoses of one or both renal arteries from atherosclerosis. The other group consists of those patients, usually of a younger age, who have fibromuscular hyperplasia of one or both arteries.[91–94] To diagnose renovascular hypertension, renal scans, renograms, split renal function studies, and renal biopsies have been utilized. However, in recent years, arteriography along with differential renal vein renin levels have proven to be satisfactory in most cases. Determining peripheral venous renin levels has not been as helpful, as these are frequently normal in the presence of documented renovascular hypertension.[93,94]

With the availability of more potent antihypertensive agents, significant disagreement exists as to which patients should be treated medically and which surgically. However, because many of these patients are relatively young and have a projected long life expectancy, and the results of operation are good, curing or significantly decreasing the hypertension in over three quarters of patients, many cases undoubtedly should be treated operatively. In addition, it has been noted that in those patients with decreased renal function, revascularization has brought about improvements in renal function.[94] In the patient with a unilateral lesion on arteriogram who has a significant increase in renal vein renin level on that side, aorto-renal bypass will be very successful. Somewhat more disagreement exists in the instance of bilateral renal artery stenosis. If no differential renal vein renin levels are detected, some authorities would choose to treat the patients with antihypertensive drugs. If, however, there is a renal vein renin difference, it would appear prudent to operate on the most seriously affected side first and postoperatively repeat the renal vein renin studies. If hypertension persists and the contralateral kidney now has increased renin levels, the second side can then be operated upon.[93] Most authorities agree that nephrectomy should only uncommonly be used in patients with normal renal function and renovascular hypertension, as this unnecessarily sacrifices functioning renal mass. Recently, a nonoperative means has been described of treating renal artery stenosis, namely percutaneous transluminal angioplasty by forceful dilatation of the obstructing lesion via an angiogram catheter. It remains to be determined what long-term lasting benefit this method will have.[95]

ANSWER: B.

References

1. Scott, H.W., Liddle, G.W., Mulherin, J.L., McKenna, T.J., Stroup, S.L., Rhamy, R.K.: Surgical experience with Cushing's disease. *Ann. Surg.* 185:524, 1977.
2. Wilson, C.B., Tyrrell, J.B., Fitzgerald, P.: Cushing's disease revisited. *Am. J. Surg.* 138:77, 1979.
3. Tyrrell, J.B., Brooks, R.M., Fitzgerald, P.A., Cofoid, P.B., Forsham, P.H., Wilson, C.B.: Cushing's disease: Selective transphenoidal resection of pituitary microadenomas. *N. Engl. J. Med.* 298:753, 1978.
4. Jennings, A.S., Liddle, G.W., Orth, D.N.: Results of treating childhood Cushing's disease with pituitary irradiation. *N. Engl. J. Med.* 297:957, 1977.
5. Luton, J.P., Mahoudeau, J.A., Bouchard, T., Thieblot, T., Hautecouverture, M., Simon, D., Laudat, M.H., Touitou, Y., Bricaire, H.: Treatment of Cushing's disease by *o,p*-DDD: Survey of 62 cases. *N. Engl. J. Med.* 300:459, 1979.
6. Scott, H.W., Foster, J.H., Rhamy, R.K., Klatte, E., Liddle, G.W.: Surgical management of adrenocortical tumors with Cushing's syndrome. *Ann. Surg.* 173:892, 1971.
7. Delarue, N.C., Laidlaw, J.C., Kovacs, K., Colapinto, R., Murray, F.T.: Hypertension due to primary aldosteronism: Surgical considerations. *Surgery* 80:289, 1976.
8. Herwig, K.R.: Primary aldosteronism: Experience with 38 patients. *Surgery* 86:470, 1979.
9. Hunt, T.K., Schambelan, M., Biglieri, E.G.: Selection of patients and operative approach in primary aldosteronism. *Ann. Surg.* 182:353, 1975.
10. Auda, S.P., Brennan, M.F., Gill, J.R.: Evolution of the surgical management of primary aldosteronism. *Ann. Surg.* 191:1, 1980.
11. Remine, W.H., Chong, G.C., VanHeerden, J.A., Sheps, S.G., Harrison, E.G.: Current management of pheochromocytoma. *Ann. Surg.* 179:740, 1974.
12. Scott, H.W., Oates, J.A., Nies, A.S., Berko, H., Page, D.L., Rhamy, R.K.: Pheochromocytoma: Present diagnosis and management. *Ann. Surg.* 183:587, 1976.
13. Harrison, T.S., Dagher, F.J., Beck, L., Bartlett, J.D.: Rationale and indications for preoperative adrenergic receptor blockade in pheochromocytoma. *Med. Clin. North Am.* 53:1349, 1969.
14. Himathongkam, T., Newmark, S.R., Greenfield, M., Dluhy, R.G.: Pheochromocytoma. *J.A.M.A.* 230:1692, 1974.
15. Fernandez-Herlighy, L.: The management of the surgical patient who has had corticosteroid therapy. *Surg. Clin. North Am.* 42:589, 1962.
16. Roberts, J.C.: Operative collapse after corticosteroid therapy: A survey. *Surg. Clin. North Am.* 50:363, 1970.
17. Sibbald, W.J., Short, A., Cohen, M.P., Wilson, R.F.: Variations in adrenocortical responsiveness during severe bacterial infections. *Ann. Surg.* 186:29, 1977.
18. Hubay, C.A., Weckesser, E.C., Levy, R.P. Occult adrenal insufficiency in surgical patients. *Ann. Surg.* 181:325, 1975.
19. Majewski, J.T., Wilson, S.D.: The MEN-I syndrome: An all or none phenomenon? *Surgery* 86:475, 1979.
20. Isenberg, J.I., Walsh, J.H., Grossman, M.I.: Zollinger–Ellison syndrome. *Gastroenterology* 65:140, 1973.
21. Deveney, C.W., Deveney, K.S., Jaffe, B.M., Jones, R.S., Way, L.W.: Use of calcium and secretin in the diagnosis of gastrinoma (Zollinger–Ellison syndrome). *Ann. Intern. Med.* 87:680, 1977.
22. Ganguli, P.C., Polak, J.M., Pearse, A.G.E., Elder, J.B., Hegarty, M.: Antral-gastrin-cell hyperplasia in peptic-ulcer disease. *Lancet* 1:583, 1974.

23. Davis, C.E., Vansant, J.H.: Zollinger–Ellison syndrome: Spontaneous regression of advanced intra-abdominal metastases with 20 year survival. *Ann. Surg.* 189:620, 1979.
24. Passaro, E., Gordon, H.E.: Malignant gastrinoma following total gastrectomy. *Arch. Surg.* 108:444, 1974.
25. Stadil, F., Stage, G., Rehfeld, J.F., Efsen, F., Fischerman, K.: Treatment of Zollinger–Ellison syndrome with streptozotocin. *N. Engl. J. Med.* 294:1440, 1976.
26. McCarthy, D.M.: Report on the United States experience with cimetidine in Zollinger–Ellison syndrome and other hypersecretory states. *Gastroenterology* 74:453, 1978.
27. Kaplan, E.L., Peskin, G.W., Deveney, C., Way, L., Jaffe, B.: Ulcer disease, metabolic alkalosis, and hyperparathyroidism: A mechanism of interrelationship? *Ann. Surg.* 180:549, 1974.
28. Welbourn, R.B.: Current status of the apudomas. *Ann. Surg.* 185:1, 1977.
29. Case 20-1975, Case records of the Massachusetts General Hospital: Weekly clinicopathologic exercises. *N. Engl. J. Med.* 292:1117, 1975.
30. Higgins, G.A., Recant, L., Fischman, A.B.: The glucagonoma syndrome: Surgically curable diabetes. *Am. J. Surg.* 137:142, 1979.
31. Ingemansson, S., Holst, J., Larsson, L.I., Lunderquist, A.: Location of glucagonomas by catheterization of the pancreatic veins and with glucagon assay. *Surg. Gynecol. Obstet.* 145:509, 1977.
32. Danforth, D.N., Triche, T., Doppman, J.L., Beazley, R.M., Perrino, P.V., Recant, L.: Elevated plasma pro glucagon like component with a glucagon secreting tumor: Effect of streptozotocin. *N. Engl. J. Med.* 295:242, 1976.
33. Bloom, S.R.: Vasoactive intestinal polypeptide, the major mediator of the WDHA pancreatic cholera syndrome. *Digestive Diseases* 23:373, 1978.
34. Ebeid, A.M., Murray, P.D., Fischer, J.E.: Vasoactive intestinal polypeptide and the watery diarrhea syndrome. *Ann. Surg.* 187:411, 1978.
35. Jaffe, B.M., Kopen, D.F., Deschryver-Kecskemeti, K., Gingerich, R.L., Greider, M.: Indomethacin responsive pancreatic cholera. *N. Engl. J. Med.* 297:817, 1977.
36. Jaffe, B.M., Condon, S.: Prostaglandins E and F in endocrine diarrheagenic symdromes. *Ann. Surg.* 184:516, 1976.
37. Elias, E., Bloom, S.R., Welbourn, R.B., Kuzio, M., Polak, J.M., Pearse, A.G.E., Booth, C.C., Brown, J.C.: Pancreatic cholera due to production of gastric inhibitory polypeptide. *Lancet* 2:791, 1972.
38. Friesen, S.R., Kimmel, J.R., Tomita, T.: Pancreatic polypeptide as screening marker for pancreatic polypeptide apudomas in multiple endocrinopathies. *Am. J. Surg.* 139:61, 1980.
39. Kahn, C.R., Levy, A.G., Gardner, J.D., Miller, J.V., Gordon, P., Schein, P.S.: Pancreatic cholera: Beneficial effects of treatment with streptozotocin. *N. Engl. J. Med.* 292:941, 1975.
40. VanHeerden, J.A., Edis, A.J., Service, F.J.: The surgical aspects of insulinomas. *Ann. Surg.* 189:677, 1979.
41. Kaplan, E.L., Rubinstein, A.H., Evans, R., Lee, C.H., Klementschitsch, P.: Calcium infusion: A new provocative test for insulinomas. *Ann. Surg.* 190:501, 1979.
42. Harrison, T.S., Child, C.G., Fry, W.J., Floyd, J.C., Fajans, S.S.: Current surgical management of functioning islet cell tumors of the pancreas. *Ann. Surg.* 178:485, 1973.
43. Ingemansson, S.G., Lunderquist, A., Lundqvist, I., Loudahl, R., Tibblin, S.: Portal and pancreatic vein catheterization with radioimmunologic determination of insulin. *Surg. Gynecol. Obstet.* 141:705, 1975.
44. Schwartz, S.S., Horwitz, D.L., Zehfus, B., Langer, B.G., Kaplan, E.: Continuous monitoring and control of plasma glucose during operation for removal of insulinomas. *Surgery* 85:702, 1979.

45. Thomas, C.G., Underwood, L.E., Carney, C.M., Dolcourt, J.L., Whitt, J.J.: Neonatal and infantile hypoglycemia due to insulin excess: New aspects of diagnosis and surgical management. *Ann. Surg.* 185:505, 1977.
46. Shermeta, D.W., Mendelsohn, G., Haller, J.A.: Hyperinsulinemic hypoglycemia of the neonate associated with persistent fetal histology and function of the pancreas. *Ann. Surg.* 191:182, 1980.
47. Carney, C.N.: Congenital insulinoma (nesidioblastoma). *Arch. Pathol. Lab. Med.* 100:352, 1976.
48. Edis, A.J., Beahrs, O.H., VanHeerden, J.A., Akwari, O.E.: "Conservative" versus "liberal" approach to parathyroid neck exploration. *Surgery* 82:466, 1977.
49. Paloyan, E., Lawrence, A.M., Baker, W.H., Straus, F.H.: Near total parathyroidectomy. *Surg. Clin. North Am.* 49:43, 1969.
50. Clark, O.H., Way, L.W., Hunt, T.K.: Recurrent hyperparathyroidism. *Ann. Surg.* 184:391, 1976.
51. Block, M.A., Frame, B., Jackson, C.E., Horn, R.C.: The extent of operation for primary hyperparathyroidism. *Arch. Surg.* 109:798, 1974.
52. Block, M.A., Frame, B., Kleerekoper, M., Rao, D.S.: Surgical management of persistence or recurrence after subtotal parathyroidectomy for primary hyperparathyroidism. *Am. J. Surg.* 138:561, 1979.
53. Perzik, S.L.: Total thyroidectomy in the management of Graves' disease: A review of 282 cases. *Am. J. Surg.* 131:284, 1976.
54. Safa, A.M., Schumacher, O.P., Rodriguez-Antunez, A.: Long-term follow-up results in children and adolescents treated with radioactive iodine (^{131}I) for hyperthyroidism. *N. Engl. J. Med.* 292:167, 1975.
55. DeGroot, L., Paloyan, E.: Thyroid carcinoma and radiation. A Chicago epidemic. *J.A.M.A.* 225:487, 1973.
56. Favus, M.J., Schneider, A.B., Stachura, M.E., Arnold, J.E., Ryo, U.Y., Pinsky, S.M., Colman, M., Arnold, M.J., Frohman, L.A.: Thyroid cancer occurring as a late consequence of head and neck irradiation. *N. Engl. J. Med.* 294:1019, 1976.
57. Paloyan, E., Lawrence, A.M., Brooks, M.H., Pickleman, J.R.: Total thyroidectomy and parathyroid autotransplantation for radiation-associated thyroid cancer. *Surgery* 80:70, 1976.
58. Heimann, P.: Should hyperthyroidism be treated by surgery? *World J. Surg.* 2:281, 1978.
59. Greer, M.A., Kammer, H., Bouma, D.J.: Short-term antithyroid drug therapy for the thyroid toxicosis of Graves' disease. *N. Engl. J. Med.* 297:173, 1977.
60. Lee, T.C., Coffey, R.J., Mackin, J., Cobb, M., Routon, J., Canary, J.J.: The use of propranalol in the surgical treatment of thyrotoxic patients. *Ann. Surg.* 177:643, 1973.
61. Bewsher, P.D., Pegg, C.A.S., Stewart, D.J., Lister, D.A., Michie, W.: Propranalol in the surgical management of thryotoxicosis. *Ann. Surg.* 180:787, 1974.
62. Starling, J.R., Thomas, C.G.: Experience with the use of propranalol in the surgical management of thyrotoxicosis. *World J. Surg.* 1:251, 1977.
63. RèMine, W.H., McConahey, W.M.: Management of thyroid nodules. *Surg. Clin. North Am. 57:523, 1977.*
64. Hoffman, G.L., Thompson, N.W., Heffron, C.: The solitary thyroid nodule. *Arch. Surg.* 105:379, 1972.
65. Refetoff, S., Harrison, J., Karanfilski, B.T., Kaplan, E.L., DeGroot, L.J., Bekerman, C.: Continuing Ooccurrence of thyroid carcinoma after irradiation to the neck in infancy and childhood. *N. Engl. J. Med.* 292:171, 1975.
66. Spitalnik, P.F., Straus, F.H.: Patterns of human thyroid parenchymal reaction following low dose childhood irradiation. *Cancer* 41:1098, 1978.

67. Thompson, N.W., Harness, J.K.: Complications of total thyroidectomy for carcinoma. *Surg. Gynecol. Obstet.* 131:861, 1970.
68. Russell, W.O., Ibanez, M.L., Clark, R.L., White, E.C.: Thyroid carcinoma. *Cancer* 16:1425, 1963.
69. Block, M.A., Miller, J.M., Horn, R.C.: Thyroid carcinoma with cervical lymph node metastasis: Effectiveness of total thyroidectomy and node dissection. *Am. J. Surg.* 122:458, 1971.
70. Harness, J.K., Thompson, N.W., Sisson, J.C., Beierwaltes, W.H.: Differentiated thyroid carcinomas: Treatment of distant metastases. *Arch. Surg.* 108:410, 1974.
71. Mazzaferri, E.L., Young, R.L., Oertel, J.E., Kemmerer, W.T., Page, C.P.: Papillary thyroid carcinoma: The impact of therapy in 576 patients. *Medicine* 56:171, 1977.
72. Katz, A.D., Bronson, D.: Total thyroidectomy: The indications and results of 630 cases. *Am. J. Surg.* 136:450, 1978.
73. Aldinger, K.A., Samaan, N.A., Ibanez, M., Hill, C.S.: Anaplastic carcinoma of the thyroid. *Cancer* 41:2267, 1978.
74. Kyriakides, G., Sosin, H.: Anaplastic carcinoma of the thyroid. *Ann. Surg.* 179:295, 1974.
75. Maloof, F.: Case 37-1979, Case records of the Massachusetts General Hospital. *N. Engl. J. Med.* 301:600, 1979.
76. Braverman, L.E.: Case 29-1975, Case records of the Massachusetts General HOspital. *N. Engl. J. Med.* 293:186, 1975.
77. Thomas, C.G., Buckwalter, J.A.: Poorly differentiated neoplasms of the thyroid gland. *Ann. Surg.* 177:632, 1973.
78. Rossi, R., Cady, B., Meissner, W.A., Sedgwick, C.E., Werber, J.: Prognosis of undifferentiated carcinoma and lymphoma of the thyroid. *Am. J. Surg.* 135:589, 1978.
79. Norton, J.A., Froome, L.C., Farrell, R.E., Wells, S.A.: Multiple endocrine neoplasia type IIB: The most aggressive form of medullary thyroid carcinoma. *Surg. Clin. North Am.* 59:109, 1979.
80. Sizemore, G.W., Carney, J.A., Heath, H.: Epidemiology of medullary carcinoma of the thyroid gland: A five year experience. *Surg. Clin. North Am.* 57:633, 1977.
81. Graze, K., Spiler, I.J., Tashjian, A.H.: Natural history of familial medullary thyroid carcinoma. *N. Engl. J. Med.* 299:980, 1978.
82. Wells, S.A., Baylin, S.B., Linehan, W.M., Farrell, R.E., Cox, E.B., Cooper, C.W.: Provocative agents in the diagnosis of medullary carcinoma of the thyroid gland. *Ann. Surg.* 188:139, 1978.
83. Freier, D.T., Thompson, N.W., Sisson, J.C., Nishiyama, R.H., Freitas, J.E.: Dilemmas in the early diagnosis and treatment of multiple endocrine adenomatosis, type II. *Surgery* 82:407, 1977.
84. Carney, J.A., Sizemore, G.W., Tyce, G.M.: Bilateral adrenal medullary hyperplasia in multiple endocrine neoplasia, type II: The precursor of bilateral pheochromocytoma. *Mayo Clin. Proc.* 50:3, 1975.
85. Patient Management Problem #3, SESAP III. American College of Surgeons Surgical Education and Self Assessment Program. Chicago, Illinois, 1979.
86. Block, M.A., Jackson, C.E., Tashjian, A.H.: Management of parathyroid glands in surgery for medullary thyroid carcinoma. *Arch. Surg.* 110:617, 1975.
87. Jackson, C.E., Tashjian, A.H., Block, M.A.: Detection of medullary thyroid cancer by calcitonin assay in families. *Ann. Intern. Med.* 78:845, 1973.
88. Block, M.A., Jackson, C.E., Tashjian, A.H.: Management of occult medullary thyroid carcinoma. *Arch. Surg.* 113:368, 1978.
89. Skeggs, L.T., Dorer, F.E., Kahn, J.R., Lentz, K.E., Levine, M.: The biochemistry of the renin angiotensin system and its role in hypertension. *Am. J. Med.* 60:737, 1976.

90. Fraley, E.E., Feldman, B.H.: Renal hypertension. *N. Engl. J. Med.* 287:550, 1972.
91. Stanley, J.C., Fry, W.J.: Renovascular hypertension secondary to arterial fibrodysplasia in adults. *Arch. Surg.* 110:922, 1975.
92. Perry, M.O.: Fibromuscular dysplasia. *Surg. Gynecol. Obstet.* 139:97, 1974.
93. Foster, J.H., Dean, R.H., Pinkerton, J.A., Rhamy, R.K.: Ten years experience with the surgical management of renovascular hypertension. *Ann. Surg.* 177:755, 1973.
94. Stanley, J.C., Fry, W.J.: Surgical treatment of renovascular hypertension. *Arch. Surg.* 112:1291, 1977.
95. Millan, V.G., Mast, W.E., Madias, N.E.: Nonsurgical treatment of severe hypertension due to renal artery intimal fibroplasia by percutaneous transluminal angioplasty. *N. Engl. J. Med.* 300:1371, 1979.

9
BREAST

9.1. A 35-year-old woman gives a 3-week history of a painful right breast lump. At the time of examination, she is menstruating. A hard, smooth, nonfixed, 3-cm mass is noted in the upper outer quadrant of the breast. Two soft 0.5-cm right axillary nodes are palpable, and the skin overlying the breast mass is normal. The next step in the management of this patient should be:

A. Aspiration of the mass.
B. Excision under local anesthesia.
C. Needle biopsy of the mass.
D. Mammography.
E. Thermography.

In all likelihood, this patient harbors a cyst; the presence of pain plus a hard smooth nonfixed mass is quite suggestive of this diagnosis. Small axillary nodes are frequently found in many patients without any demonstrable breast pathology.

It is obviously impractical to hospitalize every woman with a dominant breast mass. Even excision performed in an out-patient setting is very costly and time-consuming. In a mass that possesses none of the characteristics of a carcinoma, needle aspiration is safe, quick, and yields immediate information. With the obtaining of fluid, not only will the patient be immediately relieved, but the lesion will have been definitively managed in the majority of cases. In one series of 1500 cysts treated by aspiration, 88% disappeared completely with one aspiration, and only 12% required two or more aspirations to effect complete disappearance.[1] Following a local anesthetic injection into the skin overlying the mass, a needle is inserted and the mass aspirated until no fluid can be obtained. Although cytologic evaluation has been attempted, it is not necessary if certain criteria for subsequent biopsy are followed.[2,3] If serosanguineous fluid is obtained, or if no fluid is aspirated, indicating a solid mass, subsequent excisional biopsy is indicated. The presence of a residual mass on palpation after the aspiration or persistent recurrence of a cyst after successful aspiration represent additional indications for excisional biopsy. Using this technique, patients may be definitively managed during their initial visit with a significant saving of time, money, and anxiety.

ANSWER: A.

9.2. A 38-year-old woman undergoes a modified radical mastectomy for an infiltrating ductal carcinoma. The final pathology report discloses 28 lymph nodes, six of which are involved by tumor. She should be advised that:

A. No further treatment is indicated at this time.
B. She should undergo oophorectomy.
C. She should receive adjuvant chemotherapy.
D. She should receive estrogens.
E. She should receive antiestrogens (Tamoxifan).

There is increasing evidence that the standard operative therapy of breast carcinoma is inadequate in the management of most patients if they have systemic disease at the time of presentation. In one multi-institution cooperative study, 76% of all patients with positive nodes had evidence of recurrent disease at ten years. Within this group, 38% of those women with one to three positive nodes survived 10 years, but only 13% of those women with greater than four positive axillary nodes survived this long.[4]

Because of this, numerous trials employing adjuvant chemotherapy have been instituted for this high-risk group of patients, the assumption being that those women with negative axillary nodes have a sufficiently good chance for surgical cure that the potential risks of chemotherapy are not warranted. Both single- and multiple-drug chemotherapeutic regimens have been instituted and followed for short periods of time. L-Phenylalanine mustard (L-Pam) has been used alone, and cyclophosphamide, methotrexate, and fluorouracil have been used in combination. Similar results have been obtained, and several generalizations seem apparent.[5,6] First of all, the disease-free interval, or the time until first evidence of tumor recurrence, seems to be definitely prolonged in premenopausal women compared to postmenopausal women. In addition, although the initial studies did not show any increased survival, more recent follow-ups of the same patients have begun to indicate that survival might be enhanced.

The rationale of adjuvant chemotherapy appears to be more than to bring about a "chemical oophorectomy." Historically, controls who underwent surgical or radiation oophorectomy had lower incidences of response that the chemotherapy group. Also, some studies have shown a response rate, albeit a lower one, for postmenopausal women.

So, at the present time, it would appear to be good practice to offer adjuvant chemotherapy to any woman with more than four positive lymph nodes, especially if she is premenopausal at the time. Estrogen therapy would be contraindicated in premenopausal women, as its administration might enhance tumor growth. The new antiestrogen compound Tamoxifan may prove to be of future value, but data are still very preliminary.

ANSWER: C.

9.3. A 54-year-old woman 7 years postmenopause undergoes a modified radical mastectomy for breast carcinoma; the pathology report discloses an infiltrating ductal carcinoma with two of 28 nodes positive. The tissue is sent for estrogen receptor determination, and it is strongly positive. A bone scan is normal. No further treatment is given, and 3 years later she begins to have rib and low back pain. A bone scan at this time discloses multiple areas of metastatic disease. Treatment should consist of:

A. Local radiotherapy to the painful bone lesions.
B. Oophorectomy and adrenalectomy.
C. Oophorectomy.
D. Tamoxifan administration.
E. Multiple drug chemotherapy.

With the discovery of the presence of estrogen receptors in certain breast cancers, new options have become available for the clinician treating a patient with metastatic disease. This test relies on the fact that certain breast cancers are dependent upon estrogen for their growth. The amount of binding of estrogen to the tumor can be measured, and therefore the tumor responsiveness can be determined. The process of measuring estrogen receptor (ER) activity in tumor tissue is a complicated one, and careful attention must be paid to the obtaining of and prompt preparation of the tissue if valid results are to be secured. It has been found that ER activity may be present in many breast cancers and also in a wide variety of other carcinomas. ER activity can be present in breast cancers of pre- and postmenopausal women, but it is found more frequently in postmenopausal women, presumably owing to the endogenous circulating estrogen levels found in premenopausal women and the resultant saturation of tumor binding sites.[7] No correlation has been found with regard to ER positivity and the histologic type of breast carcinoma.

It is important to perform the estrogen receptor analysis at the time of initial excision of the breast carcinoma. At least an 80% correlation exists between ER positivity in primary and metastatic lesions in the same patient,[8] and because metastatic lesions may not be amenable to biopsy, the information gained from analysis of the primary lesion is critical. The differing ER positivity between certain primary and metastatic breast cancers in the same patient and among metastatic lesions in the same patient, may be due to the presence of a mixed group of neoplastic cells, some of which are ER-positive and some of which are negative.[9]

In general, women with ER-positive tumors have a better overall prognosis than those with ER-negative tumors.[10] No clear correlation has been demonstrated between ER status and subsequent response to chemotherapy in patients with metastatic carcinoma. However, when hormonal manipulations are performed in patients with metastatic breast cancer, the ER status of the patient is strongly predictive. At least 60% of patients with ER-positive tumors will undergo an objective response to hormonal manipulation, either additive or ablative, whereas less than 5% will respond to these manipulations if the tumors are ER-negative.[7] In the patient presented, an oophorectomy–adrenalectomy should be carried out at this time. An oophorectomy alone would not be effective in a postmenopausal woman, as the adrenal glands would still produce significant quantities of estrogens. The antiestrogen Tamoxifan may well prove effective in this setting, however, but at the present time it appears that the response rates to estrogen or antiestrogen administration are below those encountered with major hormonal ablation.

ANSWER: B.

9.4. A 45-year-old woman undergoes an excisional biopsy of a 1.5-cm breast mass noted during a routine physical examination. The final pathology report discloses noninvasive intraductal carcinoma. She should be advised that:

A. Further treatment is unnecessary at this time.
B. The surrounding quadrant of the breast should be removed.
C. A total (simple) mastectomy should be performed.
D. A total (simple) mastectomy and biopsy of the contralateral breast should be performed.
E. A modified radical mastectomy should be performed.

With an increased awareness of breast disease and wider use of mammography in questionable cases, many women with minimal breast cancer or noninvasive breast cancers are being detected. Even in the earlier noninvasive forms of carcinoma, mammography will show suspicious changes in nearly 90% of cases, making this a useful adjunct in the evaluation of a woman with a questionable breast mass.[11] The importance of proper initial treatment is highlighted by a report of women who harbored noninvasive intraductal carcinoma, were treated by excisional biopsy alone, and were subsequently followed for up to 20 years. Carcinoma, often of the invasive variety, occurred in 39% of these women during the follow-up period.[12] Several studies have indicated a high incidence of multicentricity within the same breast and bilaterality in women harboring intraductal or other forms of noninvasive carcinoma. One study disclosed carcinoma in other quadrants of the involved breast in 33% of mastectomy specimens in women who harbored an intraductal carcinoma, and an 80% incidence of carcinoma in other quadrants of the breast in women who harbored lobular carcinoma in situ.[13] None of these patients harbored positive axillary nodes. Another study of 53 patients with minimal breast cancer treated by radical mastectomy noted no positive axillary nodes in any of the patients. However, biopsy of the contralateral breast disclosed involvement in 40% of these women.[14]

Because of these data, most authorities today recommend total mastectomy for the woman found to have a noninvasive intraductal carcinoma. Whether or not a sampling of the lower axillary nodes is advisable is unclear, but perhaps this should be carried out for staging purposes.[13–15] In addition, it would appear wise to carry out a contralateral breast biopsy because of the significant incidence of bilateral disease.[14,16]

Alternatively, the use of radiation therapy as a primary treatment following excisional biopsy has been extensively studied and is quite successful in rendering such patients disease free over long periods of time.[17,18] It is quite likely that the use of this modality of treatment will increase in the future, making it possible to accumulate valid recurrence and survival data.

ANSWER: D.

9.5. A 65-year-old woman presents to her doctor with a "breast problem," seen in Figure 9-1. She had been aware of a left breast mass for at least 3 years. A biopsy discloses infiltrating ductal carcinoma with subdermal lymphatic invasion by tumor. Estrogen receptors are measured and found to be strongly positive. A bone scan is shown as Figure 9-2. A liver and brain scan are normal. Treatment should consist of:

A. Local radiotherapy and oophorectomy–adrenalectomy.
B. Local radiation therapy and oophorectomy.
C. Radical mastectomy and local radiotherapy.
D. Radical mastectomy.
E. Systemic multiple drug chemotherapy.

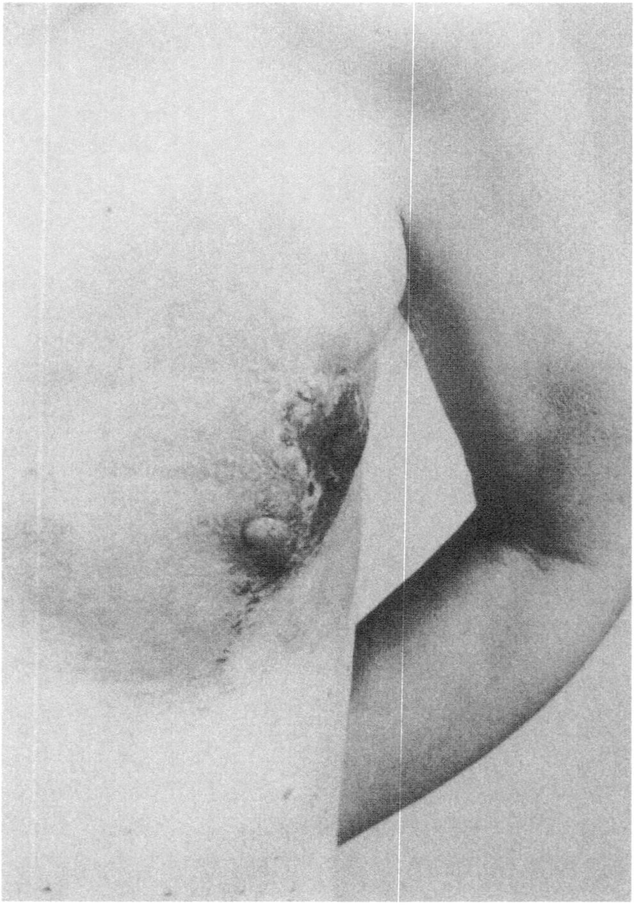

Figure 9-1

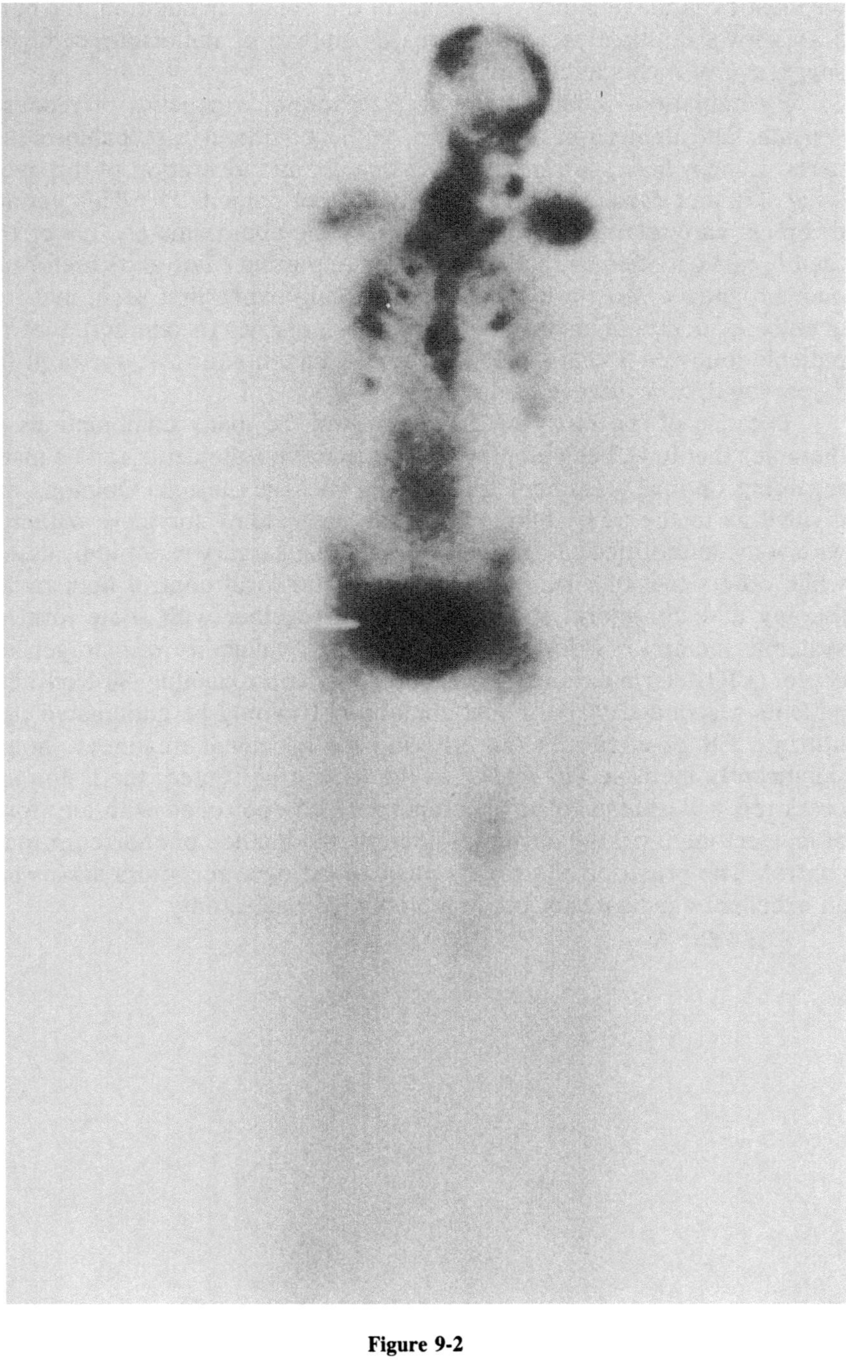

Figure 9-2

The gross appearance and microscopic description of this tumor are diagnostic of inflammatory carcinoma of the breast. In addition, the bone scan shows multiple areas of increased uptake of radioisotope, highly suggestive of metastatic disease.

By definition, inflammatory breast carcinoma consists of redness, warmth, and induration of the skin, with or without a palpable breast mass. Lymph nodes are frequently palpable, and ulceration of the overlying skin can occur in approximately 20% of patients.[19,20] This variant of breast carcinoma is quite rare, comprising approximately 1% of the total breast carcinomas that are seen. Its importance lies in its uniformly poor prognosis. Most are far advanced locally when first seen, and frequently evidence of metastatic disease is present. In one series of 63 patients followed 5 years or longer, only 2 patients, or 3%, survived for 5 years with no evidence of disease.[20]

Because of the rarity of the tumor and the many combinations of therapies that have been employed, no definitive statements can be made regarding optimal treatment for patients with this lesion. Opinions are divided as to the advisability of radical mastectomy for these patients, with some authorities categorically stating that surgery is not indicated,[20] while others feel that surgery can give better local control than radiotherapy and, therefore, should be utilized together with some form of systemic therapy.[21] Prior to the widespread availability of estrogen receptor (ER) determinations, it was noted that approximately 30% of these patients responded to hormonal ablation.[20] It would be anticipated that utilizing ER positivity as the criterion for hormonal treatment should significantly increase this figure. In the patient presented, the lesion appears too widespread to be encompassed and controlled with any form of mastectomy, making local radiotherapy the method of choice for local control. The presence of strongly positive estrogen receptors makes her an excellent candidate for oophorectomy–adrenalectomy.

ANSWER: A.

9.6. A 43-year-old woman presents with a breast lump. On examination, the mass is found to be 2.5 cm in diameter, and no axillary nodes are palpable. An excisional biopsy is performed, and a diagnosis of invasive lobular carcinoma is made. The patient should be advised that she should undergo:

A. Modified radical mastectomy.
B. Modified radical mastectomy plus contralateral breast biopsy.
C. Simple mastectomy.
D. Simple mastectomy plus contralateral breast biopsy.
E. Wide local excision of the mass and surrounding tissue.

Lobular carcinoma of the breast is one of the more uncommon varieties of breast carcinoma, occurring in from 2.5% to 5% of all women with breast carcinoma.[22,23] The lesion is unique in that it occurs in both the in situ, noninvasive form and also as an invasive tumor. Of special note is the markedly increased incidence of bilaterality of the disease in those women found to harbor a lobular carcinoma either of the invasive or of the noninvasive type. The figures of bilaterality range from 20% to 42%.[23,24] Despite frequent involvement of the contralateral breast, the clinical examination is often negative, and even such aids as xeromammography often do not detect occult disease.[24] Because of this, many authorities feel that a blind biopsy should be performed on the contralateral breast of every woman with a proven lobular carcinoma.[23] Although some authorities have indicated that they believe that the in situ variety transforms into the invasive form,[23,24] in all likelihood this does not occur, and subsequent invasive carcinomas are probably noted because of the multicentricity and frequent bilaterality of the tumor. This is also supported by the fact that the associated invasive carcinomas are often of a different histologic type.[25]

In the patient presented, an invasive carcinoma is present, and therefore some form of mastectomy and axillary dissection is required in addition to a blind biopsy of the second breast. If the excised lesion had shown only lobular carcinoma in situ, determining the necessary treatment would be significantly more difficult. Recommendations in that instance have ranged from simple mastectomy with or without contralateral biopsy to excisional biopsy only with prolonged follow-up. In one series of 21 patients with lobular carcinoma in situ, only 17% eventually developed invasive carcinoma.[26]

ANSWER: B.

9.7. A 52-year-old woman gives a 6-week history of an itching, reddened area on the areola of her right breast. No breast mass is palpable, nor are any enlarged axillary lymph nodes detected. Antibiotic salves bring about no improvement in the appearance of the lesion but do decrease the itching. A punch biopsy of the lesion is performed, and is shown as Figure 9-3. Treatment should consist of:

A. Topical corticosteroids.
B. Topical estrogens.
C. Excision of the nipple.
D. Modified radical mastectomy.
E. Simple mastectomy.

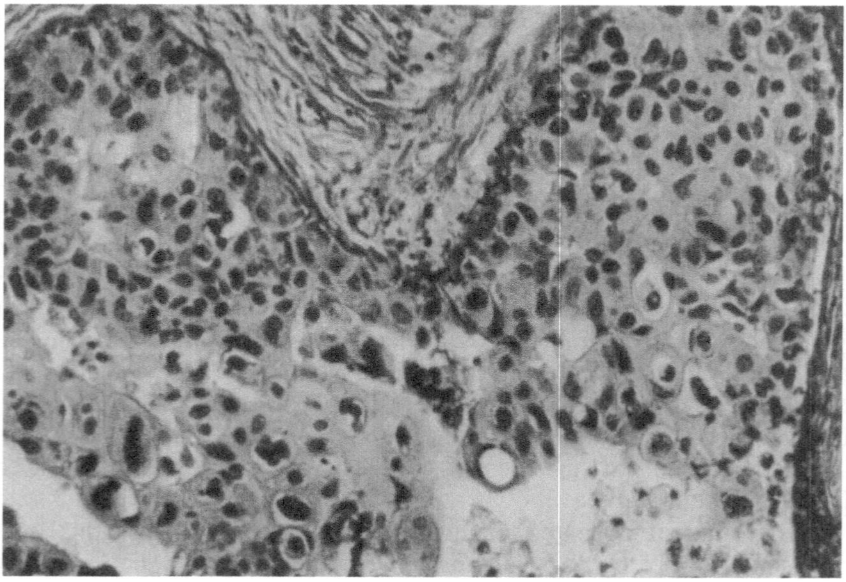

Figure 9-3

The history and biopsy specimen are typical of Paget's disease of the breast. By definition, this entity consists of the presence of malignant cells within the dermis of the nipple and areola. Even if no mass is palpable, this skin abnormality is always associated with an underlying malignancy. The incidence of Paget's disease ranges from 1.5% to 2.5% of all female breast carcinomas.[27,28]

The disease exists in three forms. In Haagensen's series of 159 cases, a mass was present along with the typical nipple changes in 29%, a mass was present without any cutaneous changes (and therefore the Paget cells were only noted microscopically) in 28%, and a typical nipple lesion was present without a mass in 43%.[27] In another series of 214 cases, 53% of patients had a palpable mass, but approximately two thirds of those women without a palpable mass were subsequently found to harbor a noninfiltrating carcinoma with negative lymph nodes.[29]

In most series of patients with Paget's disease, the disease has occurred in a similar age distribution to breast carcinoma without Paget changes, and the prognosis has been similar. Because in many cases these carcinomas are of the infiltrating variety, it is presently felt that an axillary nodal dissection is required.

ANSWER: D.

9.8. A 66-year-old man gives a 2-month history of a painless left breast lump. The mass is 3 cm in diameter and is fixed to the overlying skin. No axillary lymph nodes are palpable. A bone scan is shown as Figure 9-4. An excisional biopsy reveals infiltrating ductal carcinoma. Treatment should consist of:

A. Adrenalectomy.
B. Radical mastectomy.
C. Local radiotherapy.
D. Local radiotherapy plus systemic chemotherapy.
E. Radical mastectomy and orchiectomy.

Male breast carcinomas comprise approximately 1% of all treated breast carcinomas. In general, the same histologic varieties are noted in males and females, with similar percentages of patients with positive axillary nodes at the time of diagnosis. Differences of opinion exist regarding the prognosis of such patients, with some authorities feeling that males have roughly the same survival rate as women with breast cancer.[30] However, at least one series has shown similar survival figures at 5 years but significantly decreased 10-year survival rates for males, especially if lymph nodes were positive—an 11% figure was reported, which is significantly below comparable figures for females.[31]

In the absence of metastatic disease, men with breast carcinoma should be treated for cure by radical mastectomy. As there is usually less intervening tissue between breast cancers and the underlying pectoral muscles and fascia in men than in women, these structures tend to be involved earlier, making any procedure less than standard radical mastectomy inadvisable. A quite striking percentage of positive responses to orchiectomy have been noted, even before estrogen receptor data became available. Castration in the male has proven to be at least as effective as castration in females with metastatic breast cancer and is not age-limited, as it is in females.[32] Approximately two thirds of male patients treated with orchiectomy have shown objective responses, often for prolonged periods.[33] If a response to orchiectomy has been followed by relapse, bilateral adrenalectomy can then be expected to provide an additional response in many patients.[33,34] Additionally, there are instances where orchiectomy has not yielded an objective response but subsequent adrenalectomy has brought about a striking remission of tumor metastases.[33]

In the patient presented, local control of the tumor should be obtained with a radical mastectomy. This should be followed by an orchiectomy for control of the metastatic bone lesions. Insufficient data exist today on the role of estrogen receptors in guiding one's decision for hormonal ablation, but it is probable that this information will prove helpful.

ANSWER: E.

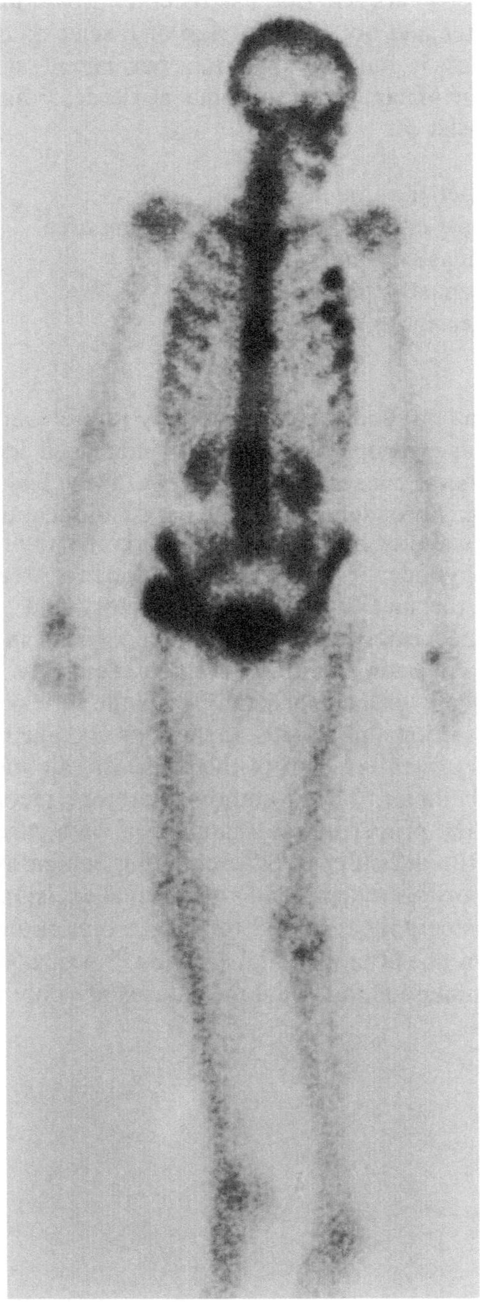

Figure 9-4

9.9. A 42-year-old woman gives a history of a breast lump that has been present for over 5 years and that has recently grown larger. The mass is 10 cm in diameter and not fixed to skin or fascia; no axillary nodes are palpable. The mass is enucleated, and the permanent pathologic specimen report reveals malignant cystosarcoma phyllodes. Management at this time should consist of:

A. No further treatment.
B. Wide local excision of the surrounding area.
C. Simple mastectomy.
D. Radical mastectomy.
E. Radiotherapy to the breast.

Cytosarcoma phyllodes is an extremely rare breast tumor that tends to occur in all age groups but is seen in increased incidence in young women. The general consensus today is that these lesions arise in many cases from benign fibroadenomas of the breast and that there is a spectrum from benign fibroadenoma to benign cystosarcoma phyllodes to malignant cystosarcoma phyllodes.[35,36] Recommendations for treatment have been complicated by the fact that the clinical history and histology of these tumors do not accurately differentiate benign from malignant, and numerous cases have been reported in which seemingly "benign" tumors later recurred locally or metastasized.[37,38] In one series of 26 patients with malignant cystosarcoma phyllodes, the lesions averaged 7 cm in diameter, and six patients ultimately died of their disease, all with lesions greater than 7 cm in diameter. These authors therefore recommended simple mastectomy as the proper initial treatment of such cases.[39]

In view of the difficulty in differentiating benign from malignant tumors, most authorities recommend a wide local excision for small tumors with simple mastectomy reserved for larger tumors or those that have evidenced recurrence after an initial excision.[36] Axillary dissection is generally not recommended, as nodal metastases are only infrequently seen with this disease.

ANSWER: C.

References

1. Abramson, D.J.: A clinical evaluation of aspiration of cysts of the breast. *Surg. Gynecol. Obstet.* 139:531, 1974.
2. Rosemond, G.P., Maier, W.P., Brobyn, T.J.: Needle aspiration of breast cysts. *Surg. Gynecol. Obstet.* 128:351, 1969.
3. Barnes, W.C.: Management of cystic disease of the breast. *Am. J. Surg.* 129:324, 1975.
4. Fisher, B., Slack, N., Katrych, D., Wolmark, N.: Ten year follow-up results of patients with carcinoma of the breast in a co-operative clinical trial evaluating surgical adjuvant chemotherapy. *Surg. Gynecol. Obstet.* 140:528, 1975.
5. Fisher, B., Carbone, P., Economou, S.G., Frelick, R., Glass, A., Lerner, H., Redmond, C., Zelen, M., Band, Katrych, D.L., Wolmark, N., Fisher, E.R.: L-phenylalanine mustard (L-Pam) in the management of primary breast cancer. *N. Engl. J. Med.* 292:117, 1975.
6. Bonadonna, G., Brusamolino, E., Valagussa, P., Rossi, A., Brugnatelli, L., Brambilla, C., Delena, M., Tancini, G., Bajetta, E., Musumeci, R., Veronasi, U.: Combination chemotherapy as an adjuvant treatment in operable breast cancer. *N. Engl. J. Med.* 294:405, 1976.
7. Block, G.E., Jensen, E.V., Polley, T.Z.: The prediction of hormonal dependency of mammary cancer. *Ann. Surg.* 182:342, 1975.
8. Hoehn, J.L., Plotka, E.D., Dixon, K.B.: Comparison of estrogen receptor levels in primary and regional metastatic carcinoma of the breast. *Ann. Surg.* 190:69, 1979.
9. Leung, B.S., Krippaehne, W.W., Fletcher, W.S.: Prognostic value of estrogen receptor to endocrine ablation in cancer of the breast. *Surg. Gynecol. Obstet.* 139:525, 1974.
10. Kern, W.H.: Morphologic and clinical aspects of estrogen receptors in carcinoma of the breast. *Surg. Gynecol. Obstet.* 148:240, 1979.
11. Westbrook, K.C., Gallager, H.S.: Intraductal carcinoma of the breast. *Am. J. Surg.* 130:667, 1975.
12. Betsill, W.L., Rosen, P.R., Liberman, P.H., Robbins, G.F.: Intraductal carcinoma: Long-term follow-up after treatment by biopsy alone. *J.A.M.A.* 239:1863, 1978.
13. Rosen, P.P., Senie, R., Schottenfeld, D., Ashikari, R.: Noninvasive breast carcinoma. *Ann. Surg.* 189:377, 1979.
14. Nevin, J.E., Pinzon, G., Moran, T.J., Baggerly, J.T.: Minimal breast carcinoma. *Am. J. Surg.* 139:357, 1980.
15. Brown, P.W., Silverman, J., Owens, E., Tabor, D.C., Terz, J.J., Lawrence, W.: Intraductal "noninfiltrating" carcinoma of the breast. *Arch Surg.* 111:1063, 1976.
16. Peters, T.G., Donegan, W.L., Burg, E.A.: Minimal breast cancer. *Ann. Surg.* 186:704, 1977.
17. Nelson, A.J., Montague, E.D.: Resectable localized breast cancer: The rationale for combined surgery and irradiation. *J.A.M.A.* 231:189, 1975.
18. Wizenberg, M.J., Brickner, T.J.: Carcinoma of the breast. *Surg. Gynecol. Obstet.* 149:321, 1979.
19. Camp, E.: Inflammatory carcinoma of the breast. *Am. J. Surg.* 131:583, 1976.
20. Robbins, G.F., Shaw, J., Rosen, P., Chu, F., Taylor, J.: Inflammatory carcinoma of the breast. *Surg. Clin. North Am.* 54:801, 1974.
21. Pollak, E.W., Getzen, L.C.: Inflammatory carcinoma of the breast. *Am. J. Surg.* 136:722, 1978.
22. Warner, N.E.: Lobular carcinoma of the breast. *Cancer* 23:840, 1969.
23. Donegan, W.L., Perez-Mesa, C.M.: Lobular carcinoma: An indication for elective biopsy of the second breast. *Ann. Surg.* 176:178, 1972.
24. Newman, W.: In situ lobular carcinoma of the breast. *Ann. Surg.* 157:591, 1963.

25. Fisher, E.R., Fisher, B.: Lobular carcinoma of the breast: An overview. *Ann. Surg.* 185:377, 1977.
26. Haagensen, C.D., Lane, N., Lattes, R., Bodian, C.: Lobular neoplasia (so-called lobular carcinoma in situ) of the breast. *Cancer* 42:737, 1978.
27. Kister, S.J., Haagensen, C.D.: Paget's disease of the breast. *Am. J. Surg.* 119:606, 1970.
28. Maier, W.P., Rosemond, G.P., Harasym, E.L., Al-Saleem, T.I., Tassoni, E.M., Schor, S.S.: Paget's disease in the female breast. *Surg. Gynecol. Obstet.* 128:1253, 1969.
29. Ashikari, R., Park, K., Huvos, A.G., Urban, J.A.: Paget's disease of the breast. *Cancer* 26:680, 1970.
30. Yap, H.Y., Tashima, C.K., Blumenschein, G.R., Eckles, N.E.: Male breast cancer. *Cancer* 44:748, 1979.
31. Heller, K.S., Rosen, P.R., Schottenfeld, D., Ashikari, R., Kinne, D.W.: Male breast cancer: A clinicopathological study of 97 cases. *Ann. Surg.* 188:60, 1978.
32. Crichlow, R.W.: Carcinoma of the male breast. *Surg. Gynecol. Obstet.* 134:1011, 1972.
33. Neifeld, J.P., Meyskens, F., Tormey, D.C., Javadpour, N.: The role of orchiectomy in the management of advanced male breast cancer. *Cancer* 37:992, 1976.
34. Houttuin, E., Prohaska, J.V., Taxman, P.: Response of male mammary carcinoma metastases to bilateral adrenalectomy. *Surg. Gynecol. Obstet.* 125:279, 1967.
35. West, T.L., Weiland, L.H., Clagett, O.T.: Cystosarcoma phyllodes. *Ann. Surg.* 173:520, 1971.
36. Al-Jurf, A., Hawk, W.A., Crile, G.: Cystosarcoma phyllodes. *Surg. Gynecol. Obstet.* 146:358, 1978.
37. Andersson, A., Bergdahl, L.: Cystosarcoma phyllodes in young women. *Arch. Surg.* 113:742, 1978.
38. Blichert-Toft, M., Hansen, J.P.H., Hansen, O.H., Schiodt, T.: Clinical course of cystosarcoma phyllodes related to histologic appearance. *Surg. Gynecol. Obstet.* 140:929, 1975.
39. Browder, W., McQuitty, J.T., McDonald, J.C.: Malignant cystosarcoma phyllodes. *Am. J. Surg.* 136:239, 1978.

10
POSTOPERATIVE COMPLICATIONS

10.1. Which of the following factors does not alter the rate of wound infection in clean surgical incisions?

A. Length of the operation.
B. Plastic wound drapes.
C. Plastic ringed wound protectors.
D. Length of preoperative hospitalization.
E. Preoperative shaving of skin.

Perhaps one of the more irrational areas of discourse among surgeons is tbe subject of the causation and prevention of wound infections. Most surgeons have little idea of their own or their hospital's infection rates and would probably be surprised at the generally stated 2%–4% infection rates in clean surgical wounds, with much higher percentages noted in clean contaminated or dirty wounds.[1]

Among the host variables that can often not be controlled but that play a significant proven role in the pathogenesis of wound infections are increasing age; the presence of malnutrition, obesity, or diabetes mellitus; and the type of operation that is required, either clean (inguinal hernia repair), clean contaminated (vagotomy and hemigastrectomy), or contaminated (appendectomy for ruptured appendix.) However, certain variables can be controlled and have been shown to affect the rate of ultimate wound infection. Several studies have shown that wound infection rates are increased with the increased duration of operating time and also the increased duration of preoperative hospitalization.[2] Preoperative shaving has also been shown to increase the incidence of wound infections. If shaving is required, it should be carried out immediately before the operative procedure, and attempts should be made to avoid cutting the skin. Electric razors and clippers along with depilatory agents have been shown to be suitable in this regard.[2,3] Another adjunct that has been shown to decrease the incidence of wound infections is the use of a ringed plastic wound protector.[2,4] These wound protectors probably act by decreasing the trauma to the subcutaneous wound during the procedure and also by preventing drying out of the wound. Plastic skin drapes (Vi-drape), although seemingly rendering the torso neater, have not been conclusively shown to decrease the incidence of wound infection.[2,4]

ANSWER: B.

10.2. For prophylactic antibiotics to be effective in decreasing the incidence of wound infection, antibiotics should be administered:

A. During the operation and for 5 days thereafter.
B. Before and during the operation and for 48 hr thereafter.
C. During the operation only.
D. Immediately after the operation for 48 hr.
E. Immediately after the operation for 5 days.

There is considerable disagreement as to the role of antibiotics in the prevention of wound infection. Hundreds of clinical and experimental studies have been performed, but few meet rigorous standards of randomization, adequate double blinding, and statistical analysis, thus rendering the conclusions in many articles subject to question.[5] In many series, infection rates in the untreated control groups are so high as to cast doubt on any conclusions. Some studies have found no benefit to prophylactic antibiotics in clean operations such as hernia repair, mastectomy, and varicose vein excisions, whereas in potentially contaminated operations, such as those involving transection at any level of the GI tract, patients have benefited from antibiotic administration.[6]

However, despite the diversity of cases that have been studied and the wide variety of antibiotics that have been used, one conclusion stands out in virtually every study, namely, that antibiotics have to be administered preoperatively so that adequate blood and tissue levels are present before the incision is made. Administering antibiotics postoperatively only has no appreciable effect on infection rates.[5,7,8] The length of time the drug must be administered is variable, but significant differences are noted using perioperative antibiotic administration with as little as 48 hr of antibiotic administration postoperatively.

ANSWER: B.

10.3. Which of the following factors does not influence the occurrence of wound dehiscence?

A. Type of incision (midline vs. paramedian vs. transverse).
B. Hypoalbuminemia.
C. Age.
D. Anemia.
E. Type of suture material.

Many local and systemic factors can contribute to the frequency of wound disruption. The incidence of this complication ranges from 0.5% to 3%. The type of abdominal incision used definitely affects the incidence of subsequent dehiscence. Midline and transverse incisions resist far more bursting force than a paramedian incision.[9] Likewise, the type of suture material used exerts a profound influence on the ultimate integrity of the wound, with materials such as plain and chromic catgut rapidly losing their initial tensile strength, thus leading to an increased incidence of fascial breakdown.[9] The presence of hypoalbuminemia, advanced age, and carcinoma all appear to be associated with an increased incidence of wound dehiscence.[10,11] Anemia, on the other hand, seems to have little effect on the incidence of wound disruptions.[10,11] Other factors, such as significant pulmonary disease leading to postoperative coughing, abdominal distention, and errors in operative technique of closure also play an important role.

ANSWER: D.

10.4. Ten days following a left hepatic lobectomy and splenectomy in a patient with idiopathic thrombocytopenic purpura and an 8-cm hepatic adenoma, the patient has a temperature of 39.4°C, with upper abdominal pain and nausea. The white blood cell count is 18,400 cells/mm^3, the platelet level is 320,000/mm^3, and the amylase content is 30 IU. A chest X ray and a right lateral decubitus abdominal X ray are shown as Figures 10-1 and 10-2. Which of the following tests would not be expected to confirm the diagnosis?

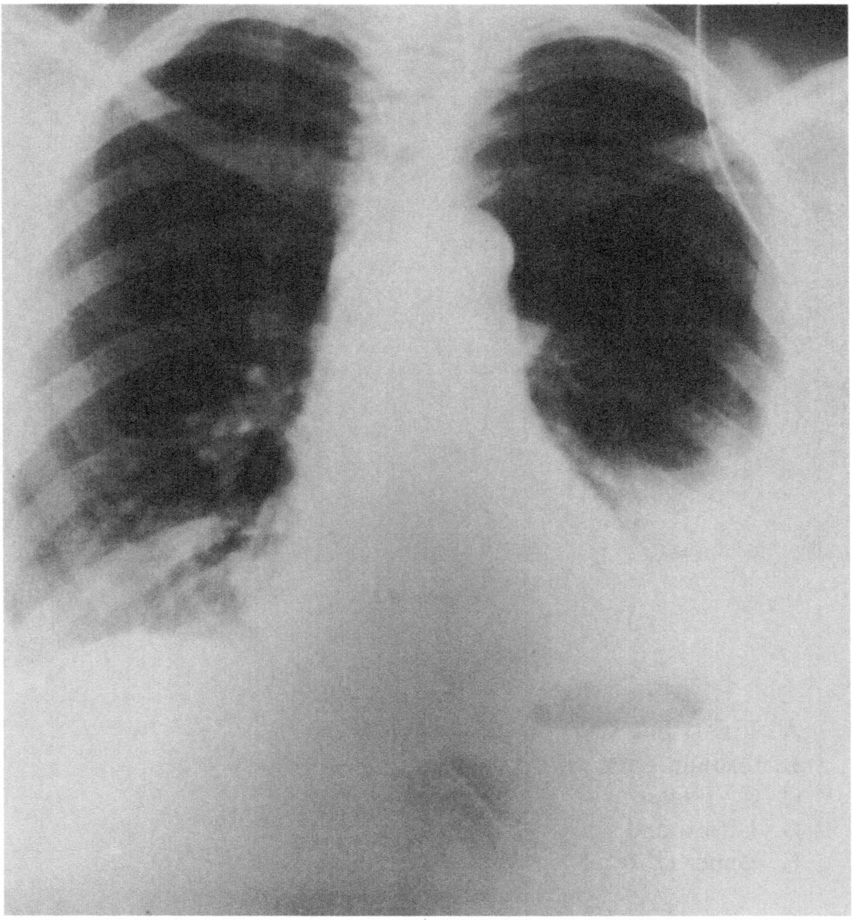

Figure 10-1

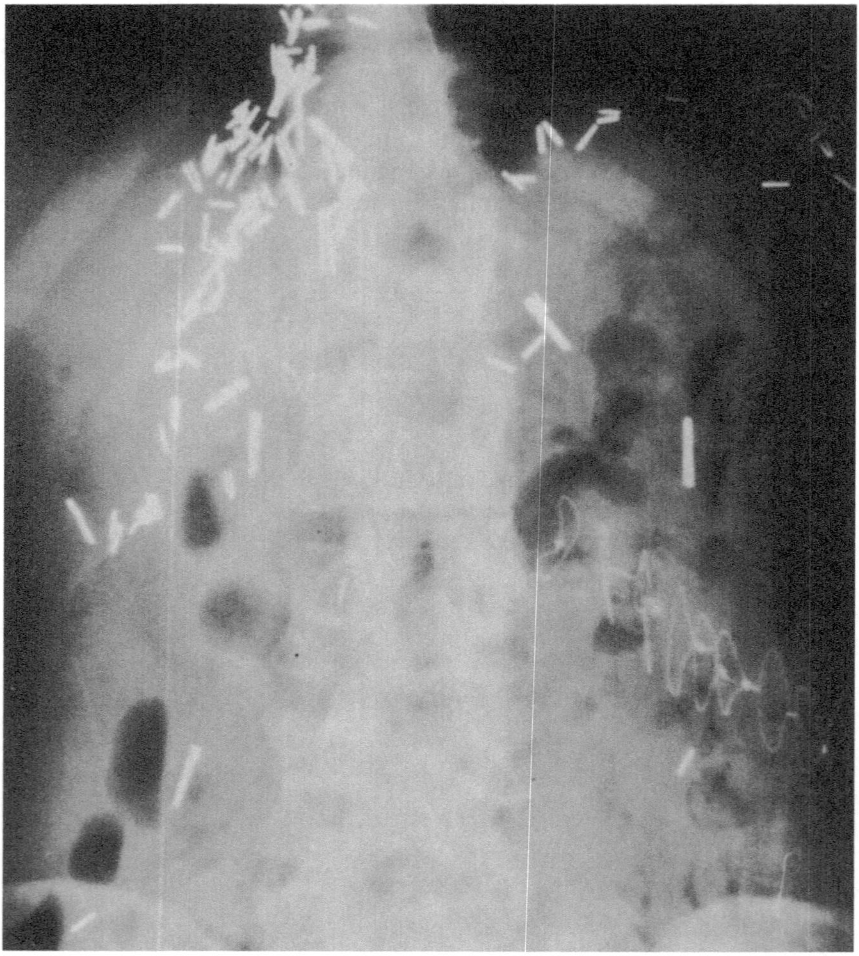

Figure 10-2

A. Liver–lung scan.
B. Gallium scan.
C. CAT scan.
D. Ultrasound.
E. Upper GI tract X ray.

Despite many improvements in patient care and the widespread use of antibiotics, subphrenic abscess following abdominal surgery remains a prominent problem. Over the years, the etiology has changed. Formerly, a ruptured appendix accounted for a large percentage of intra-abdominal abscesses. Now gastric and biliary tract operations account for perhaps half of all intra-abdominal abscesses, with colonic surgery and trauma increasing in importance.[12] Also, the bacteriology has changed with improved capabilities of culturing anaerobic bacteria. Today, *E. coli, Klebsiella, Proteus,* and *Bacteroides* account for most intra-abdominal infections. Another recent trend is the tendency for intra-abdominal abscesses to be multiple, a phenomenon that has obvious therapeutic implications. In one series, over 20% of patients had multiple intra-abdominal abscesses, and failure to appreciate this led to inadequate operations initially.[13]

It must be appreciated that some patients with intra-abdominal abscesses will not manifest fever or leukocytosis or any of the other "classical" signs and symptoms. Therefore, any postoperative patient who is failing to recover in the expected way or who has significant ileus, fever, or abdominal pain should be suspected of harboring an intra-abdominal abscess. The single most valuable diagnostic test in such a patient is abdominal X rays. Additional information can be obtained if these are repeated every few days and changes in gas patterns are noted. In most cases, more sophisticated tests are not necessary, but in case abdominal X rays are insufficient, abdominal CAT scans, ultrasound, gallium scans, and upper GI tract X rays have all proven quite effective.[14–19] In some circumstances, the use of liver–lung scanning can aid in the diagnosis of subphrenic abscesses. Surely, in right subphrenic abscesses, an increased space can be noted between the lung and liver corresponding to the abscess. In some cases of left-sided abscesses the splenic image will be seen to be displaced downward.[20] However, in the patient presented, the abscess is on the left side and the spleen is surgically absent, therefore this test would not be expected to be useful in this situation.

ANSWER: A.

10.5. A 42-year-old woman undergoes an abdominal hysterectomy for extensive endometriosis that necessitates excision of the terminal ileum and the cecum, with primary anastomosis. Seven days postoperatively, fecal material is noted to pass per vagina. A Foley catheter is inserted through the vaginal cuff, and a sinogram is taken; it is shown as Figure 10-3. The patient is afebrile, with a white blood cell count of 11,200 cells/ mm^3. During the first day, output from the vagina is 750 ml. Treatment should consist of:

A. Transvaginal oversewing of the vaginal cuff.
B. Institution of an elemental diet.
C. Institution of total parenteral nutrition.
D. Institution of a blenderized diet.
E. Celiotomy with excision of the fistula and reanastomosis of the intestine.

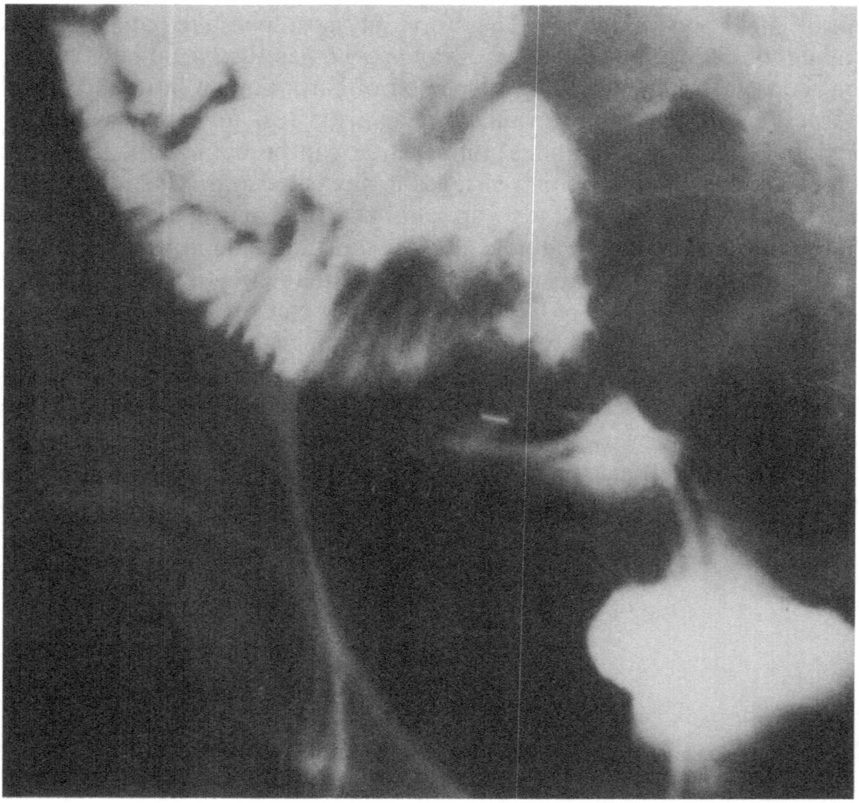

Figure 10-3

This patient clearly has an anastomotic breakdown with a small enterovaginal fistula. Most fistulas follow abdominal surgery, and many can be managed nonoperatively. Primary fistulas, on the other hand, occur in the presence of intra-abdominal carcinoma, inflammatory bowel disease, foreign bodies, or radiation therapy and will generally require operative closure.[21] When a fistula becomes evident, numerous steps must be taken if the patient is to survive. Intensive fluid and electrolyte replacement, along with blood and colloid, should be begun immediately and the infection treated by both providing adequate drainage for the fecal material and using antibiotics if necessary. Skin care is important, as the digestive enzymes will rapidly cause severe skin excoriation if allowed to remain in contact with the skin. Diagnostic studies should then be carried out with injections of water-soluble contrast material into the fistula or sinus tracts, and with upper and lower GI tract barium studies if needed. The GI tract should be defunctionalized by inserting a nasogastric tube, and then provision should be made for supplying adequate amounts of nutrition by the placement of a subclavian venous catheter and the institution of total parenteral nutrition. Utilizing this regimen, a certain number of external fistulas can be expected to close spontaneously. In one large study that compared fistula closure rates before and after the utilization of hyperalimentation, an 11% mortality rate and a 32% fistula closure rate were noted regardless of whether parenteral nutrition was utilized or not.[22] Other studies have shown similar closure rates, but have noted that in certain cases closure will be unlikely and therefore operation may be undertaken at an early stage.[23] Such situations as distal intestinal obstruction, intra-abdominal abscess, and lack of intestinal continuity at the site of the fistula all would preclude spontaneous closure. Other series of patients, on the other hand, have found far more favorable closure rates. In one study of 61 external fistulas, only 6.5% of patients died and 73% of the fistulas closed after an average of 38 days of total parenteral nutrition.[24]

In some patients with low output or distal small intestinal fistulas, elemental diets may be substituted for total parenteral nutrition with good success. The criterion for using these diets should be that they do not markedly increase fistula output.[25,26] If operation is indicated, excision and reanastomosis is the treatment of choice. Excision of the fistulous tract alone is unlikely to succeed and should not be attempted.[22]

ANSWER: C.

10.6. Which of the following statements regarding postoperative ileus is true?

A. It cannot be prevented.
B. It is caused by small intestinal hypomotility.
C. It prohibits immediate feedings following celiotomy.
D. Pharmacologic treatment is successful in most cases.
E. Effective gastric decompression will usually enable jejunal feedings to be begun immediately postoperatively.

Although varying degrees of abdominal distention regularly follow celiotomy, until recently, little has been known about its etiology, prevention, and treatment. In the past, recommendations for treatment have ranged from throwing ice water on the groin to having the patient swallow iron filings and then passing a magnet rhythmically over his abdomen. Various studies have shown that the stomach is relatively inactive postoperatively and becomes distended from swallowed air, leading to decreased motility and stasis. Normal activity returns within 48 hr. Colonic hypomotility, however, can persist for 3–5 days.[27] Small intestinal activity, on the other hand continues nearly unchanged both during and after celiotomy, with normal motility, propulsion, and absorption taking place.[28–31] Indeed, normal small intestinal motility has been documented postoperatively, even following significant peritonitis.[32]

In view of these data, many authorities have questioned the routine use of nasogastric decompression following celiotomy, and many series of patients have been published in whom this procedure was omitted with no adverse consequences. Others have gone a step further in an attempt to obviate the inevitable catabolic state that follows cessation of oral intake and have recommended immediate liquid jejunal feedings in the postoperative period.[30,31] This can be accomplished by insertion of a jejunostomy tube at the time of operation or through the use of a special double lumen tube that simultaneously decompresses the stomach while allowing instillation of liquid into the duodenum.[30]

ANSWER: E.

10.7. A 56-year-old man undergoes cholecystectomy and common bile duct exploration for acute cholecystitis and ascending cholangitis. Three days postoperatively, his temperature is 39.4°C, with a pulse rate of 120 and a respiratory rate of 26/min. His blood pressure is 130/70. Breath sounds are decreased over the right lower lung. A white blood cell count is 14,200 cells/mm^3, and a chest X ray is shown as Figure 10-4. The most likely diagnosis is:

A. Pulmonary embolus.
B. Atelectasis.
C. Aspiration pneumonia.
D. Bronchial pneumonia.
E. Right subphrenic abscess.

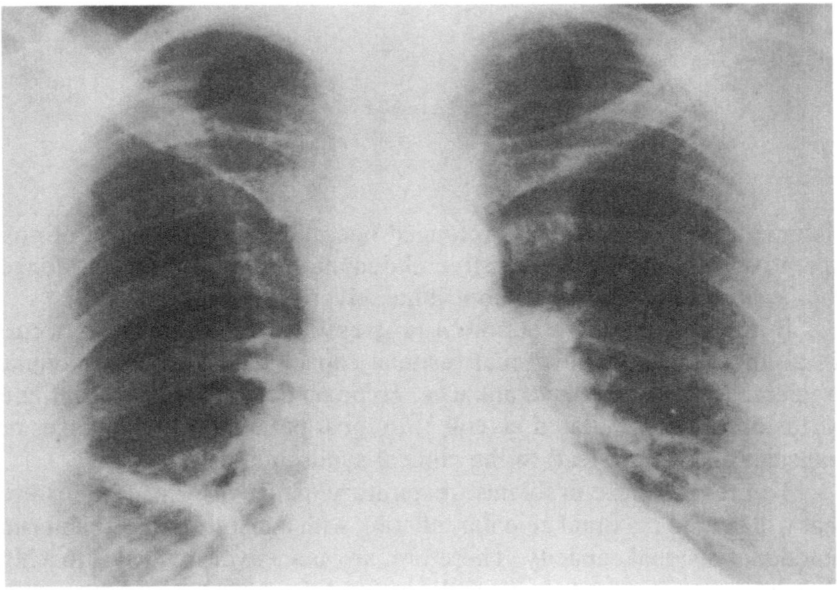

Figure 10-4

Depending upon definition, pulmonary complications occur in perhaps half of all postoperative celiotomy patients. The causes are multifactorial, but it is recognized that painful incisions, especially in the upper

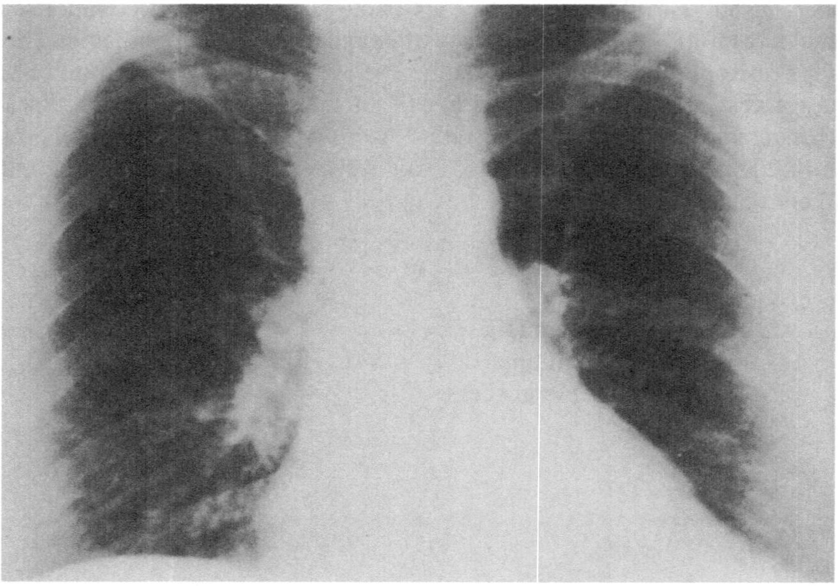

Figure 10-5

abdomen, are contributory. Prolonged operation, excessive use of postoperative narcotics, postoperative abdominal distention, and prolonged supine positioning may also contribute adversely.

In the postoperative period, a progressive alveolar collapse occurs. Total lung capacity, functional residual capacity, and residual volumes are decreased, as is lung compliance. Hypoxia occurs owing to continued perfusion of nonventilated alveoli.[33] In most patients, these changes are transient and do not lead to the clinical syndrome of atelectasis.

To prevent these problems, respiratory maneuvers must be fostered that will lead to maximal alveolar inflation with a maintenance of a normal functional residual capacity. Therefore, any maneuver that leads to a high alveolar inflating pressure carried out for a long period of time will be maximally effective. Until recent years, intermittent positive pressure breathing (IPPB) was the standard treatment utilized extensively in this country, at an estimated total annual cost of $400,000,000.[34] However, many careful studies have shown that IPPB as commonly practiced is not only ineffectual in bringing about optimal pulmonary ventilation but is also potentially dangerous.[33,34] The reasons for the general failure of IPPB are twofold. In general, the inflating volume is not measured, and the volume is controlled by the peak airway pressure. Therefore, as the functional residual capacity decreases, the volume required to reach a given pressure decreases, leading to more shallow ventilation. Additionally, supervision during IPPB treatments is usually suboptimal, thus minimizing the potential for benefit to the patient. It has been subsequently determined that maximal inhalations, as currently practiced by incentive spirometry, quickly and inexpensively overcome the major pathophysiology involved in atelectasis, and both prevent and cure the problem promptly when utilized. In most institutions, the use of incentive spirometry has completely replaced IPPB in recent years. Figure 10-5 discloses the chest X ray on the same patient 18 hr after institution of intensive incentive spirometry; the previously noted plate of atelectasis in the right lower lung field is completely resolved.

ANSWER: B.

10.8. Which of the following is the most important factor in the evolution of adult respiratory distress syndrome (ARDS)?

A. Hypovolemic shock.
B. Massive blood transfusion.
C. Oxygen toxicity.
D. Overhydration.
E. Sepsis.

The syndrome of prolonged pulmonary failure complicating severe illness is a relatively recently recognized syndrome. Many synonyms are used to describe this entity. Among these are shock lung, stiff lung syndrome, and posttraumatic pulmonary insufficiency. In general, the syndrome occurs several days after severe wounding or hypotension and is manifested by evidence of increasing respiratory difficulty with dyspnea, hypocapnia, and hypoxemia, culminating in the need for ventilatory assistance with ever increasing concentrations of oxygen to maintain P_{O_2} levels. The chest X ray that was initially normal begins to disclose diffuse infiltrates, the level of consciousness deteriorates, and evidence of sepsis usually becomes evident. Terminal hypoxia ensues despite high levels of inspired oxygen concentration, and at autopsy, the lungs are wet and heavy with fluid. Histologic changes of interstitial edema, focal interstitial and alveolar hemorrhages, and hyperplasia of the alveolar lining cells is evident.[35]

This syndrome is found in patients who have suffered severe trauma, hemorrhage, or massive transfusion. It is also seen in the presence of oxygen toxicity and fat embolism. However, the dominant factor in the causation of ARDS appears to be sepsis. It has been shown both clinically and experimentally that all of the other common etiologies alone fail to produce this syndrome, but when combined with sepsis invariably do so.[36,37]

The diagnosis of this condition is made on clinical grounds, with confirmation by serial chest X rays and measurements of the derangements in pulmonary function. In most cases, a decreased P_{O_2} is noted, with increased pulmonary artery pressures, decreased pulmonary venous admixture, and increased pulmonary shunting. Pulmonary capillary wedge pressures are often unchanged.[38]

The treatment of established posttraumatic pulmonary insufficiency depends upon the control of sepsis, ventilatory support, and careful fluid monitoring to avoid overhydration. Monitoring of pulmonary function with a Swan–Ganz catheter is essential, as it allows measurements of pulmonary artery pressures, pulmonary venous admixture, pulmonary shunt, and cardiac output. The provision of positive end expiratory pressure (PEEP) has also proven essential in maintaining oxygenation in these patients. With careful Swan–Ganz monitoring, PEEP can be used to increase pulmonary venous admixture and decrease pulmonary shunting. Contrary to some data, high levels of PEEP seem to have no adverse effects on cardiac output, nor do they lead to pulmonary oxygen toxicity.[39]

ANSWER: E.

10.9. A 32-year-old man requires continuous ventilatory support with 14-cm H_2O positive end expiratory pressure (PEEP) 10 days following celiotomy for a gunshot wound. At that time, injuries to the liver, stomach, and small intestine were repaired, and the perforated colon was exteriorized as a colostomy. The patient has a temperature of 38.5°C with periodic chills. His white blood cell count is 22,000 cells/mm^3. Suddenly, he develops a pulse of 130 associated with restlessness. Breath sounds are barely audible bilaterally, and there is hyperresonance over the left chest; P_{O_2} is 47 torr; P_{CO_2} is 64 torr. A chest X ray is shown as Figure 10-6. The patient should have immediate:

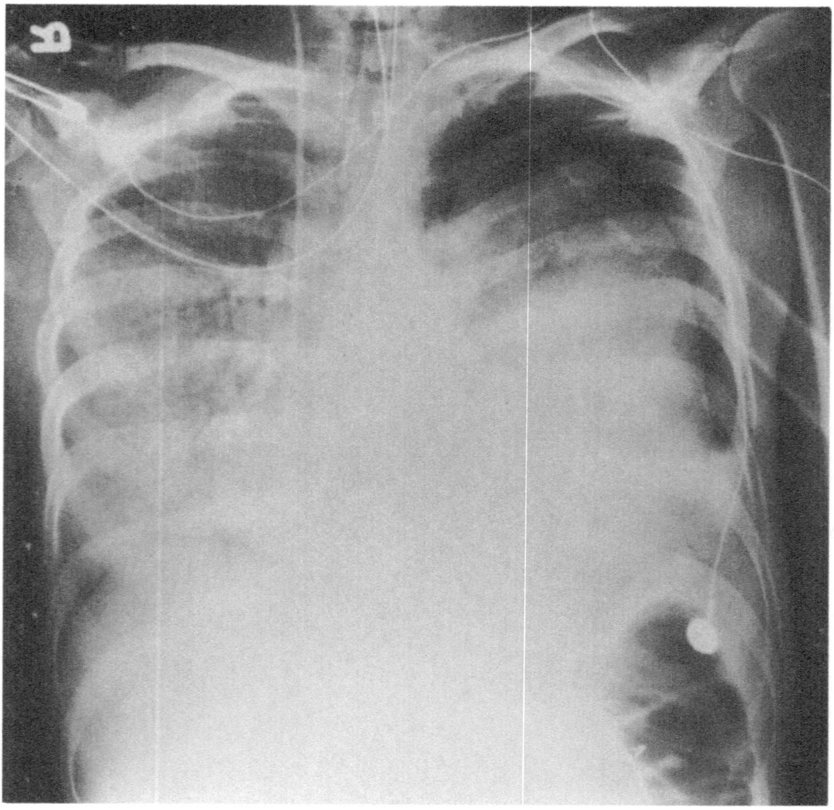

Figure 10-6

A. Increase in the level of PEEP to 20 cm H_2O.
B. Decrease in the level of PEEP to 8 cm H_2O.
C. Insertion of a Swan–Ganz pulmonary artery catheter.
D. Left tube thoracostomy.
E. Cessation of PEEP and institution of intermittent mandatory ventilation.

This patient is suffering from adult respiratory distress syndrome requiring continuous ventilatory support and high levels of PEEP to maintain oxygenation. The sudden deterioration of such a patient is often caused by the development of a pneumothorax. The clinical picture of such an event is that of a sudden and dramatic onset of tachycardia, decreased breath sounds, tachypnea, and hypotension, with a decreased P_{O_2} and increased P_{CO_2}. Subcutaneous emphysema may be present, but the mere presence of subcutaneous emphysema does not mean that a pneumothorax is present, as many patients on high levels of PEEP will manifest this finding.[39] In a series of 74 pneumothoraces complicating prolonged ventilation, the right and left sides were affected equally, and the percent of collapse was variable. Seventy-one of 74 patients, however, had tension pneumothoraces.[40] In this series, 16% of the patients died. The incidence of this complication in patients on continuous ventilatory support ranges from 12% of those patients who are not receiving PEEP to 18% of those patients receiving PEEP.[41]

Treatment of a patient with a suspected pneumothorax secondary to the administration of PEEP must be immediate tube thoracostomy. Altering the level of PEEP or performing such diagnostic maneuvers as a chest X ray or insertion of a Swan–Ganz catheter could well prove fatal, as the diagnosis must be a clinical one and rapid treatment must be instituted.

ANSWER: D.

10.10. A 42-year-old man undergoes a proctocolectomy for a toxic megacolon complicating ulcerative colitis. Six days postoperatively, his temperature is 38.6°C, with a white blood cell count of 16,200 cells/mm^3. His BUN is noted to be 86 mg%, with a creatinine level of 6.2 mg%. Urinary output for the previous 24 hr was 2400 ml; urinary sodium level is 50 mEq/liter. Urine specific gravity is 1.009, with an osmolality of 270; serum osmolality is 285. The preoperative intravenous pyelogram (IVP) was normal. The most likely diagnosis is:

A. Diabetes insipidus.
B. Inappropriate ADH secretion.
C. Nonoliguric acute renal failure.
D. Postrenal failure.
E. Prerenal azotemia.

In a postoperative patient who is found to be azotemic, the usual difficulty is differentiating nonoliguric acute renal failure from dehydration and prerenal azotemia. For this reason, careful recording of daily weight and intake and output figures is essential. In the patient presented, there is current evidence for sepsis, and it can be presumed that the patient previously might have suffered from hypovolemia, both of which are known to predispose to the development of renal failure.

In renal failure, the urine-to-plasma osmolality ratio is usually less than 1.1:1.0, whereas in prerenal azotemia, the ratio is usually greater than 2:1. The urinary sodium concentration is usually greater than 40 mEq/liter in renal failure and usually less than 20 mEq/liter in prerenal azotemia.[42] Also in prerenal azotemia, the serum BUN-to-serum creatinine ratio is usually greater than 19:1, and the urinary specific gravity is generally greater than 1.018. The patient does not manifest the excessive dilute urine excretion that would be expected in diabetes insipidus, and he obviously does not have inappropriate antidiuretic hormone secretion, in which the urinary outputs are minimal. The presence of a normal IVP preoperatively renders postoperative postrenal obstruction less likely.

The treatment of a patient with established renal failure is mainly supportive, especially in the high-output variety, in which spontaneous recovery is the rule. In oliguric cases, nutritional needs must be attended to and often peritoneal dialysis or hemodialysis will be necessary to combat the complications of fluid overload, acidosis, and hyperkalemia. Sepsis is a frequent concomitant of acute renal failure in the postoperative patient, and its source must be vigorously sought after and eradicated if the renal failure is to resolve. Despite recent advances, the mortality rate of patients with postoperative renal failure remains in excess of 50%.[42–45]

ANSWER: C.

10.11. A 62-year-old previously healthy man undergoes an emergency vagotomy and antrectomy for a bleeding duodenal ulcer. Eighteen units of blood are used, and the patient is hypotensive for 1 hr preoperatively. Halothane is utilized for the operation, and a Penrose drain is placed adjacent to the duodenal stump. Five days postoperatively, no fluid is exiting from the drain site, and the drain is removed. At that time, the following is noted: bilirubin, 19 mg%; SGOT, 220 U/ml; and alkaline phosphatase, 90 IU. His temperature is 39.8°C, and his white blood cell count is 23,000 cells/mm^3. The most likely diagnosis is:

A. Halothane hepatitis.
B. Transected common bile duct.
C. Hepatic failure due to sepsis.
D. Transfusion reaction.
E. Cirrhosis.

The appearance of jaundice during the postoperative state may be due to many factors. A modest degree of hyperbilirubinemia may result from transfusions, and this is usually noted within a few days of surgery. Halothane hepatotoxicity is rare, occurring in perhaps 1 out of 10,000 patients who receive this drug.[46] Current evidence points to an inital damage of the hepatocyte followed by a delayed-type hypersensitivity reaction. The onset of jaundice is generally several weeks after exposure to halothane unless the patient has had a prior exposure, in which case the onset may be several days postoperatively. In the patient presented, no previous operations had been performed, making halothane hepatitis in the present circumstance most unlikely.

The patient appears to have an obvious source of sepsis associated with hepatic failure. In such a setting, hepatic failure is noted frequently, especially if the patient has undergone previous operation, massive transfusions, and a period of hypotension. All of the other causes of jaundice are possible, but unlikely. In many cases of common bile duct injury or transection, the operation is noted to be excessively difficult, and there is often a drainage of bile from a drain site. Likewise, there was no other clinical evidence of a severe hemolytic transfusion reaction.

The importance of recognizing that many factors, such as shock, transfusion, operation, and sepsis, can predispose to hepatic failure lies in the necessity of searching for and treating any focus of sepsis postoperatively. In the absence of treatment of the sepsis, most of these patients will die, whereas with resolution of the septic process, a gradual improvement in liver function and also in other organ system dysfunctions, such as renal and pulmonary failure, will occur.[47–49]

ANSWER: C.

10.12. A 60-year-old woman is recovering from a left hemicolectomy and primary anastomosis performed 6 days previously for diverticulitis. She has been febrile since the operation and suddenly has a shaking chill. She complains of low abdominal pain and is noted to be pale and sweaty, with a pulse of 132 and a blood pressure of 90/40. Her temperature is 35.8°C, and her extremities are warm. The white blood cell count is 2400 cells/mm^3. Hematocrit is 40%. Serum electrolytes, BUN, and sugar levels are normal. A microscopic urinalysis and chest X ray are normal. The most likely diagnosis is:

A. Myocardial infarction.
B. Septic shock associated with anastomotic leak.
C. Hypovolemia from inappropriate fluid administration.
D. Acute gastric dilitation.
E. Pulmonary embolus.

In the clinical situation presented, the appearance of a shaking chill preceded by fever and accompanied by low abdominal pain, hypothermia, tachycardia, hypotension, and warm extremities are virtually diagnostic of early gram-negative septicemia. In this instance, this is most likely from a disrupted anastomosis, although other common sources such as urinary tract and intravenous lines should be sought. During the early phases of septic shock, arterial vasodilatation typically predominates, accompanied by an increase in pulse rate and cardiac output and warm extremities. This is subsequently followed by the more typical shock picture, including arterial vasoconstriction, decreased urinary output, and cold extremities. During this later phase, cardiac output is reduced, peripheral arterial resistance is increased, and tissue oxygenation is below normal. Anaerobic cellular metabolism occurs, with characteristic organ dysfunction and elevated blood lactate levels. Several excellent clinical and experimental studies of septic shock are available.[50–53]

Although a myocardial infarction or pulmonary embolus can likewise cause tachycardia and hypotension, the presence of previous fever, a drop in body temperature, and a low white blood cell count all point toward sepsis as the etiology in this instance. Likewise, the normal urinalysis helps in ruling out a urinary tract infection as the source. The treatment of a patient in septic shock includes intensive care monitoring, utilizing a Swan–Ganz pulmonary artery catheter and serial measurements of cardiac output and pulmonary capillary wedge pressures as a guide to restoration of fluid volume. The use of a central venous catheter alone, while suitable in some cases, will provide inaccurate data frequently enough in septic shock that it will not be as useful as a pulmonary artery catheter.[50,54] Volume expansion will increase peripheral perfusion and thus decrease the acidosis. Antibiotics should be administered immediately, and will have to be selected before any culture results are available. In this instance, drugs covering the spectrum of GI tract organisms, including aerobes and anaerobes, are essential. Gentamicin and clindamycin are a suitable choice in this regard. The use of pharmacologic doses of corticosteroids in this setting is quite controversial, but some authorities feel that they may be useful if given early in the course of septic shock. At the very least, there appears to be no short-term hazard in the use of large doses of corticosteroids, and they are therefore recommended.[50,55,56]

Following restoration of intravascular volume, if the patient still manifests evidence of vasoconstriction and oliguria, vasoactive drugs should be employed. In this instance, dopamine would probably be used, as this drug increases myocardial contractability and renal blood flow.

ANSWER: B.

References

1. Halasz, N.A.: Wound infection topical antibiotics: The surgeon's dilemma. *Arch. Surg.* 112:1240, 1977.
2. Cruse, P.J.E., Foord, R.: A five year prospective study of 23,649 surgical wounds. *Arch. Surg.* 107:206, 1973.
3. Seropian, R., Reynolds, B.M.: Wound infections after preoperative depilatory versus razor preparation. *Am. J. Surg.* 121:251, 1971.
4. Raahave, D.: Effect of plastic skin and wound drapes on the density of bacteria in open wounds. *Br. J. Surg.* 63:421, 1976.
5. Chodak, G.W., Plaut, M.E.: Use of systemic antibiotics for prophylaxis in surgery: A critical review. *Arch. Surg.* 112:326, 1977.
6. Evans, C., Pollack, A.V.: The reduction of surgical wound infections by prophylactic parenteral cephaloridine: A controlled clinical trial. *Br. J. Surg.* 60:434, 1973.
7. Stone, H.H., Hooper, C.A., Kolb, L.D., Geheber, C.E., Dawkins, E.J.: Antibiotic prophylaxis in gastric, biliary, and colonic surgery. *Ann. Surg.* 184:443, 1976.
8. Polk, H.C.: Diminished surgical infection by systemic antibiotic administration in potentially contaminated operations. *Surgery* 75:312, 1974.
9. Malt, R.A.: Abdominal incisions, suture and sacrilege. *N. Engl. J. Med.* 297:722, 1977.
10. Alexander, H.C., Prudden, J.F.: The causes of abdominal wound disruption. *Surg. Gynecol. Obstet.* 122:1223, 1966.
11. Schwartz, S.I.: Complications, in Schwartz, S.I. (ed.): *Principles of Surgery,* ed. 3. New York, McGraw–Hill, 1978, p. 496.
12. Wang, S.M.S., Wilson, S.E.: Subphrenic abscess: The new epidemiology. *Arch. Surg.* 112:934, 1977.
13. Halasz, N.A.: Subphrenic abscess: Myths and facts. *J.A.M.A.* 214:724, 1970.
14. Norton, L., Eule, J., Burdick, D.: Accuracy of techniques to detect intraperitoneal abscess. *Surgery* 84:370, 1978.
15. Daffner, R.H., Halber, M.D., Morgan, C.L., Trought, W.S., Thompson, W.M., Rice, R.P.: Computed tomography in the diagnosis of intra-abdominal abscess. *Ann. Surg.* 189:29, 1979.
16. Damron, J.R., Beihn, R.M., Deland, F.H.: Detection of upper abdominal abscesses by radionuclide imaging. *Radiology* 120:131, 1976.
17. Teates, C.D., Hunter, J.G.: Gallium scanning as a screening test for inflammatory lesion. *Radiology* 116:383, 1975.
18. Friday, R.O., Barriga, P., Crummy, A.B.: Detection and localization of intra-abdominal abscesses by diagnostic ultrasound. *Arch. Surg.* 110:335, 1975.
19. Doust, B.D., Doust, V.L.: Ultrasonic diagnosis of abdominal abscess. *Digestive Diseases* 21:569, 1976.
20. White, P.H., Hayes, M., Benfield, J.R.: Combined liver lung scanning in the management of subdiaphragmatic abscesses. *Am. J. Surg.* 124:143, 1972.
21. Halasz, N.A.: Changing patterns in the management of small bowel fistulas. *Am. J. Surg.* 136:61, 1978.
22. Reber, H.A., Roberts, C., Way, L.W., Dunphy, J.E.: Management of external gastrointestinal fistulas. *Ann. Surg.* 188:460, 1978.
23. Aguirre, A., Fischer, J.E., Welch, C.E.: The role of surgery and hyperalimentation in therapy of gastrointestinal–cutaneous fistuale. *Ann. Surg.* 180:393, 1974.
24. Macfadyen, B.V., Dudrick, S.J., Ruberg, R.L.: Management of gastrointestinal fistulas with parenteral hyperalimentation. *Surgery* 74:100, 1973.
25. Rocchio, M.A., Cha, C.M., Haas, K.F., Randall, H.T.: Use of chemically defined diets in the management of patients with high output gastrointestinal cutaneous fistulas. *Am. J. Surg.* 127:148, 1974.

26. Voitk, A.J., Echave, V., Brown, R.A., McArdle, A.H., Gurd, F.N.: Elemental diet in the treatment of fistulas of the alimentary tract. *Surg. Gynecol. Obstet.* 137:68, 1973.
27. Nachlas, M.M., Younis, M.T., Roda, C.P., Wityk, J.J.: Gastrointestinal motility studies as a guide to postoperative management. *Ann. Surg.* 175:510, 1972.
28. Rothnie, N.G., Harper, R.A.K., Catchpole, B.N.: Early postoperative gastrointestinal activity. *Lancet* 2:64, 1963.
29. Noer, T.: Roentgenological transit time through the small intestine in the immediate postoperative period. *Acta Chir. Scand.* 134:577, 1968.
30. Moss, G., Friedman, R.C.: Abdominal decompression: Increased efficiency by esophageal aspiration utilizing a new nasogastric tube. *Am. J. Surg.* 133:225, 1977.
31. Glucksman, D.L., Kalser, M.H., Warren, W.D.: Small intestinal absorption in the immediate postoperative period. *Surgery* 60:1020, 1966.
32. Mishra, N.K., Appert, H.E., Howard, J.M.: Studies of paralytic ileus. *Am. J. Surg.* 129:559, 1975.
33. Bartlett, R.H., Gazzaniga, A.B., Geraghty, T.R.: Respiratory maneuvers to prevent postoperative pulmonary complications: A critical review. *J.A.M.A.* 224:1017, 1973.
34. McConnell, D.H., Maloney, J.V., Buckberg, G.D.: Postoperative intermittent positive-pressure breathing treatments: Physiological considerations. *J. Thorac. Cardiovasc. Surg.* 68:944, 1974.
35. Pardy, B.J., Dudley, H.A.F.: Post-traumatic pulmonary insufficiency. *Surg. Gynecol. Obstet.* 144:259, 1977.
36. Fulton, R.L., Jones, C.E.: The cause of post-traumatic pulmonary insufficiency in man. *Surg. Gynecol. Obstet.* 140:179, 1975.
37. Esrig, B.C., Fulton, R.L.: Sepsis, resuscitated hemorrhagic shock, and "shock lung": An experimental correlation. *Ann. Surg.* 182:218, 1975.
38. Hirsch, E.F., Clarke, J.R., Gomez-Engler, H.E., Clowes, G.H.A.: The lung: Responses to trauma, surgery, and sepsis. *Surg. Clin. North Am.* 56:909, 1976.
39. Kirby, R.R., Downes, J.B., Civetta, J.M., Modell, J.H., Dannemiller, F.J., Klein, E.F., Hodges, M.: High level positive end expiratory pressure (PEEP) in acute respiratory insufficiency. *Chest* 67:156, 1975.
40. Steier, M., Ching, N., Roberts, E.B., Nealon, T.F.: Pneumothorax complicating continuous ventilatory support. *J. Thorac. Cardiovasc. Surg.* 67:17, 1974.
41. Lewis, F.R., Blaisdell, F.W., Schlobohm, R.M.: Incidence and outcome of post-traumatic respiratory failure. *Arch. Surg.* 112:436, 1977.
42. Griffith, G.L., Maull, K.I., Coleman, C., Baehler, R.W.: Acute reversible intrinsic renal failure. *Surg. Gynecol. Obstet.* 146:631, 1978.
43. Baek, S.M., Makabali, G.G., Shoemaker, W.C.: Clinical determinants of survival from postoperative renal failure. *Surg. Gynecol. Obstet.* 140:685, 1975.
44. Casali, R., Simmons, R.L., Najarian, J.S., von Haritizsch, B., Buselmeier, T.J., Kjellstrand, C.M.: Acute renal insufficiency complicating major cardiovascular surgery. *Ann. Surg.* 181:370, 1975.
45. Elmgren, D.T., Cheung, L.Y., Bloomer, A., Maxwell, J.G.: Acute renal failure after abdominal surgery: The importance of sepsis. *Am. J. Surg.* 128:743, 1974.
46. LaMont, J.T., Isselbacher, K.J.: Postoperative jaundice. *N. Engl. J. Med.* 288:305, 1973.
47. Kantrowitz, P.A., Jones, W.A., Greenberger, N.J., Isselbacher, K.J.: Severe postoperative hyperbilirubinemia simulating obstructive jaundice. *N. Engl. J. Med.* 276:591, 1967.
48. Norton, L., Moore, G., Eiseman, B.: Liver failure in the postoperative patient: The role of sepsis and immunologic deficiency. *Surgery* 78:6, 1975.
49. Eley, A., Hargreaves, T., Lambert, H.P.: Jaundice in severe infections. *Br. Med. J.* 2:75, 1965.

50. Shubin, H., Weil, M.H.: Bacterial shock. *J.A.M.A.* 235:421, 1976.
51. MacLean, L.D., Mulligan, W.G., McLean, A.P.H., Duff, J.H.: Patterns of septic shock in man: A detailed study of 56 patients. *Ann. Surg.* 166:543, 1967.
52. Siegel, J.H., Cerra, F.B., Coleman, B., Giovannini, I., Shetye, M., Border, J.R., McMenamy, R.H.: Physiological and metabolic correlations in human sepsis. *Surgery* 86:163, 1979.
53. Baue, A.E., Chaudry, I.H., Wurth, M.A., Sayeed, M.M.: Cellular alterations with shock and ischemia. *Angiology* 25:31, 1974.
54. DeLaurentis, D.A., Hayes, M., Matsumoto, T., Wolferth, C.C.: Does central venous pressure accurately reflect hemodynamic and fluid volume patterns in the critical surgical patient? *Am. J. Surg.* 126:415, 1973.
55. Schumer, W.: Steroids in the treatment of clinical septic shock. *Ann. Surg.* 184:333, 1976.
56. Smith, J.A., Norman, J.N.: Use of glucocorticoids in refractory shock. *Surg. Gynecol. Obstet.* 149:369, 1979.

11
THROMBOEMBOLIC DISEASE

11.1. The most accurate test that can be performed to confirm the presence of a suspected pulmonary embolus is:

A. Arterial blood gases.
B. Ventilation–perfusion lung scan.
C. Pulmonary arteriography.
D. Perfusion lung scan.
E. Electrocardiogram.

Venous thrombosis and its potentially fatal sequela, pulmonary embolus, represent a frequent source of morbidity and mortality in hospitalized populations. Although several British studies would indicate that the incidence of pulmonary emboli is increasing, this has not been noted in this country. In one series of 4600 autopsies, pulmonary emboli were found in 12.3% of all patients.[1] However, it has been repeatedly noted that certain groups are at significantly increased risk when compared to routine hospital populations. Age is a definite risk factor, with the incidence of pulmonary embolus increasing with advancing age. Patients with cancer or cardiac disease are likewise subject to an increased risk. Lastly, patients who have undergone any major abdominal operations or lower limb orthopedic procedures are at high risk.[1,2]

The clinical diagnosis of pulmonary embolism is notoriously difficult, as the signs and symptoms are quite similar to those of other cardiorespiratory disorders. Even in a patient with the classic symptoms of dyspnea, tachypnea, tachycardia, chest pain, hemoptysis, and hypotension, subsequent laboratory evaluation will often not document the presence of a pulmonary embolus. In addition, only a small percentage of patients with documented pulmonary emboli will have clinical evidence of deep venous thrombosis of the legs.[1,2] Because of these problems, a wide variety of tests are routinely performed in the patient suspected of having sustained a pulmonary embolus. The chest X ray is characteristically normal during the acute phase. Pulmonary vascular markings may be decreased in the presence of a massive embolus, but this is inconstant, and therefore the chest X ray is of minimal help, at least until radiologic evidence of pulmonary infarction has occurred days later. The electrocardiogram will show changes in less than a quarter of patients with pulmonary embolus.[2] Likewise, the presence of arterial hypoxia has been thought to correlate strongly with the diagnosis of pulmonary embolus. Unfortunately, many patients who are hospitalized will have a lowered P_{O_2}, and the mere demonstration of this does not indicate that a pulmonary embolus is present. Even the finding of P_{O_2} levels greater than 90 torr does not definitely rule out the presence of a pulmonary embolus.[3] Perfusion lung scanning utilizing the intravenous injection of radioisotopes likewise has serious limitations. A correlation with a recent chest X ray should always be made, as asthma, emphysema, and pneumonia can all produce perfusion defects. A negative pulmonary scan, however, will be quite significant in excluding the presence of a pulmonary embolus, whereas a positive scan will require much more careful interpretation. Recently, the addition of inhalation Xenon scanning to standard perfusion lung scans has given additional aid in diagnosing pulmonary emboli. Ideally, a pulmonary embolus would be manifest by an area of decreased perfusion but normal ventilation utilizing the ^{133}Xe ventilation scan. However, since pulmonary emboli may also produce bronchoconstriction, thereby reducing the amount of air delivered to the embolized portion of the lung, even this can be misleading.[2,3]

In view of all the preceding limitations, it is obvious that definite anatomic information concerning the pulmonary arterial circulation can be gained only by direct study via a pulmonary arteriogram. This undoubtedly represents the most accurate method in the diagnosis of pulmonary embolism and should be utilized much more frequently than is currently practiced in most hospitals. The morbidity is minimal, and the positive or negative results obtained enable the clinician to proceed with nearly absolute confidence to withhold or administer anticoagulants.[2,3]

ANSWER: C.

11.2. A 58-year-old woman with a previous coronary artery bypass is 5 days postoperative following a radical hysterectomy for uterine carcinoma. While walking in the hall, she becomes dyspneic and weak. On examination, she is pale and sweaty. Her pulse is 130, with a blood pressure of 110/60. Examination of the heart is normal. Wheezes are heard bilaterally on auscultation of the lungs. A chest X ray and pulmonary arteriogram are shown as Figures 11-1 and 11-2. Treatment should consist of:

A. Incentive spirometery.
B. Intermittent positive pressure breathing (IPPB).
C. Pulmonary embolectomy.
D. Intravenous heparin.
E. Chest physiotherapy.

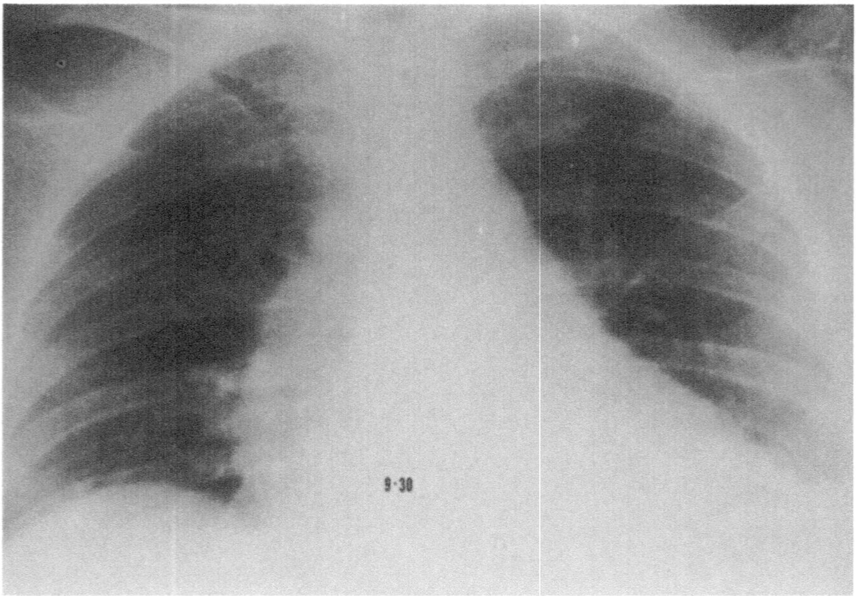

Figure 11-1

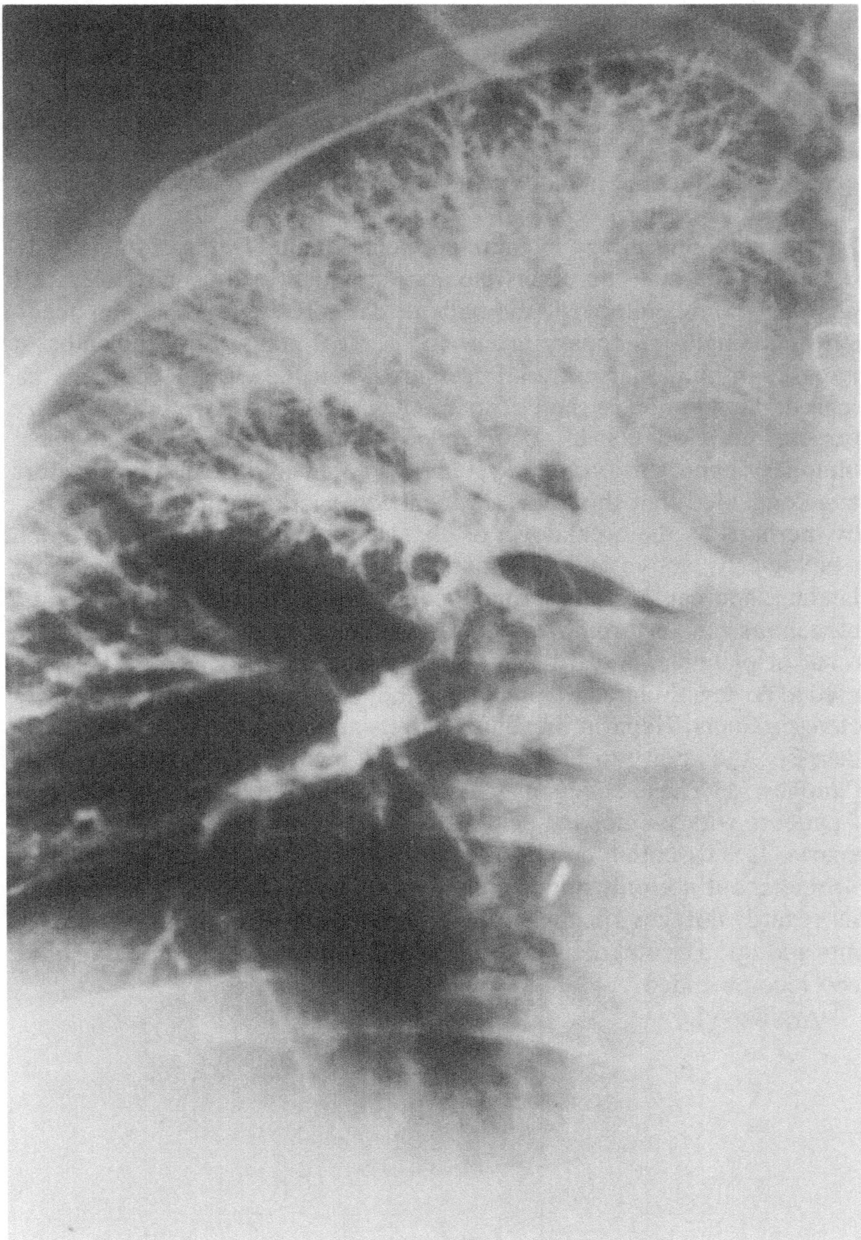

Figure 11-2

This patient's clinical picture is compatible with that of an acute pulmonary embolus, and this is confirmed by the pulmonary angiogram, which discloses a massive right pulmonary arterial blockage. Incentive spirometery, IPPB, and chest physiotherapy, while perhaps helpful for the patient with atelectasis, would be of no benefit in such a patient. Likewise, there is no indication for emergency pulmonary embolectomy, because the patient is hemodynamically stable. The treatment of choice is intravenous heparin.

The pathophysiology in acute pulmonary embolism is of interest. In the clinical situation, an otherwise normal patient will usually tolerate a pneumonectomy quite well, and patients can tolerate total balloon occlusion of a single pulmonary artery for several hours with only modest increases in pulmonary arterial pressure when the cardiac output is increased.[2] In addition to the effects of mechanical blockage of pulmonary arteries, reflex effects do occur and can be manifested by tachypnea, pulmonary hypertension, and systemic hypotension. Some investigators have concluded that this reflex bronchoconstriction is mediated humorally, perhaps by the breakdown of platelets, which are known to be rich in biologically active amines. For instance, serotonin is liberated from platelets, and can produce bronchoconstriction. In animal experiments, autogenous venous thrombi that are embolized to the lungs rapidly acquire a coat of platelets, and if these are examined microscopically, they are noted to be degranulated, implying that they had released their biologically active products. Heparin, in addition to its anticoagulant properties, also possesses the ability to prevent this breakdown of platelets and release of amines.[2,4,5] These effects may account for the often dramatic response of patients with pulmonary emboli to the intravenous administration of heparin. It is essential, however, that the dosage of heparin be sufficient to bring about not only anticoagulation but also platelet stabilization. In this regard, dosages ranging from an immediate dose of 10,000–15,000 units and up to a total daily dose of 60,000 units during the first day have been recommended.[4]

ANSWER: D.

11.3. A 48-year-old woman is 5 days postoperative following a radical hysterectomy for uterine cancer. While walking in the hall, she becomes dyspneic and weak. On examination, she is pale and sweaty. Her temperature is 37.2°C; her pulse is 130, with a blood pressure of 110/60. Examination of the heart is normal. Breath sounds are distant bilaterally. Arterial blood gases disclose a P_{O_2} of 64 torr and a P_{CO_2} of 38 torr. An ECG is normal. A chest X ray and a pulmonary angiogram are shown as Figures 11-3 and 11-4. Treatment should consist of:

A. Pulmonary embolectomy.
B. Intravenous heparin.
C. Incentive spirometry.
D. Chest physiotherapy.
E. Supportive care only (oxygen by mask, analgesics).

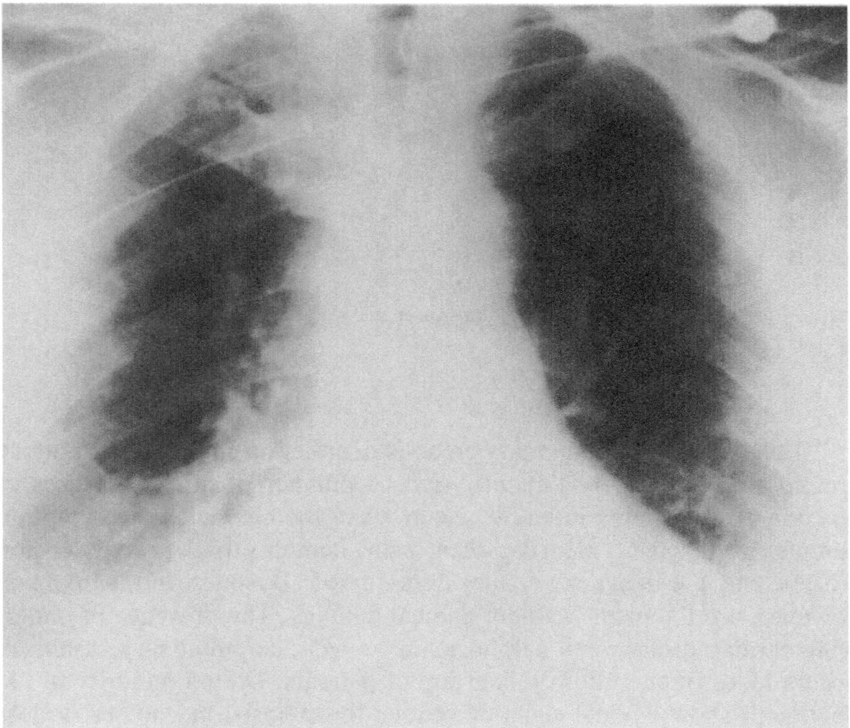

Figure 11-3

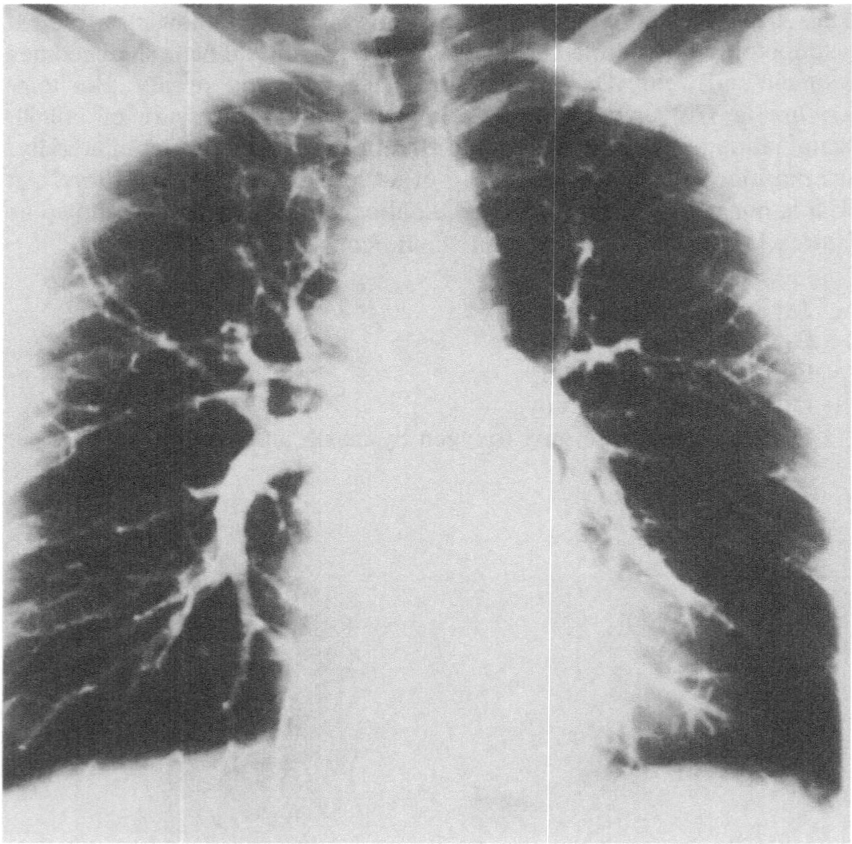

Figure 11-4

The diagnosis of pulmonary embolism, either on clinical or laboratory grounds, is notoriously difficult, since a number of other disorders of postoperative patients mimic it. Even when the characteristic symptom complex of dyspnea, pleuritic chest pain, hemoptysis, and hypotension are present, the diagnosis cannot be assumed. Dyspnea and tachypnea, however, are the most frequent clinical findings. The presence of underlying cardiac disease is a helpful guide as well, as pulmonary embolism occurs more frequently in this group of patients. Only a minority of patients will show clinical signs of venous thrombosis; in one series, less than one third of 1000 patients with documented pulmonary embolism had such leg signs, consisting of differences in leg size, leg pain, and calf tenderness.[2] In another recent study attempting to correlate clinical signs and the presence of pulmonary embolism, it was shown that tachycardia, tachypnea, and the P_{CO_2} had some discriminatory value in diagnosing patients with pulmonary embolism. In contrast, clinical evidence of deep venous thrombosis, P_{O_2}, chest X rays, and cardiograms were not helpful.[6]

Pulmonary scanning utilizing the intravenous injection of radioisotopes allows delineation of the pulmonary arterial distribution within the lungs, and theoretically at least, should demonstrate most major perfusion defects. The drawback to perfusion lung scanning, however, is that these defects are nonspecific, and lesions such as pneumonitis, atelectasis, bullae, or neoplasms may appear similar to pulmonary emboli on scanning. Classically, it has been assumed that a normal chest X ray and an abnormal perfusion scan gave a high degree of probability that a pulmonary embolus was present. However, this is not the case.[2,3] The recent addition of combined ventilation–perfusion scanning utilizing the inhalation of ^{133}Xe has proven to be an additional aid in interpreting perfusion scans. Ideally, a patient with a pulmonary embolus would be expected to have a defect on perfusion scanning but none on inhalation scanning. However, this ideal is unrealized sufficiently commonly that the only way to definitely diagnose pulmonary embolism is by pulmonary angiography.[2,3,6] Earlier fears concerning the safety of this technique have proven unwarranted, and it can be performed with minimal morbidity.

In the patient presented, the chest X ray, and pulmonary arteriogram are normal, thus effectively ruling out the presence of pulmonary embolism. Since the patient is afebrile and has no clinical evidence of atelectasis, supportive care only is indicated.

ANSWER: E.

11.4. In which of the following patients with a major pulmonary embolus is vena caval interruption not indicated?

A. A 50-year-old man with hypotension improved by vasopressors.
B. A 50-year-old man admitted 4 days previously with a bleeding duodenal ulcer.
C. A 60-year-old woman in refractory shock who is scheduled for an emergency pulmonary embolectomy.
D. A 48-year-old woman whose platelet count is $40,000/mm^3$ after 5 days of heparin therapy.
E. A 60-year-old man who has had a documented pulmonary embolus while receiving full therapeutic doses of heparin.

While it is recognized that some pulmonary emboli may originate as mural thrombi in the right side of the heart, the vast majority stem from thrombosis in the lower extremities. Therefore, the concept of inferior venal caval interruption has proven appealing in the attempt to prevent pulmonary emboli. Patients with a contraindication to heparin administration, such as those with a bleeding duodenal ulcer or active ulcerative colitis, should be considered for caval interruption, as should those who have sustained heparin-induced thrombocytopenia making further administration of heparin hazardous.[7,8] Patients who have had recurrent embolization while on full therapeutic doses of heparin should likewise receive caval interruption, as should all of those patients who are undergoing pulmonary embolectomy. It should be understood that the mainstay of treatment for a patient with a pulmonary embolus is adequate heparinization, with caval interruption utilized for patients only as previously outlined.

Once the decision to interrupt the vena cava has been made, numerous methods are available. Literally hundreds of papers have been written concerning the relative merits of ligation of the inferior vena cava versus partial plication.[9] The incidence of recurrent embolization and subsequent postoperative leg swelling have been compared for these two methods, and in many instances they are similar, thus providing no clear advantage to either method. Recently, several methods of introducing caval interruption devices have been described that utilize the insertion of the device through the femoral or jugular vein.[10–12]

One possible disadvantage of vena caval ligation results from the dilatation of other venous collaterals such as the lumbar veins or the ovarian veins in females, thus providing an alternate pathway for recurrent emboli.[13] Because of this, some authorities have advocated ligation of the ovarian veins in females. Others have denied that this is a frequent enough complication to warrant the additional surgery.[14]

At the other extreme are those authorities who feel that virtually every recurrent embolus is due to inadequate heparinization and that with closer attention to the details and dosage of heparin administration, the indications for caval interruption will be very few.[15] Another, and somewhat controversial role for caval interruption has been as a prophylactic treatment in those patients undergoing major abdominal surgery thought to predispose to a high incidence of pulmonary embolism. This has been carried out at the same time as the celiotomy with an alleged reduction in subsequent pulmonary embolization and only minimal side effects.[16,17]

ANSWER: A.

11.5. A 23-year-old woman who is taking birth control pills collapses at home and is rapidly transported to the emergency room. Her pulse is 160 and her blood pressure is 50/0. Her abdomen is soft and nontender. A chest X ray discloses no vascular markings bilaterally. Treatment with fluids and vasopressors brings about no change in her vital signs in one half hour. Treatment at this time should consist of:

A. Pulmonary arteriography and pulmonary embolectomy if a massive pulmonary embolus is noted.
B. Large doses of heparin.
C. Fibrinolytic therapy.
D. Pulmonary embolectomy with extracorporeal circulation.
E. Pulmonary embolectomy without extracorporeal circulation.

The key to management of this patient rests with the rapid clinical assessment of her condition and an appreciation of the high likelihood of rapid death unless definitive treatment is immediately undertaken. In an otherwise healthy young woman, the presence of refractory shock in the absence of any evidence of blood loss raises the possibility of a massive pulmonary embolus. The history of taking birth control pills further substantiates this impression, because of the known increased association with thrombotic problems in users of these medications. Immediate treatment with fluids and vasopressors have brought about no improvement in her condition, and death is imminent. Under less critical circumstances, pulmonary arteriography for confirmation of the embolus would be suitable. However, in the situation presented, the added hours this procedure would entail are contraindicated. The patient must be operated on immediately, utilizing extracorporeal circulation. In the past, embolectomy without extracorporeal circulation, as first performed by Trendelenburg in 1908, has been attempted, but most series of patients treated by this means have very high mortality rates associated with this operation in the absence of cardiopulmonary bypass.[2,18]

Attempts at anticoagulation or fibrinolytic therapy in this critically ill patient are probably contraindicated, although there are authorities who maintain that any patient who survives long enough to arrive in the operating room for a pulmonary embolectomy might well have survived without the surgery, whereas those patients who truly require the surgery probably do not live long enough to get to the operating room. While this controversy can obviously not be settled to everyone's satisfaction, it is clear that there are many patients in an agonal situation from a massive pulmonary embolus who have been saved by prompt embolectomy, and, therefore, this operation should continue to be used in carefully selected critically ill patients.

ANSWER: D.

11.6. Fibrinolytic agents (streptokinase and urokinase):

A. Are ineffective in treating pulmonary emboli.
B. Are ineffective in treating deep venous thrombosis of the legs.
C. Are useful in the treatment of postoperative deep venous thrombosis.
D. Are associated with a greater incidence of bleeding complications than is heparin.
E. Do not lower pulmonary artery pressure in patients with an acute pulmonary embolus.

Streptokinase and urokinase are fibrinolytic activators and exert their effect by converting plasminogen into plasmin, the active fibrinolytic enzyme. Streptokinase is an enzyme produced by group C beta hemolytic streptococci. Urokinase is derived from human urine through an elaborate and quite expensive process.

Both agents have been studied in a wide variety of thrombotic disorders and have been found to be quite effective. In the patient with an acute pulmonary embolus, the administration of fibrinolytic agents brings about a prompt resolution of the angiographically demonstrated clot and an improvement in cardiopulmonary function within several hours. Significant reductions in right atrial, right ventricular, and pulmonary artery pressures are noted.[19,20] There is still no agreement, however, as to the superiority of this form of treatment over emergency pulmonary embolectomy in a patient with a massive pulmonary embolus with hypotension.

Thrombolytic therapy has been likewise successful in treating patients with deep venous thrombosis. Rapid clinical resolution is generally noted, and subsequent venograms have demonstrated high venous patency rates, especially when treatment was begun early after the onset of the thrombosis.[19–21]

The fibrinolytic state produced by these drugs interferes with normal hemostasis. Therefore, many patients will manifest contraindiations to fibrinolytic therapy. A generalized bleeding disorder, an operation within the previous 10 days, severe hypertension, active gastrointestinal ulceration, and recent cerebrovascular accidents are all considered contraindications. In general, bleeding complications have been much more frequent after fibrinolytic therapy than with heparin, but many of these complications have been rather minor bleeding from venous and arterial puncture sites. However, in several major trials utilizing these agents, numerous patients were withdrawn from the study because of major bleeding complications and often required subsequent transfusions.[20]

ANSWER: D.

11.7. The incidence of deep venous thrombosis of the legs cannot reliably be reduced in postoperative general surgery patients by:

A. Administration of Coumadin.
B. Administration of low doses of heparin.
C. Administration of Dextran.
D. External pneumatic compression stockings.
E. Early ambulation postoperatively.

Despite numerous published articles, many of the evangelical variety, that attest to the dire consequences of deep venous thrombosis and subsequent pulmonary embolism, there is no universal agreement as to how important a clinical problem these complications represent. On the one hand are studies that show extremely high rates of pulmonary embolism, ranging from 5% to 12%.[22,2] However, these studies have looked at all hospital deaths, including both medical and surgical patients. Other studies have shown an extremely low incidence of fatal pulmonary embolus postoperatively. One multi-institution restrospective study disclosed a 0.2% incidence of fatal pulmonary embolism in over 300,000 major surgical procedures performed over a 10-year period.[23] Also, the largest study of minidose heparin published to date, although noting a decreased incidence of fatal pulmonary embolism in treated patients, still had only a 0.5% incidence in the control group of untreated patients.[24]

Despite this debate, a wide variety of physical measures and antithrombotic drugs have been employed in an attempt to decrease the incidence of deep venous thrombosis of the calves. The assumption has been that by a decrease in calf vein thrombosis, propagation into the iliofemoral system will be prevented, with a resultant decrease in pulmonary emboli. Low-dose or minidose heparin has received the most publicity. There is no question that subcutaneous heparin in doses of 5000 units every 8 or 12 hr decreases the incidence of calf vein thrombosis, as diagnosed by ^{125}I fibrinogen scanning. The rate of this complication is about 25%, whereas in those patients who receive low-dose heparin, this figure is reduced to about 6%.[2,24] There are, however, some cautions regarding the use of heparin even in this reduced dosage. In some studies, the incidence of postoperative wound hematoma has been increased,[24] and recently heparin-induced thrombocytopenia with subsequent thrombosis has been described in as many as 5% of patients taking the drug.[8]

Warfarin has likewise been studied and found to be highly effective, expecially in elderly patients undergoing lower-extremity orthopedic procedures. However, its use leads to signifiantly increased bleeding complications, making it unsuitable for use in many general surgical patients.[25]

The use of Dextran is somewhat more controversial, but in general has likewise shown an ability to decrease the incidence of deep venous thrombosis, although not to as great a degree as has heparin. This decreased effectiveness, as well as occasional allergic reactions and problems of fluid overload, have limited the use of this drug.

External pneumatic compression of the calves is highly effective in preventing deep venous thrombosis, achieving results similar to that obtained with low-dose heparin. The problem with this method is that it is cumbersome and somewhat uncomfortable for the patient.

Early ambulation of general surgical patients is an ideal seldom achieved clinically. The usual end result of early ambulation of the high-risk patient with numerous tubes and monitoring devices attached to him is two or three steps from the bed to the chair, where the patient will remain slumped with his legs in a dependent position for a period of an hour, followed by a rapid trip back to bed. Also, studies utilizing ^{125}I fibrinogen have demonstrated that leg clots form preoperatively and intraoperatively, thus rendering postoperative ambulation less important.[26,27]

ANSWER: E.

11.8. A 50-year-old man is recovering 7 days postoperatively after a vagotomy and antrectomy for a bleeding duodenal ulcer. He begins to complain of severe left leg pain. The leg is noted to be purplish and blotchy and is visibly swollen from the inguinal ligament downward (Figure-11-5). A dorsalis pedis pulse is audible with a Doppler examination. The left calf is 6 cm greater in circumference than the right; the left thigh is 9 cm greater in circumference than the right. Urine output for the past 8 hr has been 40 ml. Venography confirms a diagnosis of iliofemoral thrombosis, and full doses of heparin are begun. The leg is unchanged 4 hr later, but the pain has increased, and the patient can no longer dorsiflex his foot. Treatment should consist of:

A. Increased doses of heparin.
B. Administration of fibrinolytic drugs.
C. Inferior vena cava ligation.
D. Saphenous vein ligation.
E. Iliofemoral thrombectomy.

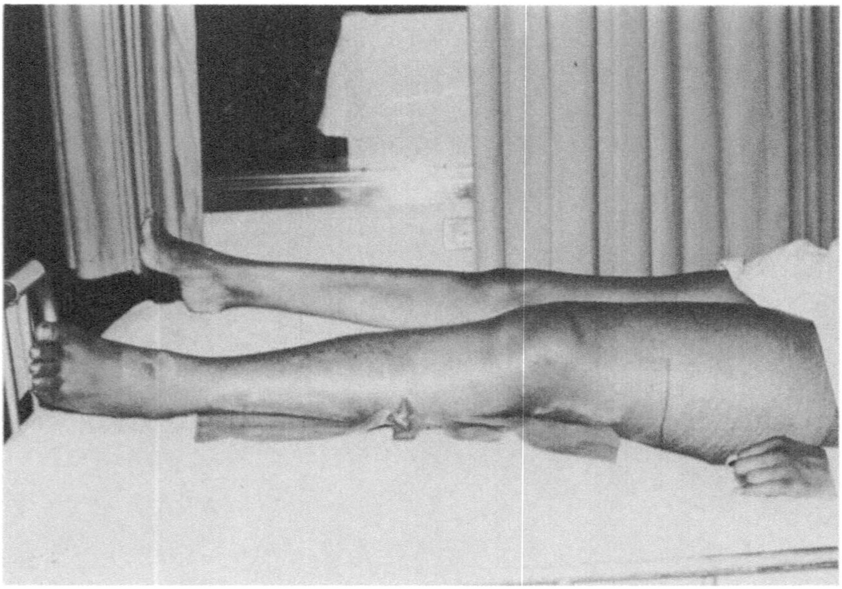

Figure 11-5

The clinical picture is that of a phlegmasia cerulea dolens with marked hypovolemia owing to third-space fluid losses in the leg and resultant oliguria. Currently, the two treatment options in such a patient are reliance upon anticoagulation alone or venous thrombectomy. This latter approach has had numerous supporters on and off over the past 30 years, and, at present, there is no clear-cut evidence of the superiority of the surgical treatment. In the early 1960s there was some enthusiasm for venous thrombectomy.[28] However, follow-up of this same group of patients disclosed no improvement regarding the sequelae of chronic lower limb venous insufficiency.[29]

Several studies have shown a 40%–80% incidence of postphlebitic syndrome following iliofemoral thrombosis, and because of this, a more aggressive management has been advocated.[30] Using an early approach, before the iliofemoral clot has organized and become adherent, good results have been obtained, with immediate relief of pain and edema, a low incidence of recurrent pulmonary embolus, and long-term prevention of incompetent veins. For any patient in whom thrombectomy is advocated, a definitive diagnosis using a venogram is essential. In the patient presented, a phlegmasia cerulea dolens is present, and this has progressed to the point of lower limb ischemia manifested by pain and an anterior compartment syndrome with loss of dorsiflexion of the foot. If not promptly treated, a permanent foot drop might be anticipated. While some might argue that a continuation of anticoagulants with the performance of a fasciotomy is indicated in this instance, if there is a role for venous thrombectomy it would surely be in such a severe instance. Fibrinolytic drugs such as steptokinase or urokinase would be contraindicated in any postoperative patient, as bleeding would probably be precipitated in the operated areas. Likewise, ligation of the inferior vena cava or saphenous vein ligation would do nothing to relieve the symptoms of the compartment syndrome.

ANSWER: E.

References

1. Coon, W.W.: The spectrum of pulmonary embolism: 20 years later. *Arch. Surg.* 111:398, 1976.
2. Sabiston, D.C.: Pathophysiology, diagnosis, and management of pulmonary embolism. *Am. J. Surg.* 138:384, 1979.
3. Menzoian, J.O., Williams, L.F.: Is pulmonary angiography essential for the diagnosis of acute pulmonary embolism? *Am. J. Surg.* 137:543, 1979.
4. Thomas, D.P.: The management of pulmonary embolic disease. *Am. J. Med. Sci.* 259:157, 1970.
5. Woolverton, W.C., Hyman, A.L.: The pulmonary hemodynamic effects of lung thromboemboli in dogs. *Surgery* 73:572, 1973.
6. Goodall, R.J.R., Greenfield, L.J.: Clinical correlations in the diagnosis of pulmonary embolism. *Ann. Surg.* 191:219, 1980.
7. Nelson, J.C., Lerner, R.G., Goldstein, R., Cagin, N.A.: Heparin induced thrombocytopenia. *Arch. Intern. Med.* 138:548, 1978.
8. Kapsch, D.N., Adelstein, E.H., Rhodes, G.R., Silver, D.: Heparin-induced thrombocytopenia, thrombosis, and hemorrhage. *Surgery* 86:148, 1979.
9. Eberlein, T.J., Carey, L.C.: Comparison of surgical management for pulmonary emboli. *Ann. Surg.* 179:836, 1974.
10. Greenfield, L.J., Scher, L.A., Elkins, R.C.: KMA–Greenfield filter placement for chronic pulmonary hypertension. *Ann. Surg.* 189:560, 1979.
11. Lawrence, G.H., Beebe, H.G.: An evaluation of the Mobin–Uddin umbrella in the prevention of pulmonary thromboembolism. *Am. J. Surg.* 132:204, 1976.
12. Hunter, J.A., Dye, W.S., Javid, H., Najafi, H., Goldin, M.D., Serry, C.: Permanent transvenous balloon occlusion of the inferior vena cava. *Am. Surg.* 186:491, 1977.
13. Grollman, J.H., Marx, F.W.: The importance of bilateral ovarian vein ligation in the control of thromboembolic disease. *Surgery* 71:352, 1972.
14. Gardner, A.M.N., Askew, A.R., Harse, H.R., Wilmshurst, C.C., Turner, M.J.: Partial occlusion of the inferior vena cava in the prevention of fatal pulmonary embolism. *Surg. Gynecol. Obstet.* 138:17, 1974.
15. Silver, D., Sabiston, D.C.: The role of vena caval interruption in the management of pulmonary embolism. *Surgery* 77:1, 1975.
16. Rosenthal, D., Cossman, D., Matsumoto, G., Callow, A.D.: Prophylactic interruption of the inferior vena cava. *Am. J. Surg.* 137:389, 1979.
17. Lindenauer, S.M.: Prophylactic staple plication of the inferior vena cava. *Arch. Surg.* 107:669, 1973.
18. Heimbecker, R.O., Keon, W.J., Richards, K.U.: Massive pulmonary embolism: A new look at surgical maangement. *Arch. Surg.* 107:740, 1973.
19. Porter, J.M., Godnight, S.H.: The clinical use of fibrinolytic agents. *Am. J. Surg.* 134:217, 1977.
20. Fratantoni, J.C., Ness, P., Simon, T.L.: Thrombolytic therapy: Current status. *N. Engl. J. Med.* 293:1073, 1975.
21. Tsapogas, M.J., Jindal, P.K.: Fibrinolytic therapy for deep venous thrombosis. *Contemp. Surg.* 10:29, 1977.
22. Coon, W.W.: Risk factors in pulmonary embolism. *Surg. Gynecol. Obstet.* 143:385, 1976.
23. Bell, W.R., Zuidema, G.D.: Low-dose heparin; Concern and perspectives. *Surgery* 85:469, 1979.
24. Kakkar, V.V., Corrigan, T.P., Fossard, D.P.: Prevention of fatal postoperative pulmonary embolism by low doses of heparin. *Lancet* 2:45, 1975.

25. Salzman, E.W., Davies, G.C.: Prophylaxis of venous thromboembolism. *Ann. Surg.* 191:207, 1980.
26. Kakkar, V.V.: The I^{125} labeled fibrinogen test and phlebography in the diagnosis of deep vein thrombosis, in Foster, C.S. (ed.): *The Epidemiology of Venous Thrombosis*. Millbank Memorial Fund Quarterly 50(1):206, 1972.
27. Heatley, R.V., Morgan, A., Hughs, L.E., Okwonga, W.: Preoperative or postoperative deep vein thrombosis. *Lancet* 1:437, 1976.
28. Haller, J.A., Abrams, B.L.: Use of thrombectomy in the treatment of acute iliofemoral venous thrombosis in 45 patients. *Ann. Surg.* 158:561, 1963.
29. Lansing, A.M., Davis, W.M.: Five year follow-up study of iliofemoral venous thrombectomy. *Ann. Surg.* 168:620, 1968.
30. Kistner, R.L., Sparkuhl, M.D.: Surgery in acute and chronic venous disease. *Surgery* 85:31, 1979.

12
TRAUMA

12.1. A 26-year-old male is the driver of an automobile that swerved off the road. On admission, he is intoxicated and smells of alcohol. Central nervous system examination is otherwise normal. His pulse is 120; his blood pressure is 110/40. Chest examination is normal. There is a large contusion over the midabdomen. The abdominal examination is difficult to perform owing to the patient's uncooperative status, but it seems to disclose tenderness and guarding throughout. Which of the following studies is most likely to benefit this patient?

A. Chest and abdominal X rays.
B. Abdominal angiography.
C. Liver–spleen scan.
D. Peritoneal lavage.
E. Abdominal CAT scan.

This item addresses the common problem of the evaluation of an abdominal injury in an unconscious or intoxicated trauma victim. A wide variety of adjuncts to physical examination have been utilized with rather inconstant success in the evaluation of the trauma victim. All have their own peculiar limitations and must be interpreted in view of the patient's history and physical findings. Dependence upon a lowered hemoglobin level and a lowered hematocrit as guides to the presence of significant hemorrhage is notoriously misleading, for with rapid transport of the trauma victim to the hospital, hemodilution often has not occurred, and these determinations can be normal. Likewise, the serum amylase level may be misleading. In the past, it was thought that elevations of this enzyme after trauma indicated the presence of a pancreatic injury, which mandated immediate operation. However, this has not been shown to be the case. In one study, only 8% of patients with abdominal trauma and an elevated amylase concentration had a pancreatic injury, and fully 33% of trauma patients with an elevated serum amylase level had no significant intra-abdominal injury at all.[1]

In a stable patient, it is often helpful to obtain four views of the abdomen and chest. This will disclose a number of unsuspected injuries in blunt trauma, and at the same time if there is any question of renal damage, either because of hematuria or injury in the area of the kidneys, an intravenous pyelogram can be carried out. Angiography of the abdominal viscera has been advocated in the past in the management of the patient with multiple injuries,[2–4] but the current management utilizing peritoneal lavage for these patients has largely supplanted this, except in specialized instances. One absolute indication for angiography exists, in the patient found to have a widened mediastinum on chest X ray following blunt trauma to the chest, giving rise to the suspicion of a ruptured aorta. Abdominal ultrasound and CAT scanning have also been used, but less frequently, are not routinely available, and tend to be less helpful with many intra-abdominal injuries than with solid organ or retroperitoneal injuries. A liver–spleen scan will reliably detect any major splenic injury, but may miss smaller liver injuries. The major usefulness of this study lies in the evaluation of these organs in the stable patient during the days following the accident, when delayed hemorrhage and rupture of the spleen can occur.

Probably the single most important advance made in the diagnostic evaluation of the trauma victim in recent years has been the emergence of peritoneal lavage as a highly accurate method of determining significant intra-abdominal injury in blunt trauma. Recognizing the poor correlation between physical findings and the presence of intra-abdominal injury,[5] many trauma centers have perfected the technique of peritoneal lavage and have performed this maneuver in large numbers of patients with minimal complications and excellent accuracy. In general, no more than 3% false negative and false positive results have been obtained in most series of patients. If anything, the problem has arisen whereby this technique is too sensitive and will detect small amounts of intra-abdominal bleeding that are not associated with any significant intra-abdominal injury. Because of this, various quantitative criteria have evolved. The finding of a white blood cell count in the peritoneal lavage fluid return greater than 500 cells/mm^3, a red blood cell count greater than 100,000 cells/mm^3, or an amylase concentration of greater than 100 units/100 cc of lavage fluid have all correlated significantly with the presence of intra-abdominal injury requiring laparotomy.[6–11] This collected experience has indicated that peritoneal lavage should be attempted in any case of serious blunt abdominal trauma in which obvious signs of visceral injury are not present. This procedure is also strongly recommended in patients who are either intoxicated or have a clouded sensorium resulting from head injury. Complications of the procedure have been infrequent and, in general, related to faulty technique. Perforations of major vessels and hollow viscera have been described but can be virtually eliminated with adherence to certain technical steps, especially the avoidance of direct puncture of the skin and fascia. The preferred method utilizes a small skin and fascial incision and the opening of the peritoneum under direct vision. The dialysis catheter is inserted through this hole. If bloody return is obvious, the procedure is terminated. Otherwise, approximately 1 liter of lactated Ringers solution or normal saline is run into the abdomen and after several minutes is allowed to run out by gravity. Contraindications to peritoneal lavage include multiple abdominal scars with presumed intra-abdominal adhesions, the presence of a gravid uterus, the presence of significantly dilated intestine, or the hemodynamically unstable patient, in whom the test is probably not indicated in any event.

ANSWER: D.

12.2. A 28-year-old man is brought to the emergency room following a fight. He reports being stabbed in the abdomen with a knife approximately 6 in. long 1 hr previously. His pulse is 90 and his blood pressure is 140/80. He has pain around the entrance wound, which is located 1 cm above the umbilicus. His abdomen is otherwise soft and nontender. Proper treatment should be:

A. Immediate celiotomy.
B. Observation.
C. Digital exploration of the wound.
D. Sinogram of the wound.
E. Peritoneal lavage.

While it might seem obvious that all patients with a penetrating wound of the abdomen require celiotomy, extensive clinical experience has shown that this is not the case. The physician should first recognize the anatomical limits of the peritoneal cavity. Basically, it is possible for any penetrating instrument entering below the nipples or above the gluteal crease to enter the peritoneal cavity.[12] There is little disagreement concerning the treatment of a patient with penetrating abdominal trauma who has evidence of shock or peritoneal signs. This patient requires immediate celiotomy. However, because of the significant morbidity and mortality that attend the performance of a negative celiotomy for abdominal trauma,[13,14] many surgeons in trauma centers have endeavored to select out those patients who are unlikely to have significant intra-abdominal injury and who could be observed safely without operation. This selective observation of patients with penetrating abdominal trauma has been utilized for both gunshot and stab wounds with considerable success.[15-19] Using these treatment protocols, patients with obvious blood loss or peritoneal signs are operated upon immediately, and the remainder are observed with frequent examinations and determinations of serial blood counts. If any clinical deterioration occurs, these patients are then operated upon immediately. By this method, the number of negative celiotomies has been reduced markedly and there has been little or no increase in morbidity in that small group of patients who had to be operated upon after an observation period. However, because of the greater chance of peritoneal penetration and intraperitoneal damage in the gunshot victim, it would seem wise to immediately operate upon this group of patients. However, it has been repeatedly noted that approximately one third of all stab wounds of the abdomen do not penetrate the peritoneal cavity, and of those that do penetrate, approximately one half are unassociated with any significant intra-abdominal injury. This means that approximately two thirds of all abdominal stab wounds do not require any operation.[15,18]

ANSWER: B.

12.3. A 60-year-old woman undergoes gastroscopy for an upper GI tract hemorrhage. She vomits during the procedure, which is then completed without incident. A duodenal ulcer is noted, and bleeding has ceased at the time of the endoscopy; 6 hr later, she complains of substernal pain and pain in the left chest on deep inspiration. Temperature is 37.8°C, her lungs are clear to auscultation, her abdomen is soft and nontender. Crepitus is felt in her neck 24 hr later. The white blood cell count is 12,400 cells/mm^3, and a chest X ray and esophagogram are obtained and are shown as Figures 12-1 and 12-2. Treatment should consist of:

A. Antibiotics and observation.
B. Immediate left thoracotomy.
C. Immediate celiotomy.
D. Cervical esophagostomy and gastrostomy.
E. Left tube thoracostomy.

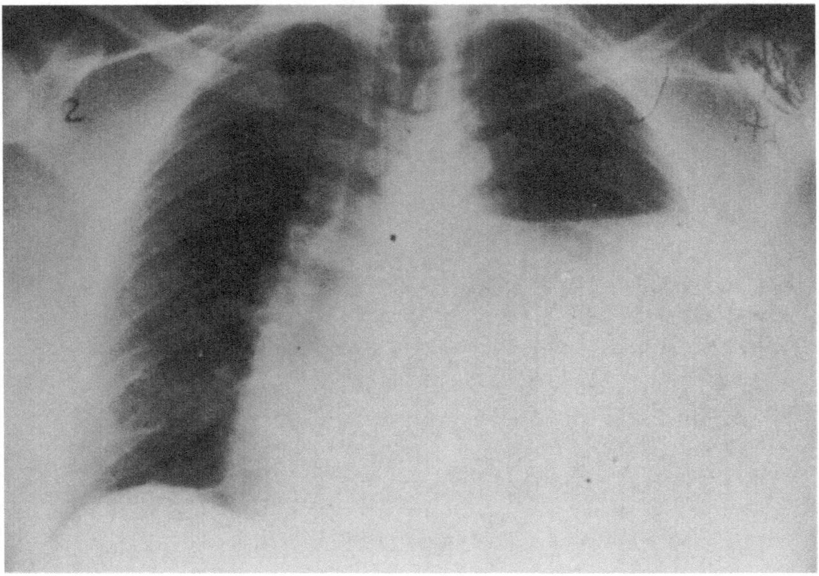

Figure 12-1

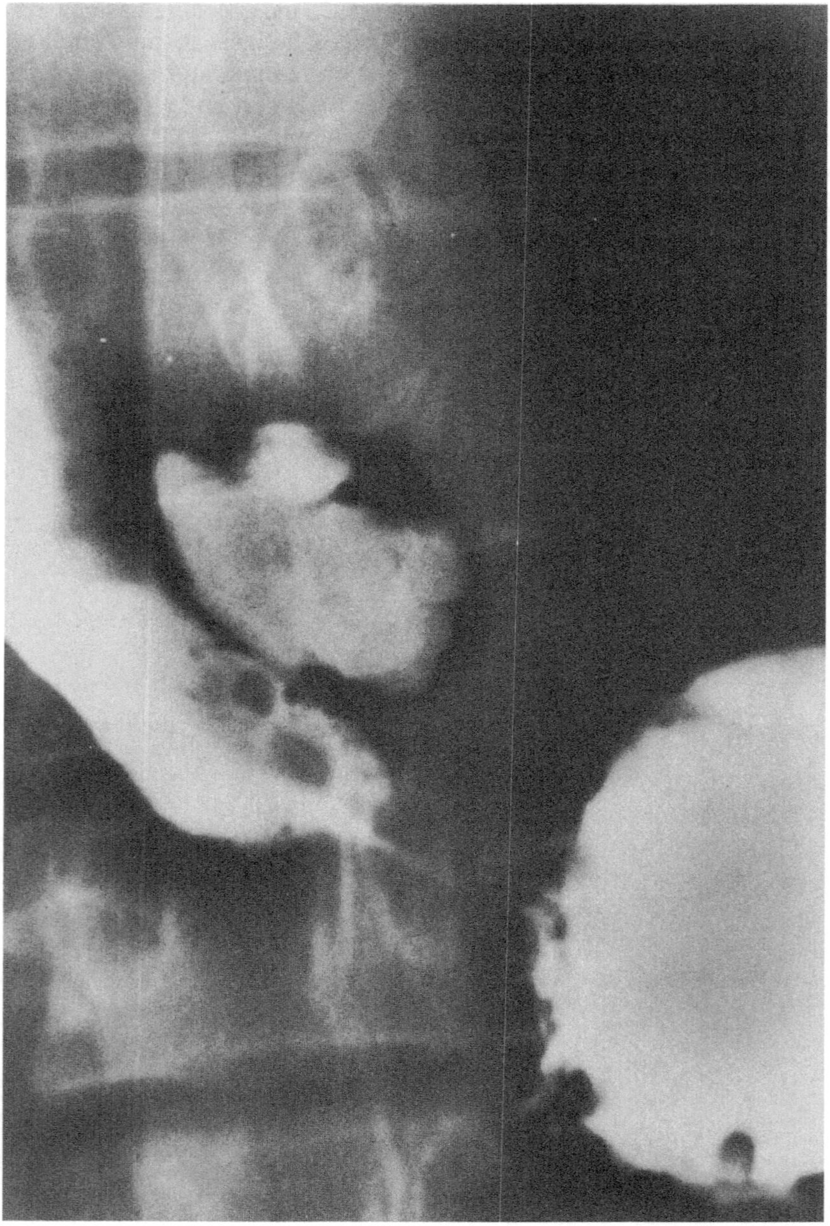

Figure 12-2

This patient has an obvious perforation of the distal esophagus with pneumomediastinum and a left pleural effusion. The contrast study clearly demonstrates the esophageal leak. Perforation of the esophagus is an uncommon event with diverse etiologies. Endoscopic injury is probably the most frequent cause, followed by spontaneous or emetogenic rupture of the esophagus. In addition, the esophagus may be injured by forceful dilitation, ingestion of foreign bodies, perforating and blunt trauma, and during operations around the esophageal hiatus, especially in the performance of truncal vagotomy. If spillage of GI contents occurs into the free peritoneal cavity, symptoms are immediate and peritonitis is readily evident. However, in many cases, leakage occurs into the mediastinum with the progressive onset of pain, dysphagia, and sepsis. In general, gunshot and stab wounds usually involve the cervical esophagus, whereas instrumental perforations usually involve the distal esophagus. The key to managing esophageal perforations lies in suspicion of their presence and the prompt institution of diagnostic measures soon after the injury. X rays of the neck and thorax will often show air in the neck or mediastinum, and this strongly suggests the diagnosis. Contrast studies using water-soluble contrast media should be performed, and these will accurately localize the perforation in most cases. In questionable cases, esophagoscopy should be performed, as this has been shown to be highly accurate and associated with no additional morbidity.[20] For all patients with esophageal injuries, vigorous fluid resuscitation is indicated, along with broad-spectrum antibiotic treatment. In addition, the institution of total parenteral nutrition should be considered, as many of these patients will require long term parenteral nutritional support. With the advent of improved supportive care, a controversy has evolved regarding the treatment of instrumental perforations of the esophagus manifested by air in the mediastinum associated with a small perforation. Some authorities advocate nonoperative management of these patients unless evidence of sepsis occurs. However, a considerable clinical experience would support vigorous resuscitation followed by immediate operation, and this has yielded excellent results.[21–24] Surely, there is little to debate in the case of an esophageal perforation associated with pleural or peritoneal involvement. Immediate left thoracotomy or celiotomy is indicated. The management of perforation of the esophagus associated with extensive esophageal tissue loss is more controversial. In these instances, primary repair is often doomed to failure, and some form of staged operation may be required.[25] For extensive perforations at the distal esophagus, it is often possible by an abdominal approach to repair the perforation primarily, drain it, and then perform a wrap of gastric fundus around the perforation. This so-called fundic patch will be successful in the majority of cases.[26]

ANSWER: B.

12.4. A 12-year-old boy falls from his bicycle, striking his upper abdomen. He is seen shortly afterward by his family physician, who assures his mother that there is no evidence of significant injury. Three days later, he begins to feel bloated in the upper abdomen and to vomit undigested food and bilious material. He is admitted to the hospital. His temperature is 37.4°C. His abdomen is tender in the epigastrium. No organs or masses are palpable. His white blood cell count is 11,200 cells/mm^3; the hematocrit is 33%. An upper GI tract X ray is obtained and is shown as Figure 12-3. This presentation is diagnostic of:

A. Retroperitoneal duodenal rupture.
B. Ruptured right kidney.
C. Stress ulcer of the duodenum.
D. Pancreatic pseudocyst.
E. Intramural hematoma of the duodenum.

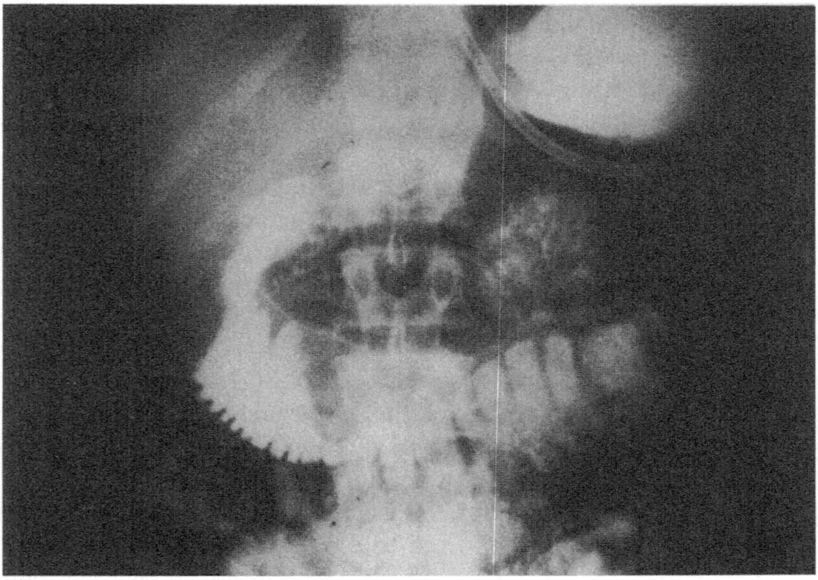

Figure 12-3

Treatment should consist of:

A. Nasogastric suction and total parenteral nutrition.
B. Excision and repair of duodenal injury.
C. Celiotomy and evacuation of duodenal hematoma.
D. Nasogastric instillation of enzymes.
E. Pancreaticoduodenectomy.

The X ray demonstrates compression and partial obstruction of the second portion of the duodenum, typical of an intramural duodenal hematoma. This injury is an uncommon sequela of abdominal trauma, and less than 200 cases have been reported in the literature. Over 75% of these cases have been due to blunt abdominal trauma, and most cases have been reported in children or young adults. Additional etiologies that have been described include complications of anticoagulation or blood dyscrasias and association with pancreatitis and alcoholism.

Typically, symptoms do not become apparent until 24 to 48 hr postinjury. At that time, pain and vomiting occur. Melena is rarely present. The patients are often febrile and dehydrated, and in 40% of cases a tender mass is palpable. No abdominal distention is present and bowel sounds are normal. A gastric succussion splash is usually present. Anemia is present in about 25% of these patients, and leukocytosis is characteristic.[27] Abdominal X rays may demonstrate a gastric dilatation, an air fluid level in the duodenum, or an absent right psoas shadow. Upper GI tract X rays will confirm the diagnosis, in many cases showing the classic "coiled spring" effect in the duodenum.

Operative treatment has traditionally been recommended. In a review of the 179 reported cases in the literature, 135 were operated upon while 44 were treated nonoperatively with nasogastric suction and intravenous fluid therapy. Twenty-five percent of the nonoperative group died. Operation consisted mainly of evacuation of the hematoma through a serosal incision in the duodenum. In those cases in whom the obstruction did not appear to be relieved, a gastrojejunostomy was also added. A few patients required reoperation for persistent obstruction.[28] However, a recent review of 14 patients disclosed 11 in whom nonoperative treatment was successful, but the average duration of nonoperative therapy before resolution of symptoms was 4 days, and this is considerably shorter than the time required for resolution in other reported series.[29] It is, therefore, unclear at this time whether nonoperative treatment can be employed in the majority of cases. It would seem that the appropriate treatment for a patient with intramural duodenal hematoma includes intravenous therapy, nasogastric suction, and careful radiologic studies to rule out associated injuries or duodenal lacerations. In those patients who have minimal evidence of obstruction or in whom a clotting disorder is present, nonoperative management can be attempted. Many of these patients will require maintenance of nutrition with parenteral hyperalimentation. All other patients should be promptly operated upon with evacuation of the hematoma. A bypass of the obstructed duodenal segment with gastrojejunostomy should be reserved for those patients in whom evacuation of the hematoma does not relieve the obstruction.

Although blunt torso trauma can result in rupture of the stomach, the usual gastric perforation is caused by penetrating trauma. The diagnosis is generally not difficult, as the patient will present with signs of severe peritonitis, often with shock. Primary repair of the injured area is almost always possible, and the only pitfall lies in failing to search for associated perforations of the posterior aspect of the stomach by opening the lesser omental bursa. The duodenum, on the other hand, is one of the more commonly injured viscera in both blunt and penetrating abdominal injuries. Perforation of the duodenum can occur with massive spillage of upper GI tract contents into the free peritoneal cavity making the diagnosis fairly easy. More difficult are the situations associated with blunt trauma in which the duodenum is ruptured in it's retroperitoneal portion, and the symptoms of the ruptured viscus are more delayed. In this circumstance, diagnosis can be obscure for several days, with ongoing retroperitoneal soilage. In many of these instances, abdominal X rays will verify the presence of retroperitoneal gas. However, up to 30% of these hidden injuries are missed at celiotomy.[30] Associated intra-abdominal injuries are common,[31] leading to an overall mortality in duodenal injuries of approximately 15% to 20%.[30,32]

There are several different types of injury to the duodenum and each must be managed individually. In its simple form, the injury is a simple laceration, and this can be primarily repaired after the edges have been debrided. An important adjunct at this time is adequate drainage of the duodenal area, as those repairs are prone to break down, leading to the common complications of intra-abdominal abscess and duodenal fistula.[32] If there is further concern with the integrity of the duodenal closure, a tube duodenostomy inserted through a separate incision in the duodenum can afford effective internal decompression of the duodenum. Even transections of the duodenum may be handled by primary repair along with internal and external drainage in selective cases.

Another form of duodenal injury occurs when large lacerations of the duodenum are present with extensive devitalization of the duodenal wall. For these types of injuries, when it is felt that primary repair is not feasible, a jejunal serosal patch may be utilized by swinging up a loop of jejunum and suturing it circumferentially around the defect.[33-35] For yet more extensive injuries, even for those combined with some element of pancreatic injury, a technique known as duodenal diverticulization has been described and can be effective. A vagotomy and a hemigastrectomy are carried out, with a Billroth II reconstruction, an oversewing of the duodenal stump, and primary repair of the duodenal lacerations. In addition, a tube duodenostomy is placed along with external drains. This effectively isolates the area of duodenal injury.[36]

ANSWERS: E; A.

12.5. A 36-year-old man sustains an abdominal gunshot wound. At celiotomy 6 hr later, several small bowel perforations are identified and primarily repaired. There is a 6-cm defect in the transverse colon from which extensive amounts of stool have leaked. Treatment should consist of which of the following:

A. Primary repair of the laceration.
B. Primary repair of the laceration plus cecostomy.
C. Primary repair of the laceration plus ileostomy.
D. Exteriorization of the injured segment.
E. Resection of the colon segment and primary anastomosis.

The treatment of penetrating wounds of the intra-abdominal colon is very controversial. In the past, treatment consisted of exteriorizing the area of injury as a colostomy. This was associated with significant morbidity and mortality, and of course necessitated a second operation. Because of dissatisfaction with this method of treatment, many surgeons began to attempt primary repair of colon lacerations, usually without proximal diversion of fecal contents, and a number of reports have attested to its safe and effective utilization.[37–39]

However, it is recognized that more severe injuries can be better treated with exteriorization of the injured segment. Excellent surgical judgment is necessary in these cases, and such determinants as age and general status of the patient, time of delay before operation, the amount of fecal spillage, and the extent of the colon injury all enter into the decision. If it is judged that the colon cannot be primarily repaired, it is advisable to exteriorize the injured segment. Controversy here revolves around whether the colon should be primarily repaired and exteriorized in the hopes that the repair will remain intact or whether the injured segment should be exteriorized as a colostomy. Several reviews have indicated that primary healing of such an exteriorized repair is unlikely. However, a recent review disclosed healing of the anastomosis in 70% of the patients in whom this was attempted.[40]

Injuries of the extraperitoneal rectum require special consideration, for it is well recognized that proximal fecal diversion alone will be unsuccessful in the majority of cases. Four basic principles must be adhered to if satisfactory results are to be achieved. First is proximal diversion of the fecal stream with a completely diverting sigmoid colostomy. Second is irrigation of the rectal segment through a tube inserted in the anus so that the entire rectum and distal colon are free of stool. Third is presacral drainage of the rectum, and fourth is repair of the rectal defect itself.

Utilization of these four principles will lead to successful treatment of most rectal injuries. One exception to this will be the massively destroyed rectum sometimes seen as a result of an explosion injury. In such a case of extensive devascularization and/or gangrene of the rectal segment, nothing short of abdomino-perineal resection will be life-saving.[41]

ANSWER: D.

12.6. A 3-year-old child is struck by an automobile. A peritoneal lavage performed in the emergency room reveals bloody fluid. At celiotomy, the only significant injury noted is a 3-in. profusely bleeding laceration of the outer surface of the spleen. Treatment should consist of:

A. Splenectomy.
B. Splenic artery ligation.
C. Application of hemostatic agents such as bovine crystalline collagen.
D. Debridement and primary repair of the defect.
E. Splenic artery ligation and direct pressure until the bleeding ceases.

A great deal of recent controversy exists regarding the proper treatment of a patient who sustains trauma to the spleen. In past years, splenectomy was routinely advocated, and there was little discussion of treatment alternatives. However, reports of serious infections following splenectomy began to occur in the literature in the 1950s, and this has led to a complete reappraisal of the management of splenic trauma.

Unfortunately, at present, there is still controversy regarding the exact incidence of postsplenectomy sepsis. However, certain general observations appear to be valid. The increased incidence of postsplenectomy sepsis seems to be related to several variables:

1. The age of the patient at the time of splenectomy. The younger the patient, the higher the risk of subsequent sepsis.
2. The time since splenectomy. Patients are at greatest risk within the year following splenectomy and at decreased risk from then onwards.
3. The reason for which splenectomy was performed. Those patients who have serious underlying hematologic or immunologic diseases for which splenectomy was required have a far greater incidence of postsplenectomy sepsis than those patients in whom the spleen was removed for trauma.[42]

However, several large reviews have disclosed no increased incidence of postsplenectomy sepsis in children who did not harbor significant underlying disease.[43,44] In contrast to these reports, a recent report has documented a disturbingly high incidence of postsplenectomy infections in "normal" asplenic patients.[45]

When these infections occur, *Pneumococcus* tends to be the infecting organism in greater than 50% of cases. Other commonly encountered organisms are the *Meningococcus, Streptococcus,* and *Hemophilus influenzae*. The infections tend to be associated with a mortality rate as high as 70%.[45] The infections are characterized by an abrupt onset in a patient with no obvious focus of infection elsewhere. A fulminant course is noted, often with associated disseminated intravascular coagulation and pneumococcal bacteremia, leading rapidly to death. These infections have stimulated a reappraisal of the role of the spleen in combating infection. The spleen is known to clear foreign particulate matter from the circulation by phagocytosis and also to elaborate an early appearing antibody in response to an intravenous challenge by particulate antigens such as bacteria.[46] Splenic phagocytosis appears to be important when there is a lack of opsonizing antibody. It is hypothesized that a patient can contract a pneumococcal infection of a serologic type against which he has not previously acquired opsonizing antibodies. Another theory for the increased incidence of infection is the deficiency of the phagocytosis-promoting peptide tuftsin that is seen in asplenic hosts.[47]

In summary then, it is well accepted that the asplenic child is susceptible to an increased incidence of overwhelming postsplenectomy infections, while there is a suspicion that the asplenic adult may also be at risk. Because of this, a wide variety of approaches to the patient with splenic trauma have been advocated. At one extreme are the clinicians who fear the specter of postsplenectomy sepsis to such a degree that they choose to treat children with documented splenic rupture without operation, merely transfusing the patient as much as is necessary in the hope that splenic hemorrhage will cease spontaneously.[48–50] However, in view of the relatively low incidence of postsplenectomy infection in otherwise normal children and the significant risk associated with nonoperative management of splenic rupture, this approach seems unwise unless the most careful observation of these patients is carried out. Another approach that has been utilized quite successfully is surgical repair of the ruptured spleen at the time of laparotomy. Several series of patients have been published in which primary repair has been carried out successfully with the placement of hemostatic sutures, and it would appear at this time that this is the treatment of choice for all children with a ruptured spleen if the nature of the splenic defect lends itself to repair.[51,52] Another approach that likewise emphasizes the benefits to be derived from early operation is the application of bovine crystalline collagen to the raw splenic defect.[53,54] In the patient presented, application of this material would be unlikely to work owing to the profuse nature of the bleeding.

Other authors have recognized the desirability of splenectomy for splenic trauma but have advocated long-term prophylactic antibiotic therapy as a means of preventing postsplenectomy infectious complications.

At this time, while it is probably true that young children should receive long-term prophylactic antibiotics, it is far more debatable whether this should be carried out in adults.[55] Perhaps the most promising recent approach has been the use of specific polyvalent pneumococcal polysaccharide vaccines. In several large series, these have been proven to initiate specific antibodies, and the incidence of subsequent infections has been reduced.[56,57] Another method of attempting to protect the asplenic individual from subsequent infection has been the induction of splenosis at the time of splenectomy. Splenosis is the condition whereby fragments of spleen left free in the peritoneal cavity or abdominal incision regenerate and form histologically normal splenic tissue.[58,59] It has been hoped that the implantation and subsequent regeneration of splenic tissue would provide some of the lost immunity following spenectomy. At least one experimental report in mice suggests that this may be so.[60] However, at the present time it is questionable whether splenic implants in animals or humans confer immunologic protection to the host and if so whether this would be sufficient to prevent postsplenectomy sepsis.

ANSWER: D.

12.7. A 36-year-old man is the driver of an automobile that strikes a tree. On admission to the emergency room, his blood pressure is 70/40 and his pulse is 140. A peritoneal lavage yields grossly bloody return, and celiotomy is performed after rapid volume repletion. A deep stellate bursting injury is present on the dome of the right lobe of the liver and is the only injury noted. Profuse bleeding is present from the depths of the liver laceration. Compression of the hepatic artery leads to a marked reduction in bleeding, and direct ligation of individual bleeding vessels within the liver is possible. However, on release of the hepatic artery clamp, severe bleeding ensues. Treatment at this point should consist of:

A. Right hepatic lobectomy.
B. Deep mattress sutures to close the defect.
C. Packing of the defect with an omental pedicle.
D. Application of bovine crystalline collagen (Avitene).
E. Hepatic artery ligation.

Which of the following should not be used as an adjunct at this time?

A. Antibiotics.
B. Insertion of a T tube into the common duct.
C. Administration of total parenteral nutrition.
D. Penrose and sump drainage of the liver.
E. Postoperative treatment with albumin and 10% glucose and water.

The liver is one of the most frequently injured organs in both blunt and penetrating trauma of the abdomen. In most large series of patients with liver trauma, the overall mortality rate has ranged between 10% and 15%, with no major improvements in this figure being recognized in recent years.[61–63] Regardless of the nature of the injury, three basic principles must be adhered to if complications are to be prevented. These general principles are: (1) the insuring of adequate hemostasis, (2) the debridement of all devitalized liver tissue, and (3) provision of adequate postoperative drainage to allow egress of blood or bile from the peritoneal cavity.

In the situation presented, hepatic artery occlusion was effective in temporarily controlling the bleeding while an attempt was made to individually ligate vessels in the depths of the liver wound. However, the bleeding recurred upon release of the hepatic artery occlusion. At this point the surgeon is faced with the decision of whether to proceed with a formal right hepatic lobectomy or to ligate a branch of the hepatic artery. Surely, in some instances of massive destruction of the liver, hepatic lobectomy will be required, but despite the fact that this procedure has been championed by some, its performance in liver trauma is attended by a mortality of approximately 50%, making it a poor initial choice for therapy.[61]

Given this situation, the technically easier expedient of hepatic artery ligation has gained popularity, although once again there is some evidence that it has been overenthusiastically used in some institutions, when perhaps lesser means would have sufficed. Classic teaching in surgery held that if the hepatic artery was ligated, death was sure to result.[64] However in recent years, it has become quite accepted that the main hepatic artery or either of its major branches may be safely ligated in nearly all patients with a previously healthy liver, resulting in dramatic hemostasis and minimal complications.[65] In addition, studies have demonstrated the rapid development of collateral arterial flow after hepatic artery interruption, accounting for the lack of liver failure after this procedure.[66,67] When ligation of the hepatic artery is thought to be necessary, efforts should be made to place the ligature as close to the liver as possible (in one of the branches of the hepatic artery rather than the main hepatic artery) so as to devascularize as little as possible of the hepatic parenchyma. In addition, physiologic support of the patient is essential postoperatively. Glycogen stores are rapidly depleted after this procedure, leading to hypoglycemia. This can be combated by the administration of 10% glucose for about a week postoperatively. In addition, because the liver is depending upon portal venous flow for its oxygen, the patient should be fasted for a week in order to increase the oxygenation of the portal vein. Shock and low flow states must be rapidly corrected so that portal venous flow remains at normal levels. Also, intravenous albumin should be administered, as the synthesis of protein by the liver is reduced.

Other adjuncts in the treatment of liver injuries should be mentioned at this point. In the 1960s, it was accepted that biliary decompression by either a cholecystostomy or an indwelling T tube in the common duct was beneficial following liver trauma.[68] However, more recently it has been shown that the use of routine biliary decompression after hepatic trauma leads to an increased incidence of septic complications and upper GI tract hemorrhage, and for this reason, this technique should not be routinely used.[69–71] In those instances where massive hemorrhage is occurring and temporary occlusion of the hepatic artery does not result in cessation of bleeding, it must be suspected that an injury to the hepatic veins has occurred. This injury is nearly always fatal,[61] but on rare occasions a caval shunt bypassing the liver can be successfully utilized, resulting in salvage of the patient.[72] The use of deep mattress sutures to obtain hemostasis should be avoided if possible, but there are instances where this type of treatment may be successfully utilized. This may, of course, result in a certain amount of devitalized liver tissue and can predispose to late abscess formation. Recently, the application of Avitene (microcrystalline collagen) to the raw bleeding liver surface has been advocated, and this can be successful in stopping modest but not major liver bleeding. As sepsis is a common complication of major liver trauma, the prophylactic use of antibiotics should be considered. In addition, as many of these patients will suffer septic complications and require reoperation for hemorrhage, sepsis, or biliary fistula, total parenteral nutrition should be instituted as soon as possible in the postoperative period.

ANSWERS: E; B.

12.8. A 40-year-old woman strikes her torso against the steering column when her car runs off the road. On admission to the emergency room 1 hr later, her pulse is 96 and her blood pressure is 140/90. She complains of severe epigastric pain. A peritoneal lavage is performed, which returns blood-tinged fluid. The serum amylase level is 86 units/ml (normal is 4–20 units/ml). The hematocrit is 41% and the white blood cell count is 12,200 cells/mm^3. At celiotomy, she is noted to have a complete transection of the pancreas at the level of the mesenteric vessels. Operative treatment should consist of:

A. Pancreaticoduodenectomy (Whipple procedure).
B. Pancreatic duct ligation and drainage of the laceration.
C. Sump drainage only.
D. Roux-en-Y longitudinal pancreaticojejunostomy (Puestow procedure).
E. Roux-en-Y pancreaticojejunostomy to distal stump plus oversewing of the proximal pancreas.

Despite its retroperitoneal location, injuries to the pancreas are frequent from both blunt and penetrating abdominal trauma. Complications of pancreatic injury are frequent, and the mortality rate of such injuries remains about 20%.[73–75] Because of the retroperitoneal location of the organ, pancreatic injuries may be difficult to diagnose. Significant pancreatic injury can exist in the presence of a normal serum amylase concentration, and an elevated serum amylase level is only an inconstant indicator of pancreatic injury.[1,76,77] However, diagnosis should be easily accomplished with an increased awareness of the frequency of pancreatic trauma, careful physical evaluation, a judicious interpretation of the serum amylase level, and the use of peritoneal lavage.

Most of the complications of pancreatic trauma are the results of the uncontrolled leakage of pancreatic contents and include severe pancreatitis, pancreatic abscess, fistula, pseudocyst, and sepsis with multiple organ system failure. Because of this, many diverse and innovative methods have been proposed in the management of pancreatic trauma. In the situation presented, a blunt injury gave rise to a complete transection at the midbody of the pancreas at the level of the superior mesenteric vessels and the vertebral column. Methods for dealing with this type of injury have ranged from drainage only to Roux-en-Y anastomoses to both proximal and distal pancreatic segments. Drainage only in this type of wound is virtually certain to lead to many of the complications listed above, while oversewing of the proximal end of the pancreas with ligation of the pancreatic duct in the distal segment has been associated with fistula formation in a significant number of cases.[78] Some authorities have championed distal pancreatectomy, while others have advocated the retention of the distal transected pancreas, claiming that sacrifice of this remnant led to an unacceptable incidence of diabetes mellitus and pancreatic exocrine insufficiency in the future. These authors also have noted that it is scarcely easier to perform a distal pancreatectomy and splenectomy than it is to bring up a Roux-en-Y loop to the distal pancreas.[75] However, several large series of patients with this injury have been published in which the proximal pancreas was oversewn along with a performance of a distal pancreatectomy, with excellent results.[74,78] One series has been reported with 60 patients in whom this treatment was carried out with only a 12% mortality and one case of pancreatic insufficiency in the future. There were no cases of diabetes mellitus.[79] Therefore, it is likely that either of these two methods is suitable in the management of a patient with a transected pancreas, and the choice should depend upon the experience and abilities of the surgeon along with the exact findings at the time of laparotomy. A longitudinal pancreaticojejunostomy (Puestow procedure) is useful for treatment of patients with incapacitating pain from chronic calcific pancreatitis. It has not been used in patients with a transected pancreas. There would be no indication for a pancreaticoduodenectomy in this type of injury. Only when extensive devitalization of the pancreatic head is present with duct disruption or when there is major hemorrhage from the head of the pancreas or serious combined pancreatic and duodenal injuries is this form of treatment truly necessary.[74] When treating any form of pancreatic injury, it is essential to provide adequate drainage of the pancreas. Drains should be of the sump variety, as simple soft rubber drains have been associated with a much higher incidence of local postoperative complications.[80] Another adjunct that can prove most useful is the early use of total parenteral nutrition in these patients, in whom the resumption of oral intake is often delayed for many weeks.

ANSWER: E.

12.9. An 18-year-old woman falls off a horse, landing on her back. When seen in the emergency room 2 hr later, she has severe left flank pain and microscopic hematuria. An intravenous pyelogram (IVP) is obtained and is shown as Figure 12-4. Treatment should consist of:

A. Bedrest and antibiotics.
B. Exploration of the left kidney and primary repair of the laceration.
C. Left tube nephrostomy.
D. Left nephrectomy.
E. Exploration of the left kidney and partial nephrectomy.

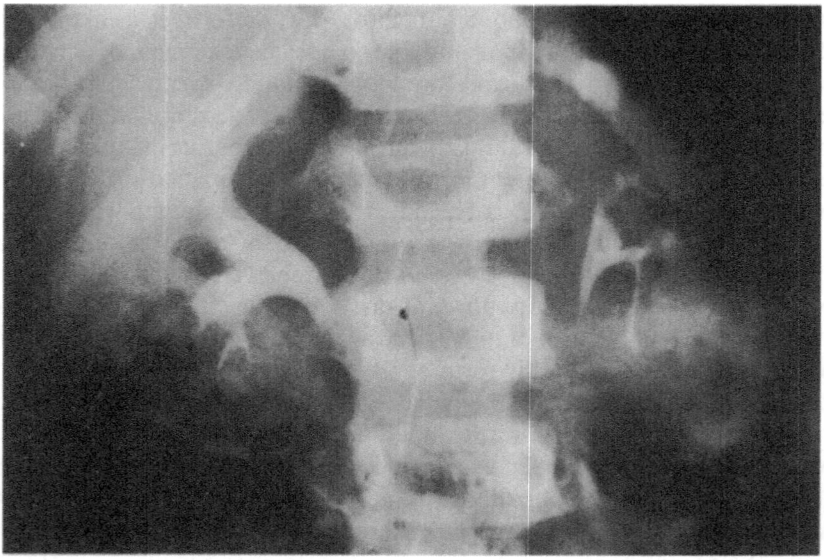

Figure 12-4

The IVP on this patient discloses a minor degree of parenchymal damage associated with minimal urinary extravasation. It has been found in recent years that it is quite safe to treat such patients nonoperatively. Utilizing nonoperative management, one large series of patients noted that over 86% of all injured kidneys were normal on IVP 6 months after the injury.[81] Using this conservative approach to renal trauma, the nephrectomy rate today is less than 4%. However, a certain amount of selectivity is required in order to determine which patients require renal arteriography or exploratory celiotomy. The complications of renal trauma, such as loss of functioning renal tissue, infection, hypertension, and prolonged or delayed hemorrhage, are directly related to the initial judgments made in the trauma victim. Injuries to the kidney may include minimal contusions of the renal parenchyma, lacerations of the parenchyma with perirenal extravasation of blood, major disruptions of the kidney with leakage of urine into the perirenal spaces, or complete shattering and disruption of the kidney with or without renal vessel disruption. The mere demonstration of extravasation of urine is not an indication for operation, as it has been noted that the leakage of the normally sterile urine into the perirenal tissues is not harmful, at least for periods of up to 24–36 hr.[81]

By far the most important study in a patient with suspected renal trauma is a drip infusion IVP. This will not only give information as to the extent of the injury but will also provide crucial information as to the functional state of the contralateral kidney. The role of arteriography in renal trauma is more controversial. Surely, a stable patient who has a nonvisualized kidney on IVP or in whom the suspicion of renal vascular damage exists should have an arteriogram. However, other patients will be deteriorating clinically at such a rapid rate that the time spent on this procedure would be ill advised.

The treatment, therefore, of minor renal injuries is admission to the hospital with observation, strict bedrest, analgesics, hydration, and antibiotics.[81] The patient is observed for evidence of perirenal infection along with evidence of continued bleeding, such as an expanding flank mass or a falling hematocrit. These patients should undergo an IVP prior to hospital discharge and should be followed up over the next few months to rule out the development of renal hypertension from renal vascular compromise. If the patient's clinical course dictates celiotomy, it is essential to gain control of the renal vessels as they arise from the aorta and vena cava. Following this, Gerota's fascia may be opened and any retroperitoneal hematoma explored.[82] With adequate exposure and preliminary vascular control, it will be possible in the majority of cases to avoid nephrectomy and to accomplish primary repair of lacerations or partial nephrectomy in more serious injuries.

ANSWER: A.

12.10. A 60-year-old male pedestrian is struck by an automobile. When first seen in the emergency room 30 min later, his pulse is 130 and his blood pressure is 90/40. There is no obvious injury to the chest; the abdomen is distended but not tender. Rectal examination is normal. There is severe pain in the pelvis on compression. A pelvic X ray is shown as Figure 12-5. He receives 6 units of whole blood over the next 8 hr. At that time, his pulse is 120, blood pressure is 100/50, and hematocrit is 26%. His urine output has been 200 cc over the last 8 hr. Treatment should consist of:

A. Celiotomy and bilateral hypogastric artery ligation.
B. Celiotomy and direct control of bleeding retroperitoneal vessels.
C. Arteriography and embolization of bleeding retroperitoneal vessels.
D. Systemic vasopressors.
E. Continued transfusions only.

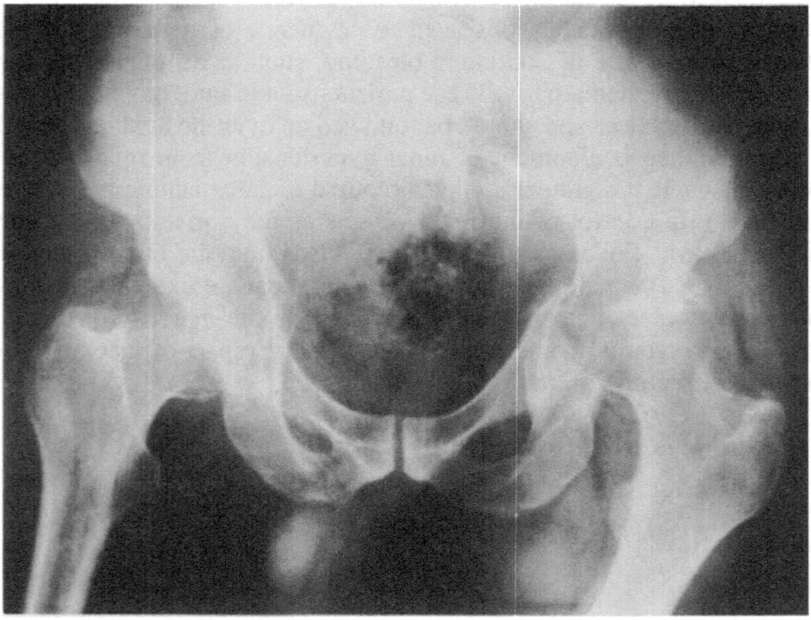

Figure 12-5

The X ray demonstrates a fracture through the left acetabulum and fractures of the pubis. This man has persistent massive bleeding secondary to disruption of retroperitoneal vessels as a consequence of his fractures. Although some authorities advocate transfusion only for this type of injury, it must be recognized that 60% of all deaths from pelvic fractures are secondary to hemorrhage and its consequences.[83] Because of this, other means of treatment have evolved that attempt to directly control the bleeding that may come from minor pelvic vessels or from disruption of the major pelvic arteries and veins.

Until recently, operation was felt to be indicated in such patients if bleeding did not stop with multiple transfusions. One advantage of this approach is that many of these patients harbor injuries to intra-abdominal viscera that require operative repair. Injuries to the spleen and liver are often noted, as are ruptures of the diaphragm, leading to acute diaphragmatic herniation.[84] The problem with attempted direct control of massive pelvic hematomas lies in the loss of the tamponade effect once the hematoma is entered. This can lead to uncontrollable bleeding, and it is rarely possible to gain control of individually bleeding vessels under such circumstances. Hypogastric artery ligation has been recommended under such circumstances, and there are reports of dramatic cessation of bleeding when this is employed.[85] However, bilateral hypogastric artery ligations have been carried out in many other patients with no discernable effect on the hemorrhage. Therefore, it is unrealistic to rely on this method of control in most patients.[86] If angiographic facilities are available, it would seem that the best way to attempt control of pelvic hemorrhage is by means of arteriography. This can localize any areas of arterial bleeding, and then these areas can be selectively embolized with either autologous clot or some other substance such as oxidized cellulose (Gelfoam).[83,86] Another method that has been successful in arresting hemorrhage secondary to pelvic fractures is selective balloon occlusion of individual bleeding vessels via arteriographic control.[87]

Using continued transfusion with whole blood and fresh frozen plasma, most bleeding from pelvic injuries should cease. In those situations where it does not, arteriography should be resorted to promptly. If a bleeding site is demonstrated, control should be attempted with one of the above methods. If no arteriographic abnormality is noted and the bleeding continues, venography can be used. This technique can localize areas of major venous disruption, and although no method exists for stopping this type of hemorrhage except operation, the surgeon can at least proceed with knowledge of the exact segment of vein that is involved.[83] If operation is required because of the presence of associated intra-abdominal injuries, it is best to leave small nonenlarging pelvic hematomas undisturbed.[88] A recent innovative approach to the problem of massive hemorrhage associated with pelvic fractures has been the application of a G suit. This consists of a wrap-around vinyl bag extending from the ankles to the epigastrium into which air is inflated. This can cause a marked decrease in the amount of hemorrhage and can also maintain blood pressure at high levels. It would seem, however, that the chief use of this device will be during the transport of an accident victim to the hospital.[89]

ANSWER: C.

12.11. A 48-year-old man falls asleep while driving, and his car runs off the road. On examination in the emergency room 1 hr later, he is inebriated but appears neurologically intact. He complains of anterior rib pain. Vital signs are normal. A chest X ray and arch aortogram are obtained and are shown as Figures 12-6 and 12-7. Treatment should consist of:

A. Observation only.
B. Immediate thoracotomy.
C. Bilateral tube thoracostomy.
D. Pericardiocentesis.
E. Aortic repair after a 2- to 3-week stabilization.

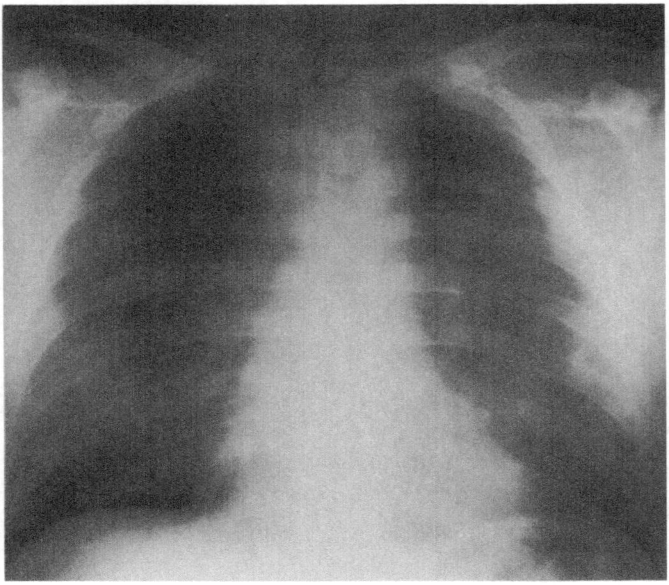

Figure 12-6

The chest X ray clearly shows a widened mediastinum and a downward depression of the left apical pleura by blood, leading to the suspicion that a ruptured thoracic aorta is present. This is confirmed on the aortogram, where a tear is noted in the aortic wall distal to the left subclavian artery. Ruptured thoracic aorta is seen commonly as a result of high-speed automobile accidents. It has been estimated that in over one out

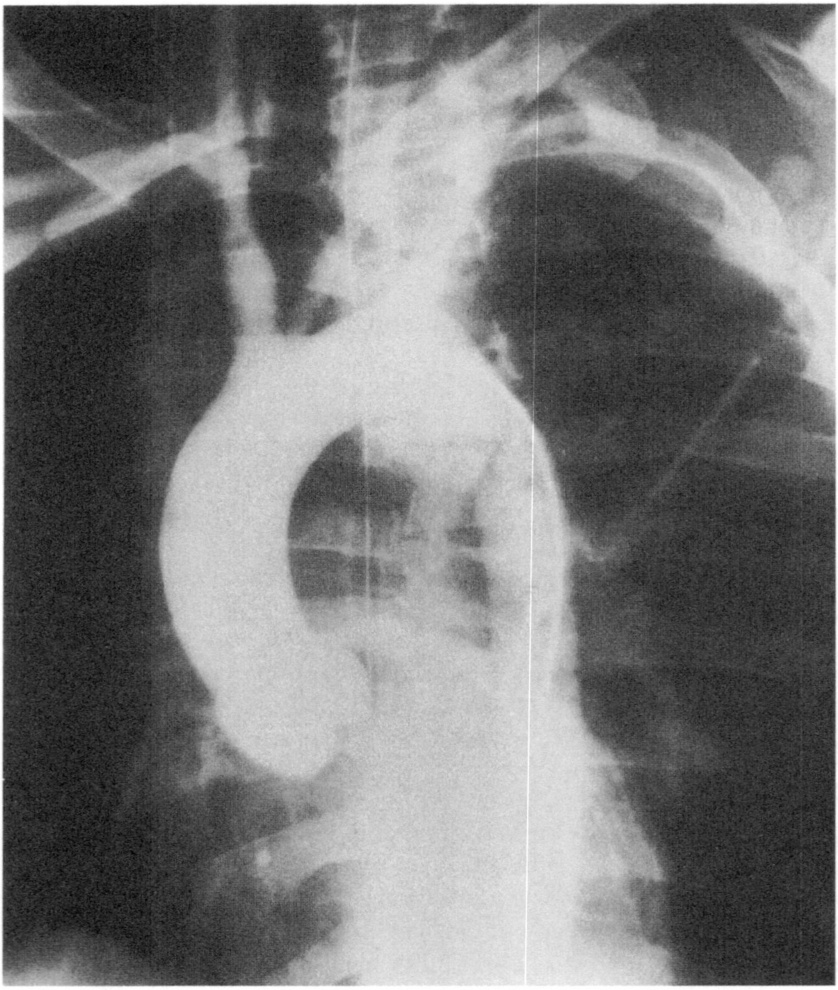

Figure 12-7

of ten fatal automobile accidents a ruptured thoracic aorta is present. The injury is caused by a horizontal deceleration of different parts of the aorta at points of fixation leading to a rupture at the aortic isthmus just distal to the left subclavian artery in the majority of cases. The injury may range from a small tear to a complete transection of the aorta. Eighty to 90% of patients with such an injury die immediately. The remainder survive for varying periods of time, as the aortic blood is contained by the adventitia, the pleura, and mediastinal tissue. In one review of 125 cases of aortic rupture, 20% of patients survived more than 1 hr after injury. Of these, 30% died within 6 hr, 49% within 24 hr, 72% within 8 days, and 90% by 4 months.[90] These observations make it imperative to suspect this injury in any patient who has sustained a deceleration accident. Symptoms and signs are inconsistent. Some patients will complain of chest pain, some will manifest upper extremity hypertension thought to be due to a coarctationlike picture, and some will manifest a systolic murmur thought to be caused by turbulent flow through the injured area.[91] In any patient in whom significant deceleration or thoracic injury has taken place, a good-quality upright chest X ray is essential. In nearly 100% of cases of traumatic thoracic aorta rupture, a widened superior mediastinum or abnormal aortic contour will be noted.[91] In any such patient, the next step must be immediate aortography, which will localize the tear. The only patients who should not undergo aortography are those whose clinical signs are rapidly deteriorating and who cannot safely undergo aortography while awaiting surgery. Immediately following aortography, a left thoracotomy is performed. It is generally possible to accomplish repair of the defect using a bypass shunt without extracorporeal circulation. In some instances, a small tear can be directly repaired; in other instances, replacement of a segment of aorta with a Dacron graft will be necessary. Utilizing these rapid diagnostic and therapeutic means, surgeons have been able to obtain survival in as many as 70% of patients presenting with a ruptured thoracic aorta.[91]

For those patients in whom diagnosis has been delayed and who present later with evidence of a posttraumatic aneurysm of the thoracic aorta, repair is likewise advised for those patients who are good operative risks. In one series of 12 patients with chronic aneurysms, 8 of these patients either became symptomatic or manifested aortic enlargement during prolonged periods of observation. Surgical excision was carried out in this group of patients with good results.[92]

ANSWER: B.

12.12. A 26-year-old man is shot in the forearm with a handgun. A minimal amount of blood is oozing from the skin wounds, but the area is swollen and tender. A bruit is present over the injured area, distal pulses are present, and movement of the distal extremity is normal. An arteriogram is obtained and is shown as Figure 12-8. Treatment should consist of:

A. Observation, and operation only if ischemic symptoms develop.
B. Repair of the artery only; vein ligation.
C. Primary repair of the artery and the vein.
D. Ligation of the artery and the vein.
E. Repair of the vein with ligation of the artery.

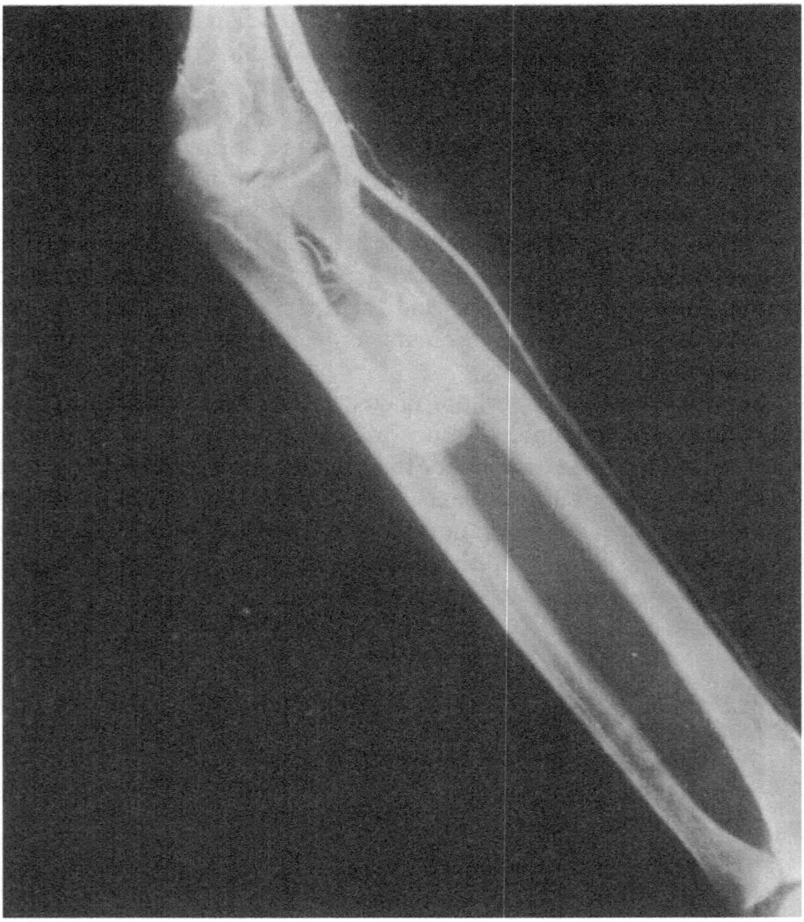

Figure 12-8

The arteriogram demonstrates a large false aneurysm at the site of injury. Although not seen on this study, an arteriovenous (AV) fistula was present, as anticipated from the presence of the bruit. The physician caring for a patient with a penetrating wound of the extremities (i.e., distal to the clavicle or the inguinal ligament) can sometimes have difficulty in determining if major vascular injury is present. It is well recognized that the presence of distal pulses do not rule out serious arterial injury.[93] In one series of 128 patients with major vascular trauma of the extremities, 27% of patients had palpable distal pulses.[94] Other clinical signs that tend to suggest arterial bleeding are a history of persistent arterial bleeding, a large or expanding hematoma, hypotension, a bruit at or distal to the site of injury, injury to nearby nerves, or even the anatomic proximity of the wound to a major artery. It is important to understand that the presence of distal ischemia invariably implies major vascular injury and should not be misinterpreted as merely arterial spasm.[95]

The role of preoperative angiography in the diagnosis of arterial injury is controversial. Certain authorities have maintained that if the clinical examination is normal, no arteriogram is indicated.[96] However, data from various trauma centers have indicated that arteriography is extremely accurate in the detection of arterial injury. One study has shown only one false negative arteriogram in 183 patients with vascular injuries, leading to the conclusion that a normal arteriogram nearly excludes the presence of arterial injury.[97] If the decision to operate is made based upon the presence of any of the above clinical signs and any arteriographic abnormality, few if any cases that require exploration will be ignored. The importance, of course, of prompt exploration of these injuries lies in their capacity to develop the late complications of false aneurysm or AV fistula.[97] In the case presented, an obvious false aneurysm is present, along with an AV fistula. At the time of operation, both the arterial and any concomitant venous injury should be repaired.[95,98] Repair of both vessels is technically easier at this time than if performed in the future for late complications. Also, if the major venous injury is not repaired, it contributes to stasis and phlebitis and can compromise the success of the arterial repair. Another technical point in a combined arterial and venous injury is that no ipsilateral vein should be used as a donor graft if one is required.[95] An additional adjunct at this time is the use of operative angiography to detect technical errors and thus preclude many early failures of the vascular repair.[97] The postoperative care of the patient with vascular trauma is exceedingly important and stresses the need for maintenance of circulating blood volume and frequent evaluation of the revascularized extremity so that any early failures may be reoperated upon promptly.

ANSWER: C.

12.13. A 28-year-old man develops left calf pain after strenuous exercise. When examined 6 hr later, there is swelling and tenderness to palpation of the left calf, and the patient cannot dorsiflex any of his toes. Pedal pulses are palpable. Treatment should consist of:

A. Bed rest and leg elevation.
B. Heparin.
C. Fasciotomy.
D. Warm compresses.
E. Venous thrombectomy.

This patient has an anterior compartment syndrome with increased compartmental pressure and compression of the anterior compartmental muscles and the anterior tibial nerve, leading to a foot drop. This syndrome can result from many causes, such as a leg fracture, arterial thrombosis or embolus, acute venous occlusion, leg trauma, or severe or unaccustomed exercise. All of these etiologies have in common the production of an increased anterior compartment tissue pressure leading to decreased tissue perfusion and resultant ischemic necrosis of the muscles contained within the compartment. The differential diagnosis of this syndrome is exceedingly important, owing to the severe sequelae of an untreated compartment syndrome. Such conditions as cellulitis, thrombophlebitis, tibial stress fractures, tenosynovitis, osteomyelitis, and the more mild ''shin splints'' must be considered.

The clinical presentation of these patients is typical, with pain, swelling, and tenderness over the anterior compartment and weakness or paralysis of the compartmental muscles, along with hypoesthesia in the first interdigital cleft. Depending upon the etiology of the compartment syndrome, pedal pulses may or may not be present. The anterior tibial compartment is a space surrounded by rigid bony and fascial boundaries. Therefore, any increase in size of any of the enclosed structures cannot be accomodated within the compartment. The compartment contains the anterior tibial muscle and the extensor muscles to all of the toes. In addition, the anterior tibial nerve passes through this compartment, and this nerve is motor to the compartmental muscles. One of the terminal branches of this nerve is sensory to the dorsal surface of the first interdigital cleft, accounting for the hypoesthesia in this area in a compartmental compression syndrome. The compartment also contains the anterior tibial artery. A diagram of the anterior compartment is shown as Figure 12-9.

In view of this rigidly enclosed space, the only practical way to lower pressure within the compartment is by means of a fasciotomy. This can usually be easily managed by making a long incision over the anterior compartment down to and through the superficial fascia. Attempts at

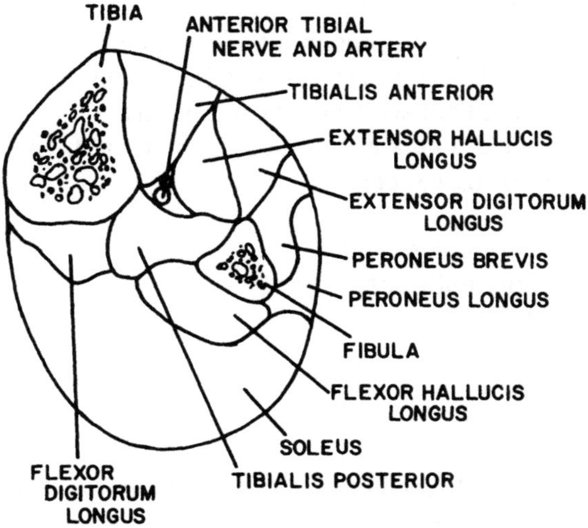

Figure 12-9

lesser degrees of compartmental decompression may fail because of compression at the skin level, so therefore a full length skin and fascial incision is indicated. Another effective way of decompressing the anterior and all other compartments of the leg is with a partial fibulectomy, but this is far more treatment than most of these patients require. Fasciotomy is, however, not without its own complications, as infection can occur in the underlying ischemic muscles and necessitate amputation.[99]

Most authorities are in agreement that as soon as a definite diagnosis of anterior compartment syndrome is made, fasciotomy is indicated. In a review of 137 cases from the literature, only 13% were relieved by fasciotomy if foot drop was already present.[99] Another series of 46 cases demonstrated that only 8% of patients regained normal leg and foot function if fasciotomy was performed late.[100] However, it is recognized that lesser degrees of compartment compression are treatable without fasciotomy and complete recovery can be expected. It is for this reason that measurements of tissue pressure within the compartment have gained some importance. By utilizing a relatively simple manometer and pressure-recording device, absolute tissue pressures and serial changes in tissue pressure can be noted, and fasciotomy can be carried out if pressures are noted to increase.[101–103] However, it is equally clear that tissue pressure measurements are of little value in the patient with evidence of muscular weakness. In such a patient, the delay may be critical and prompt fasciotomy is required.

ANSWER: C.

12.14. A 60-year-old man enters the hospital with painful neck and back spasms and is unable to open his mouth or swallow; 3 hr later, he has a generalized seizure. His wife relates that he cut his arm with an ax 12 days previously but did not seek medical attention at that time. The wound is minimally reddened and is not draining pus. Treatment should consist of each of the following except:

A. Wound debridement.
B. Gas gangrene antitoxin.
C. Tetanus antitoxin.
D. Penicillin.
E. Tracheostomy.

This patient has a clinically obvious case of tetanus. Unlike clostridial gas gangrene, which is a complication of severe or neglected wounds, tetanus may occur in individuals with superficial or very minor wounds. The bacterium responsible for tetanus is an anaerobic spore-forming rod, *Clostridium tetani,* and symptoms are caused by the formation of an exotoxin produced by the multiplying bacteria within devitalized tissue. This toxin has been named tetanospasmin and acts on four areas of the nervous system: the motor end plates in skeletal muscle, the spinal cord, the brain, and the sympathetic nervous system.[104] The spinal cord effects account for the severe spasms characteristic of the disease; the cerebral involvement accounts for seizures; the sympathetic disturbances account for hypertension, tachycardia, peripheral vasoconstriction, cardiac arrhythmias, and profuse sweating.

The incubation period of tetanus is usually 3 to 21 days. However, much longer periods have been recorded. The prognosis is directly related to the length of incubation and to the length of the period between the onset of symptoms and the full picture of tetanus. The longer the period is, the better the prognosis.[105]

The diagnosis of tetanus is a clinical one. The characteristic gram-positive rods are only infrequently recovered from wounds, and the spinal fluid is normal. The mortality rate in generalized tetanus is greater than 50% and has shown little improvement over the past 70 years.[104,105] Deaths occur most commonly from respiratory failure, cardiac arrest, or complications of tracheostomy.

Prevention is the key to the tetanus problem. Active immunization is fully protective and extremely safe. In one series of over two and one half million tetanus immunizations, no deaths were recorded.[106] Similarly, in the prevention of the disease, judicious use of human antitoxin is indicated in all previously unimmunized patients and in some immunized patients who have significantly contaminated wounds and are beyond 5 years from their last toxoid dose. Treatment of an established case includes wound care with extensive debridement, irrigation, and avoidance of wound closure so that anaerobic conditions are not present. Administration of tetanus human globulin in a dose of 3000 to 6000 units IM will also neutralize toxin that is already formed, although there is some question whether toxin fixed in the central nervous system can be neutralized. Systemic antibiotics are recommended not only to prevent multiplication of *C. tetani* in the wound with further toxin production but also to decrease secondary bacterial infection in the wound. Penicillin is recommended in a dose of one million units every 6 hr for 10 days. General supportive measures are extremely important, and excellent nursing care is essential. Control of muscle spasms and convulsions is essential. Many drugs have been employed, and diazepam (Valium) intravenously appears able to control most of these symptoms. Maintenance of nutrition with parenteral hyperalimentation is a recent important advance, as many of these patients cannot open their mouths for prolonged periods of time. Early tracheostomy can also be life-saving. Most authorities agree that routine tracheostomy in every patient is not required, but most patients will require tracheostomy. Surely after the first generalized seizure this should be instituted.[104,105] Treatment must also include completion of active tetanus immunization.

ANSWER: B

References

1. Olsen, W.R.: The serum amylase in blunt abdominal trauma. *J. Trauma* 13:200, 1973.
2. Lim, R.C., Glickman, M.G., Hunt, T.K.: Angiography in patients with blunt trauma to the chest and abdomen. *Surg. Clin. North Am.* 52:551, 1972.
3. Freeark, R.J.: Role of angiography in the management of multiple injuries. *Surg. Gynecol. Obstet.* 128:761, 1969.
4. Love, L., Greenfield, G.B., Braum, T.W., Moncada, R., Freeark, R.J., Baker, R.J.: Arteriography of splenic trauma. *Radiology* 91:96, 1968.
5. Olsen, W.R., Redman, H.C., Hildreth, D.H.: Quantitative peritoneal lavage in blunt abdominal trauma. *Arch. Surg.* 104:536, 1972.
6. Perry, J.F., Strate, R.G.: Diagnostic peritoneal lavage in blunt abdominal trauma: Indications and results. *Surgery* 71:898, 1972.
7. Ahmad, W., Polk, H.C.: Blunt abdominal trauma: A prospective study with selective peritoneal lavage. *Arch. Surg.* 111:489, 1976.
8. Thal, E.R., Shires, G.T.: Peritoneal lavage in blunt abdominal trauma. *Am. J. Surg.* 125:64, 1973.
9. Sachatello, C.R., Bivins, B.: Technic for peritoneal dialysis and diagnostic peritoneal lavage. *Am. J. Surg.* 131:637, 1976.
10. Civetta, J.M., Williams, M.J., Richie, R.E.: Diagnostic peritoneal irrigation: A simple and reliable technique. *Surgery* 67:874, 1970.
11. Parvin, S., Smith, D.E., Asher, W.M., Virgilio, R.W.: Effectiveness of peritoneal lavage in blunt abdominal trauma. *Ann. Surg.* 181:255, 1975.
12. Freeark, R.J.:Penetrating wounds of the abdomen. *N. Engl. J. Med.* 291:185, 1974.
13. Lowe, R.J., Boyd, D.R., Folk, F.A., Baker, R.J.: The negative laparotomy for abdominal trauma. *J. Trauma* 12:853, 1972.
14. Forde, K.A., Ganepola, G.A.P.: Is mandatory exploration for penetrating abdominal trauma extinct? The morbidity and mortality of negative exploration in a large municipal hospital. *J. Trauma* 14:764, 1974.
15. Nance, F.C., Cohn, I.: Surgical judgment in the management of stab wounds of the abdomen: A retrospective and prospective analysis based on a study of 600 stabbed patients. *Ann. Surg.* 170:569, 1969.
16. Nance, F.C., Wennar, M.H., Johnson, L.W., Ingram, J.C., Cohn, I.: Surgical judgment in the management of penetrating wounds of the abdomen: Experience with 2212 patients. *Ann. Surg.* 179:639, 1974.
17. Richter, R.M., Zaki, M.H.: Selective conservative management of penetrating abdominal wounds. *Ann. Surg.* 166:238, 1967.
18. Wilder, J.R., Lotfi, M.W., Jurani, P.: Comparative study of mandatory and selective surgical intervention in stab wounds of the abdomen. *Surgery* 69:546, 1971.
19. Netterville, R.E., Hardy, J.D.: Penetrating wounds of the abdomen: Analysis of 155 cases with problems in management. *Ann. Surg.* 166:232, 1967.
20. Spenler, C.W., Benfield, J.R.: Esophageal disruption from blunt and penetrating external trauma. *Arch. Surg.* 111:663, 1976.
21. Rosoff, L., White, E.J.: Perforation of the esophagus. *Am. J. Surg.* 128:207, 1974.
22. Sheely, C.H., Mattox, K.L., Beall, A.C., DeBakey, M.E.: Penetrating wounds of the cervical esophagus. *Am. J. Surg.* 130:707,1975.
23. Sawyers, J.L., Lane, C.E., Foster, J.H., Daniel, R.A.: Esophageal perforation an increasing challenge. *Ann. Thorac. Surg.* 19:233, 1975.
24. Loop, F.D., Groves, L.K.: Esophageal perforations. *Ann. Thorac. Surg.* 10:571, 1970.
25. Urschel, H.C., Razzuk, M.A., Wood, R.E., Galbraith, N., Pockey, M., Paulson, D.L.:

Improved management of esophageal perforation: Exclusion and diversion in continuity. *Ann. Surg.* 179:587, 1974.
26. Loop, F.D.: Trauma to the esophagus. *Cleve. Clin. Q.* 42:175, 1975.
27. Jones, W.R., Hardin, W.J., Davis, J.T., Hardy, J.D.: Intramural hematoma of the duodenum: A review of the literature and case report. *Ann. Surg.* 173:534, 1971.
28. Margolis, I.B., Carnazzo, A.J., Finn, M.P.: Intramural hematoma of the duodenum. *Am. J. Surg.* 132:779, 1976.
29. Fullen, W.D., Selle, J.G., Whitely, D.H., Martin, L.W., Altemeier, W.A.: Intramural duodenal hematoma. *Ann. Surg.* 179:549, 1974.
30. King, W.L.M., Provan, J.L.: Diagnosis and management of duodenal injuries. *Can. J. Surg.* 15:269, 1972.
31. Corley, R.D., Norcross, W.J., Shoemaker, W.C.: Traumatic injuries to the duodenum: A report of 98 patients. *Ann. Surg.* 181:92, 1975.
32. Morton, J.R., Jordan, G.L.: Traumatic duodenal injuries: Review of 131 cases. *J. Trauma* 8:127, 1968.
33. Bender, H.W., Sebor, J., Zuidema, G.D.: Serosal patch grafting for closure of posterior duodenal defects. *Am. J. Surg.* 115:103, 1968.
34. Jones, S.A., Gazzaniga, A.B., Keller, T.B.: The serosal patch: A surgical parachute. *Am. J. Surg.* 126:186, 1973.
35. McInnis, W.D., Aust, J.B., Cruz, A.B., Root, H.D.: Traumatic injuries of the duodenum: A comparison of 1° closure and the jejunal patch. *J. Trauma* 15:847, 1975.
36. White, E.J., Yellin, A.E., Berne, C.J., Donovan, A.J.: Duodenal "diverticulization" for duodenal and pancreatic injury. *Am. J. Surg.* 127:503, 1974.
37. Beall, A.C., Bricker, D.L., Alessi, F.J., Whisennand, W.W., DeBakey, M.E.: Surgical considerations in the management of civilian colon injuries. *Ann. Surg.* 173:971, 1971.
38. Josen, A.S., Ferrer, J.M., Forde, K.A., Zikria, B.A.: Primary closure of civilian colorectal wounds. *Ann. Surg.* 176:782, 1972.
39. LoCicero, J., Tajima, T., Drapanas, T.: A half century of experience in the management of colon injuries: Changing concepts. *J. Trauma* 15:575, 1975.
40. Kirkpatrick, J.R.:The exteriorized anastomosis: Its role in surgery of the colon. *Surgery* 82:362, 1977.
41. Getzen, L.C., Pollak, E.W., Wolfman, E.F.: Abdominoperineal resection in the treatment of devascularizing rectal injuries. *Surgery* 82:310, 1977.
42. Winkelstein, J.A.: Splenectomy and infection. *Arch Intern. Med.* 137:1516, 1977.
43. Eraklis, A.J., Filler, R.M.: Splenectomy in childhood: A review of 1413 cases. *J. Pediatr. Surg.* 7:382, 1972.
44. Eraklis, A.J., Kevy, S.V., Diamond, L.K., Gross, R.E.: Hazard of overwhelming infection after splenectomy in childhood. *N. Engl. J. Med* 276:1225, 1967.
45. Gopal, V., Bisno, A.L.: Fulminant pneumococcal infections in "normal" asplenic hosts. *Arch Intern. Med.* 137:1526, 1977.
46. Ellis, E.F., Smith, R.T.: The role of the spleen in immunity with special reference to the post-splenectomy problem in infants. *Pediatrics* 37:111, 1966.
47. Constantopoulos, A., Najjar, V.A., Wish, J.B., Necheles, T.H., Stolbach, L.L.: Defective phagocytosis due to tuftsin deficiency in splenectomized subjects. *Am. J. Dis. Child.* 125:663, 1973.
48. Ein, S.H., Shandling, B., Simpson, J.S., Stephens, C.A., Bandi, S.K., Biggar, W.D., Freedman, M.H.: The morbidity and mortality of splenectomy in childhood. *Ann. Surg.* 185:307, 1977.
49. Douglas, G.J., Simpson, J.S.: The conservative management of splenic trauma. *J. Pediatr. Surg.* 6:565, 1971.
50. Shandling, B.: Splenectomy for trauma: A second look. *Arch. Surg.* 111:1325, 1976.

51. Burrington, J.D.: Surgical repair of a ruptured spleen in children. *Arch. Surg.* 112:417, 1977.
52. Mishalany, H.: Repair of the ruptured pleen. *J. Pediatr. Surg.* 9:175, 1974.
53. Morgenstern, L.: Microcrystalline collagen used in experimental splenic injury. *Arch. Surg.* 109:44, 1974.
54. Morgenstern, L.: The avoidable complications of splenectomy. *Surg. Gynecol. Obstet.* 145:525, 1977.
55. Dickerman, J.D.: Bacterial infection and the asplenic host: A review. *J. Trauma* 16:662, 1976.
56. Ammann, A.J., Addiego, J., Wara, D.W., Lubin, B., Smith, W.B., Mentzer, W.C.: Polyvalent pneumococcalpolysaccharide immunization of patients with sickle cell anemia and patients with splenectomy. *N. Engl. J. Med.* 297:897, 1977.
57. Smit, P., Oberholzer, D., Hayden-Smith, S., Koornhof, H.J., Hilleman, M.R.: Protective efficacy of pneumococcal polysaccharide vaccines. *J.A.M.A.* 238:2613, 1977.
58. Brewster, D.C.: Spenosis: Report of two cases and review of the literature. *Am. J. Surg.* 126:14, 1973.
59. Widmann, W.D., Laubscher, F.A.: Splenosis: A disease or a beneficial condition? *Arch. Surg.* 102:152, 1971.
60. Shifir, M., Deysine, M., Bramis, J., Acker, P., Aufses, A.H.: Immunologic function of subcutaneous splenic implants in mice. *Surg. Forum* 28:335, 1977.
61. Walt, A.J.: The mythology of hepatic trauma—Or Babel revisited. *Am. J. Surg.* 135:12, 1978.
62. Trunkey, D.D., Shires, G.T., McClelland, R.: Management of liver trauma in 811 consecutive patients. *Ann. Surg.* 179:722, 1974.
63. Defore, W.W., Mattox, K.L., Jordan, G.L., Beall, A.C.: Management of 1590 consecutive cases of liver trauma. *Arch. Surg.* 111:493, 1976.
64. Graham, R.R., Cannell, D.: Accidental ligation of the hepatic artery. *Br. J. Surg.* 20:566, 1932.
65. Aaron, S., Fulton, R.L., Mays, E.T.: Selective ligation of the hepatic artery for trauma of the liver. *Surg. Gynecol. Obstet.* 141:187, 1975.
66. Mays, E.T., Wheeler, C.S.: Demonstration of collateral arterial flow after interruption of hepatic arteries in man. *N. Engl. J. Med.* 290:993, 1974.
67. Koehler, R.E., Korobkin, M., Lewis, F.: Arteriographic demonstration of collateral arterial supply to the liver after hepatic artery ligation. *Radiology* 117:49, 1975.
68. Merendino, K.A., Dillard, D.H., Cammock, E.E.: The concept of surgical biliary decompression in the management of liver trauma. *Surg. Gynecol. Obstet.* 117:285, 1963.
69. Lucas, C.E.: Prospective clinical evaluation of biliary drainage in hepatic trauma. *Ann. Surg.* 174:830, 1971.
70. Lucas, C.E., Walt, A.J.: Analysis of randomized biliary drainage for liver trauma in 189 patients. *J. Trauma* 12:925, 1972.
71. Bowen, J.C., Flemming, W.H.: Upper gastrointestinal bleeding associated with biliary diversion after hepatic injury. *Ann. Surg.* 177:402, 1973.
72. Schrock, T. Blaisdell, F.W., Mathewson, C.: Management of blunt trauma to the liver and hepatic veins. *Arch. Surg.* 96:698, 1968.
73. Jones, R.C., Shires, G.T.: Pancreatic trauma. *Arch. Surg.* 102:424, 1971.
74. Smith, A.D., Woolverton, W.C., Weichert, R.F., Drapanas, T.: Operative management of pancreatic and duodenal injuries. *J. Trauma* 11:570, 1971.
75. Jones, R.C.: Management of pancreatic trauma. *Ann. Surg.* 187:555, 1978.
76. Moretz, J.A., Campbell, D.P., Parker, D.E., Williams, G.R.: Significance of serum amylase level in evaluating pancreatic trauma. *Am. J. Surg.* 130:739, 1975.

77. White, P.H., Benfield, J.R.: Amylase in the management of pancreatic trauma. *Arch. Surg.* 105:158, 1972.
78. Northrup, W.F., Simmons, R.L.: Pancreatic trauma: A review. *Surgery* 71:27, 1972.
79. Yellin, A.E., Vecchione, T.R., Donovan, A.J.: Distal pancreatectomy for pancreatic trauma. *Am. J. Surg.* 124:135, 1972.
80. Anderson, C.B., Connors, J.P., Mejia, D.C., Wise, L.:Drainage methods in the treatment of pancreatic injuries. *Surg. Gynecol. Obstet.* 138:587, 1974.
81. Mitchell, J.P.: Trauma to the urinary tract. *N. Engl. J. Med.* 288:90, 1973.
82. Holcroft, J.W., Trunkey, D.D., Minagi, H., Korobkin, M.T., Lim, R.C.: Renal trauma and retroperitoneal hematomas: Indications for exploration. *J. Trauma* 15:1045, 1975.
83. Ring, E.J., Waltman, A.C., Athanasoulis, C., Smith, J.C., Baum, S.: Angiography in pelvic trauma. *Surg. Gynecol. Obstet.* 139:375, 1974.
84. Andrus, C.H., Morton, J.H.: Rupture of the diaphragm after blunt trauma. *Am. J. Surg.* 119:686, 1970.
85. Hauser, C.W., Perry, J.F.: Control of massive hemorrhage from pelvic fractures by hypogastric artery ligation. *Surg. Gynecol. Obstet.* 121:313, 1965.
86. VanUrk, H., Perlberger, R.R., Muller, H.: Selective arterial embolization for control of traumatic pelvic hemorrhage. *Surgery* 83:133, 1978.
87. Paster, S.B., VanHouten, F.X., Adams, D.F.: Percutaneous balloon catherization: A technique for the control of arterial hemorrhage caused by pelvic trauma. *J.A.M.A.* 230:573, 1974.
88. Hawkins, L., Pomerantz, M., Eiseman, B.: Laparotomy at the time of pelvic fracture. *J. Trauma* 10:619, 1970.
89. Batalden, D.J., Wickstrom, P.H., Ruiz, E., Gustilo, R.B.: Value of the G suit in patients with severe pelvic fracture: Controlling hemorrhagic shock. *Arch Surg.* 109:326, 1974.
90. Parmley, L.F., Mattingly, T.W., Manion, W.C., Jahnke, E.J.: Non-penetrating traumatic injury of the aorta. *Circulation* 17:1086, 1958.
91. Kirsh, M.M., Behrendt, D.M., Orringer, M.B., Gago, O., Gray, L.A., Mills, L.J., Walter, J.F., Sloan, H.: The treatment of acute traumatic rupture of the aorta: 1 10 year experience. *Ann. Surg.* 184:308, 1976.
92. Schwartz, M.L., Fisher, R., Sako, Y., Castaneda, A.R., Grage, T.B., Nicoloff, D.M.: Post-traumatic aneurysms of the thoracic aorta. *Surgery* 78:589, 1975.
93. Moore, C.H., Wolma, F.J., Brown, R.W., Derrick, J.R.: Vascular trauma: A review of 250 cases. *Am. J. Surg.* 122:576, 1971.
94. Drapanas, T., Hewitt, R.L., Weichert, R.F., Smith, A.D.: Civilian vascular injuries: A critical appraisal of three decades of management. *Ann. Surg.* 172:351, 1970.
95. Burnett, H.F., Parnell, C.L., Williams, G.D., Campbell, G.S.: Peripheral arterial injuries: A reassessment. *Ann. Surg.* 183:701, 1976.
96. McDonald, E.J., Goodman, P.C., Winestock, D.P.: The clinical indications for arteriography in trauma to the extremity. *Diagn. Radiol.* 116:45, 1975.
97. Snyder, W.H., Thal, E.R., Bridges, R.A., Gerlock, A.J., Perry, M.O., Fry, W.J.: The validity of normal arteriography in penetrating trauma. *Arch. Surg.* 113:424, 1978.
98. Perry, M.O., Thal, E.R., Shires, G.T.: Management of arterial injuries. *Ann. Surg.* 173:403, 1971.
99. Bradley, E.L.: The anterior tibial compartment syndrome. *Surg. Gynecol. Obstet.* 136:289, 1973.
100. Sheridan, G.W., Matsen, F.A.: Fasciotomy in the treatment of the acute compartment syndrome. *J. Bone Joint Surg. (Am.)* 58-A: 112, 1976.
101. Clayton, J.M., Hayes, A.C., Barnes, R.W.: Tissue pressure and perfusion in the compartment syndrome. *J. Surg. Res.* 22:333, 1977.

102. Matsen, F.A., Mayo, K.A., heridan, G.W., Krugmire, R.B.: Monitoring of intramuscular pressure. *Surgery* 79:702, 1976.
103. Whitesides, T.E., Haney, T.C., Morimoto, K., Harada, H.: Tissue pressure measurements as a determinant for the need of fasciotomy. *Clin. Ortho.* 113:43, 1975.
104. Weinstein, L.: Tetanus. *N. Engl. J. Med.* 289:1293, 1973.
105. Faust, R.A., Vickers, O.R., Cohn, I.: Tetanus: 2449 cases in 68 years at Charity Hospital. *J. Trauma* 16:704, 1976.
106. Furste, W., Wheeler, W.L.: Tetanus: A team disease. *Curr. Probl. Surg.*, October 1972, p. 25.

INDEX

Abdomen
  distention after celiotomy, 266
  mass in pancreatitis, 94
  radiography, *see* Radiography, abdominal
  stab wound of, 304
  surgery, major, and pulmonary embolism, 282
  trauma, blunt, 302–303
  ultrasound, *see* Ultrasound, abdominal
A bile, 86
Abscess
  appendiceal, 147–149
  in Crohn's disease, 153
  formation in diverticulitis, 145–146
  liver, and cholecystitis, 73
  pancreas, 97
    pancreatitis and, 95
    signs and symptoms of, 97
  rectum, in Crohn's disease, 152
  subphrenic
    cholecystitis and, 73
    drainage in mesenteric vein thrombosis, 115
    postoperative, 261–263
Acalculous cholecystopathy, 86–91
Acetabulum, fracture, 325
Achalasia, 14–15
  complications of, 14
  dilatation in, pneumatic, 14
ACTH
  in Crohn's disease, 154
  intravenous, in toxic megacolon, 157
Adenocarcinoma
  gastroesophageal junction, 176–177
  rectum, differentiated from carcinoma of anus, 195
  stomach, 16
Adenoma
  fibroadenoma of breast and cystosarcoma phyllodes, 254
  parathyroid, 220, 221
  rectal villous, 190
    excision of, 190
    fulguration of, 190
    resection of, 190
Adrenal
  cortical hyperplasia, 206
  crisis, 210–211
  hyperplasia, medullary, 230–231
Adrenalectomy
  bilateral, in Sipple's syndrome, 230
  in breast carcinoma
    inflammatory, 246
    metastatic, 242
  in Cushing's syndrome, 204
Adrenocorticolytic drugs in Cushing's disease, 202
Age
  pulmonary embolism and, 282
  thyroid nodule and, 224
  wound dehiscence and, 260
Alcoholic pancreatitis, 95, 98
Alcoholism and carcinoma of esophagus, 16
Aldosteronism, primary, 206
Aldosteronoma, 206
Alkaline reflux gastritis, 35–37
  pathophysiology, 35
Alkalosis, hypochloremic, in chronic duodenal ulcer, 24
Alveolar collapse in postoperative period, 268
Amebiasis
  hemagglutination test in, indirect, 163
  intestinal, 163

Ambeic colitis, 163–164
toxic megacolon and, 158
Amylase
in ascites, pancreatic, 98
levels in gallstone pancreatitis, 92
in mesenteric artery embolism, superior, 112
Anal carcinoma, 195–196
excision in, local, 195
Anal lesions in Crohn's disease, 152
Analgesics
in pulmonary embolism, suspected, 287
in renal trauma, 323
Anastomosis
in ascites, pancreatic, 99
in bowel obstruction, large, 109
in carcinoma of colon, 191
in Crohn's disease, 154
dehiscence, postoperative, with fistula, 264–265
in diverticulitis, perforated sigmoid, 142
in fistula, colovesical, 143
leak, and septic shock, 276
in volvulus, sigmoid, 118
Anemia
after gastric resection, 33
iron deficiency, after duodenal ulcer surgery, 33
pernicious, elevated gastrin in, 38
Anesthesia for cholecystostomy
in cholangitis, 77
in cholecystitis, 74
Aneurysm, false, and gunshot wound, 331
Angiography
of gastric mucosal hemorrhage, 42
of mediastinum, widened, after blunt trauma, 302
of patency after Warren shunt, 58
preoperative, in arterial injury, 331
in pulmonary embolism, 284
suspected, 287, 288
Angiotensin, 232
Antacids
in esophageal reflux, 5
in gastritis, stress, 42
Anterior compartment
diagram of, 332, 333
syndrome, 332–333
presentation of, clinical, 332
Antibiotics
in abscess
appendiceal, 148
pancreas, 97
before operation, 259
in bowel obstruction, small, 124
broad-spectrum, in amebic colitis, 163
in cholangitis, 77
in cholecystitis, 72, 74
in colitis, ischemic, 165
in common duct stone, 82
in diverticulitis with abscess, 145
in duodenal ulcer, perforated, 25
during operation, 259
in ileus, gallstone, 131
in megacolon, toxic, 158
in mesenteric vein thrombosis, 115
in pancreatitis, gallstone, 92
in phlegmon, appendiceal, 150
prophylactic
for postoperative wound infection, 259
after splenectomy, in children, 316
in renal trauma, 322
after volvulus surgery, sigmoid, 118
Anticholinergics
in bowel obstruction, small, 124
in cholecystopathy, acalculous, 86
Anticoagulants in Budd–Chiari syndrome, 62
Antigen, carcinoembryonic, role of, 192
Antitoxin, tetanus, 334
Antrectomy
in duodenal ulcer, 26
perforated, 30
in gastric ulcers, multiple, 44
Anus, *see* entries under Anal
Aorta, rupture, 327, 329
Aortography in chest trauma, blunt, 327
Aorto-renal bypass in renovascular hypertension, 232
Appendectomy
in appendiceal abscess, 148
in appendiceal phlegmon, 150
small bowel obstruction and, 124
Appendiceal abscess, 147–149
Appendiceal phlegmon, 150–151
Appendicostomy
in appendiceal abscess, 148

Appendicostomy *(cont.)*
  in appendiceal phlegmon, 150
ARDS, *see* Respiratory distress syndrome, adult
Areola in Paget's disease, 250
Arrhythmia after vasopressin, 56
Arteries
  hepatic, ligation after trauma, 317
  injury
    in gunshot wound, 330–331
    preoperative angiography in, 331
  mesenteric, *see* Mesenteric, superior
  repair in gunshot wound, 330
Arteriography
  in glucagonoma, 214
  in gunshot wound with arterial injury, 330
  hepatic, in Budd–Chiari syndrome, 62
  in insulinoma, 217
  in mesenteric artery embolism, superior, 112
  in pelvic hemorrhage and fracture, 324
  pulmonary, in embolism, 282, 284, 285
  in renovascular hypertension, 232
Arteriovenous fistula and gunshot wound, 331
Ascites
  intractable, treatment, 66–67
  pancreas, 98–99
    diagnosis, 98
    pancreatitis and, 98
Atelectasis, postoperative, 267–269
Atherosclerotic plaque and mesenteric artery embolism, superior, 112
Atony, gastric, postvagotomy, 127
Atrial fibrillation and mesenteric artery embolism, superior, 112
Atrophic gastritis, elevated gastrin in, 38
AV fistula and gunshot wound, 331
Azathioprine in Crohn's disease, 154
Azotemia and renal failure, 274

Back-diffusion of hydrogen ion and stress ulcer, 41
Bacteroides fragilis in biliary tree, 77
Baker tube, 135, 136
Balloon tamponade
  in portal vein thrombosis, 60
  for variceal hemorrhage, 54–55
Barium enema
  in bowel obstruction, large, 108
  in colitis
    granulomatous, 160, 161
    ischemic, 165–166
  in Crohn's disease, 154, 155
  in fistual
    colovesical, 143
    rectovaginal, radiation-induced, 168
  hydrostatic, in cecal volvulus, 121
  in intussusception, 137
  in phlegmon, appendiceal, 150, 151
  in volvulus
    cecal, 120
    sigmoid, 116, 117
Barium gastrointestinal study in bowel obstruction, small, postoperative, 126
Barium meal in alkaline reflux gastritis, 37
Barrett's esophagus, 4
B bile, 91
Bedrest in renal trauma, 322
Belsey repair for hiatus hernia with reflux, 5
Bernstein test, 4
Bethanechol for esophageal sphincter pressure, 5
BIDA scan in cholecystitis, 72
Bile
  A bile, 86
  B bile, 89
  duct, *see also* Common duct
    exploration in cholangitis, 77
  reflux, and gastric ulcer and gastritis, 40
  salts and common duct stone, 84
Biliary colic in cholecystopathy, acalculous, 89
Biliary excretion scan in cholecystitis, 74, 75
Biliary problems, 71–106
Biliary tract intubation in cholecystitis, 74
Biliary tree, *Bacteroides fragilis* in, 77
Billroth I anastomosis in alkaline reflux gastritis, 35
Billroth II reconstruction, gastrin elevation after, 39
Biopsy
  in adenocarcinoma of gastroesophageal junction, 176

Biopsy *(cont.)*
of breast cyst, 240
in carcinoid, small bowel, 186
in carcinoma
of anus, 195
of breast, 244
of breast, lobular, 249
in fistula, colovesical, 143
in Paget's disease of breast, 250
parathyroid, in hyperparathyroidism, 220
in reflux esophagitis, 4
"Bird's-beak" deformity in sigmoid volvulus, 118
Bladder
colovesical fistula, 143–144
fulguration in colovesical fistula, 143
repair in colovesical fistual, 143
Bleeding, *see* Hemorrhage
Blood flow
coronary, reduction by vasopressin, 56
portal, reduction by vasopressin, 56
"Blow-hole" operation in toxic megacolon, 158
Bone scan in breast carcinoma, 246, 247
in male, 252, 253
Bougie dilatation in reflux esophagitis with stricture, 2
Bouginage in Zenker's diverticulum, 18
Bowel
inflammatory disease, 141–172
large, obstruction, 108–111
obstruction, 107–140
resection in mesenteric vein thrombosis, 115
small
bypass, in carcinoid, 186
bypass, in obstruction, 133
carcinoid, 186–187
carcinoma complicating regional enteritis, 152
gangrene, in mesenteric vein thrombosis, 115
obstruction, *see below*
problems after radiotherapy, 133
resection, in carcinoid, 186
resection, in obstruction, 133
stenting of, 135
small, obstruction, 124–125
large bowel obstruction with, 111
mechanical, partial, 133–134
Bowel *(cont.)*
small, obstruction *(cont.)*
postoperative, 126–129
recurrent, 135–136
Bradycardia after vasopressin, 56
Breast, 239–256
cancer, metastatic, castration in, 252
carcinoma, *see* Carcinoma, breast
cyst
aspiration of, 240
treatment, 240
fibroadenoma, and cystosarcoma phyllodes, 254
Paget's disease of, 250–251
Bronchoconstriction, reflex, and pulmonary embolism, 286
Budd–Chiari syndrome, 62–63
Bypass
aorto-renal, in renovascular hypertension, 232
bowel, small
in carcinoid, 186
in obstruction, partial mechanical, 134
in Crohn's disease, 154

Calcific pancreatitis, Puestow procedure in, 321
Calcified gallbladder and carcinoma, 178
Calcitonin screening, 231
Calcium in hyperparathyroidism, 220
Calves, pneumatic compression, in deep venous thrombosis prevention, 295
Cancer
breast, metastatic, castration in, 252
CEA levels in, 192
colon, CEA levels in, 192
gastrointestinal, 173–199
pulmonary embolism and, 282
thyroid
anaplastic, 228–229
medullary, 230
radiation-induced, 226–227
Carcinoembryonic antigen, role of, 192
Carcinoid
bowel, small, 186–187
ileal, 186
syndrome, 186
Carcinoma
adenocarcinoma, *see* Adenocarcinoma

Carcinoma *(cont.)*
anus, 195–196
excision in, local, 195
bowel, small, complicating regional enteritis, 152
breast
chemotherapy of, adjuvant, 241
inflammatory, 246–248
intraductal noninvasive, 244–245
lobular, 249
in male, 252–253
metastases, treatment of, 242–243
CEA levels in, 192
colon, 191
relationship to polyp, 188
survival in, 193
esophagus, 16–17, 174–175
gallbladder, 178–179
hepatic duct bifurcation, 180–182
pancreas, 183–185
rectosigmoid, 110
rectum, survival in, 193
stomach
after duodenal ulcer surgery, 34
proximal, 177
thoracolaparotomy in, 16
thyroid, 224
Cardiomyotomy, Heller, in achalasia, 14
Castration in metastatic breast cancer, 252
Catheter
and embolization in gastrointestinal hemorrhage, 43
Fogarty, in mesenteric artery embolism, 113
Swan–Ganz, for lung monitoring, 270
CAT scan, abdominal
in aldosteronoma, 206
in Cushing's syndrome, 204
in endocrine neoplasia I syndrome, multiple, 212–213
in endocrine neoplasia IIA, multiple, 230
in insulinoma, 217
in pheochromocytoma, 207
CEA, 192
Cecostomy
in bowel obstruction, large, 109
in volvulus, cecal, 121
Cecum
detorsion in cecal volvulus, 121
Cecum *(cont.)*
volvulus, 120–123
signs and symptoms of, 123
Celestin tube in carcinoma of esophagus, 16, 17
Celiotomy, 9
abdominal distention after, 266
in abdominal trauma, 304
in adenocarcinoma of gastroesophageal junction, 176
in bowel obstruction, large, 109
in bowel obstruction, small, 124
in carcinoma of esophagus, 16
in colonic polyp, malignant, 188
exploratory, in diverticulitis with abscess, 145
in fistula, colovesical, 143
in ileus, gallstone, 131
in intussusception, 137
in mesenteric vein thrombosis, 115
in pancreatitis, acute, 94
in paraesophageal hernia, 10, 13
in varices secondary to splenic vein thrombosis, 64
in volvulus
cecal, 121
sigmoid, 118
Cell(s)
G, 38
hyperplasia, 39
parietal cell, *see* Vagotomy, parietal cell
Cephalosporin in cholangitis, 77
Chemotherapy
in adenocarcinoma of gastroesophageal junction, 176
adjuvant, of breast carcinoma, 241
in carcinoid, small bowel, 186
in carcinoma
of colon, 191
of esophagus, 16, 17
Chenodeoxycholic acid
in cholecystopathy, acalculous, 86
diarrhea after, 80
for gallstones, 79, 80–81
liver abnormalities after, 80
Chest
radiography, *see* Radiography, chest
trauma, blunt, 327–329
Children
hyperinsulinism in, 219

Children *(cont.)*
splenectomy in, prophylactic antibiotics after, 316
Childs plication in recurrent small bowel obstruction, 135
Cholangiography
in carcinoma
of hepatic duct bifurcation, 180
of pancreas, 183, 184
of common duct stones, 82
intraoperative
common duct stone and, retained, 84
in pancreatitis, gallstone, 92, 93
Cholangiopancreatography, endoscopic retrograde (ERCP)
in carcinoma
of hepatic duct bifurcation, 180
of pancreas, 183
in pancreatitis, chronic, 100
Cholangitis, acute ascending, 77
Cholecystectomy
in cholangitis, 77
in cholecystitis, 72, 74
in cholecystopathy, acalculous, 86
in gallstones, 78
in pancreatitis, gallstone, 92
Cholecystitis
acute, treatment, 72–76
gallstones and, 78
Cholecystoenterostomy in carcinoma of pancreas, 183
Cholecystography
after chenodeoxycholic acid for gallstones, 80
in cholecystopathy, acalculous, 86
tube, after cholecystostomy, 76
Cholecystokinin cholecystography in cholecystopathy, acalculous, 86
Cholecystopathy, acalculous, 86–91
Cholecystostomy
in cholangitis, 77
in cholecystitis, 72, 74
in pancreatitis, acute, 94
Choledochoduodenostomy
in carcinoma of pancreas, 183
in common duct stone, 82
Choledochojejunostomy, Roux-en-Y, in common duct stone, 82
Choledochotomy in common duct stone, 82
retained, 84
Cholelithiasis
carcinoma and, of gallbladder, 178
cholecystitis and, 76
Cholescintigraphy in cholecystitis, 72
Cholestyramine in gastritis, alkaline reflux, 35, 37
Cicatrix in chronic duodenal ulcer, 24
Cigarette smoking and CEA levels, 192
Cimetidine
in cholecystopathy, acalculous, 86
in duodenal ulcer, 24
in endocrine neoplasia I syndrome, multiple, 212
in gastritis, alkaline reflux, 35
in reflux esophagitis with stricture, 4
in stress hemorrhage, 43
Cineradiography in esophageal reflux, 4
Circulation, extracorporeal, in pulmonary embolism with shock, 292
Cirrhosis and mesenteric vein thrombosis, 115
Clindamycin in cholangitis, 77
Clostridium tetani, 334
Coagulation, disseminated intravascular, after intractable ascites surgery, 67
Colectomy
abdominal
in colitis, amebic, 163
in colitis, granulomatous, 160
in colitis, ischemic, 165
in megacolon, toxic, 157
subtotal, in colonic obstruction, malignant, 111
Colic, biliary, in cholecystopathy, acalculous, 91
Colitis
acute, fulminant, 163
amebic, 163–164
toxic megacolon and, 158
Crohn's, 152
granulomatous, 160–162
toxic megacolon and, 158
ischemic, 165–167
clinical course of, 166
diagnosis, 166
perforation in, 167
stricture in, 167
radiation, 169
ulcerative, 156
megacolon and, toxic, 158

Colon
cancer, CEA levels in, 192
carcinoma, *see* Carcinoma, colon
gunshot wound of, 312–313
exteriorization of injured segment, 312
interposition
in achalasia, 14
in carcinoma of esophagus, 175
involvement in proctitis, ulcerative, 156
obstruction, malignant, 111
polyp, malignant, 188–189
resection in malignant colonic polyp, 188
tumor, villous, 190
Colonoscopic polypectomy, 188
Colopexy, sigmoid, 199
Colostomy
ileo-ascending, in Crohn's disease, 154
ileotransverse, in volvulus, cecal, 123
sigmoid
in bowel obstruction, large, 109
in colitis, granulomatous, 160
in colitis, ischemic, 165
in diverticulitis, perforated sigmoid, 143
end, in diverticulitis with abscess, 145
in fistula, rectovaginal, radiation-induced, 168
transverse
in bowel obstruction, large, 109
in carcinoma of colon, 191
in colitis, granulomatous, 160
in diverticulitis with abscess, 145
in diverticulitis, perforated sigmoid, 142
in fistula, colovesical, 143
in megacolon, toxic, 157
in volvulus, cecal, 121
in volvulus, sigmoid, 118
Colotomy in malignant colonic polyp, 188
Colovesical fistula, 143–144
Common duct
stone
recurrent, treatment, 82–83
retained, treatment, 84–85
tumors, 182
Coronary blood flow reduction by vasopressin, 56
Corticosteroids
in adrenal crisis, 210
Corticosteroids *(cont.)*
in bowel obstruction, partial mechanical small, 133
intravenous, in colitis
amebic, 163
ischemic, 165
in megacolon, toxic, 157
in proctitis, ulcerative, 156
Cortisol
in Cushing's disease, 202
in Cushing's syndrome, 204
Cortisone enema
in amebic colitis, 163
in ulcerative proctitis, 156
Cricopharyngeal myotomy in Zenker's diverticulum, 18
Crohn's colitis, 152
Crohn's disease
abscess in, 153
carcinoma and, small bowel, 152
complications of, 152–153
fistula in, 153
ileocolic, 154
perforation in, 153
treatment of, 154–155
Cushing's disease
diagnosis, 202
treatment, 202–203
Cushing's syndrome, 204–205
etiology, 202
Cyclophosphamide in breast carcinoma, 241
Cyst
breast, *see* Breast, cyst
pancreatic, in ascites, 98
Cystduodenostomy in pancreatic pseudocyst, 96
Cystgastrostomy in pancreatic pseudocyst, 95
Cystjejunostomy, Roux-en-Y, in pancreatic pseudocyst, 96
Cystography in pneumaturia, 143
Cystosarcoma phyllodes, 254
Cystoscopy
in fistula, colovesical, 143
in pneumaturia, 143

Debridement
in pancreatic abscess, 97

Debridement *(cont.)*
in splenic rupture, 314
of wound in tetanus, 334
Deoxycholic acid in alkaline reflux gastritis, 35
Dextran in deep venous thrombosis prevention, 295
Diabetes mellitus
cholecystitis and, 76
gallstones and, 78–79
glucagonoma syndrome as curable form of, 215
after pancreatectomy, subtotal, 102
Diaphragmatic hernia, incarcerated traumatic, 6–9
Diarrhea
bloody, in intussusception, 137
after chenodeoxycholic acid, 80
after duodenal ulcer surgery, 27
watery, syndrome, 216
Diarrheagenic pancreatic tumor, 216
Diathesis, hemorrhagic, after intractable ascites surgery, 67
Diazepam in tetanus, 335
Dibenzyline in pheochromocytoma, 207
Diuretics in Budd–Chiari syndrome, 62
Diverticulectomy in Zenker's diverticulum, 18
Diverticulitis
with abscess formation, 145–146
sigmoid, perforated, 142
Diverticulum
Meckel's, and intussusception, 137
Zenker's, 18–19
Drainage
in diverticulitis, perforated sigmoid, 142
extraperitoneal, of abscess with diverticulitis, 145
in mesenteric vein thromobsis, 115
in pancreatic abscess, 97
in pancreatic pseudocyst, 95
Penrose, *see* Penrose drainage
sump, *see* Sump drainage
Dumping
symptoms after duodenal ulcer surgery, 27
syndrome after duodenal ulcer surgery, 33
Duodenostomy, tube, 310
Duodenum
drainage in cholecystopathy, acalculous, 86
hematoma, 308–311
lacerations, 310–311
perforation, 310
rupture, 308
ulcer, *see* Ulcer, duodenal
Duval procedure in pancreatitis, chronic, 100
Dysphagia and carcinoma of esophagus, 16

Electrocoagulation, gastroscopic, in gastrointestinal hemorrhage, 43
Electrolyte abnormalities
in duodenal ulcer, chronic, 24
in volvulus, sigmoid, 118
Embolectomy in mesenteric vein thrombosis, 115
Embolism
mesenteric artery, superior, 112–114
clinical picture in, 112
pulmonary
diagnosis, 282–283
pathophysiology, 286
shock and, treatment, 292
suspected, treatment, 287–289
symptoms of, classic, 282
thrombosis and, deep venous, 294
treatment, 284–286
vena caval interruption in, 290–291
thromboembolic disease, 281–299
Embolization
of bleeding retroperitoneal vessels, 324
with catheter in gastrointestinal hemorrhage, 43
Empyema and cholecystitis, 73
Endocrine neoplasia, multiple (MEN)
I, 212–213
IIA, 230
Endocrine surgery, 201–238
Endoscopic pancreatography
in Budd–Chiari syndrome, 62
in pancreatitis, chronic, 100
Endoscopic papillotomy, *see* Papillotomy, endoscopic
Endoscopic retrograde cholangiopancreatography, *see* Cholangiopancreatography,

Endoscopic retrograde *(cont.)*
endoscopic
retrograde
Endoscopy
in alkaline reflux gastritis, 37
injury during, 307
of varices, esophageal and gastric, 64
Enema
barium, *see* Barium enema
cortisone, *see* Cortisone enema
steroid, *see* Steroid enema
Entamoeba histolytica in amebic colitis, 163
Enteritis
radiation, 133, 169
regional, small bowel carcinoma complicating, 152
Enterolithotomy in gallstone ileus, 131
Enterovaginal fistula, 264
Epinephrine and pheochromocytoma, 207
Epithelium, columnar, in reflux esophagitis, 4
ERCP, *see* Cholangiopancreatography, endoscopic retrograde
Esophagectomy
in achalasia, 14
in adenocarcinoma of gastroesophageal junction, 176
in carcinoma of esophagus, 16, 175
Esophagogastrectomy
in achalasia, 14
in adenocarcinoma of stomach, 16
in carcinoma of esophagus, 16
in portal vein thrombosis, 60
Esophagography
in achalasia, 14
in carcinoma of esophagus, 174
in esophageal perforation, 305, 306
in Zenker's diverticulum, 18, 19
Esophagoscopy
in carcinoma of esophagus, 16, 174–175
of reflux esophagitis, 4
with stricture, 4
Esophagus, 1–21
Barrett's, 4
carcinoma, 16–17, 174–175
epithelium of, columnar, 4
laceration due to Sengstaken–Blakemore tube, 54
Esophagus *(cont.)*
manometry of, 4
in Zenker's diverticulum, 18
paraesophageal hernia, *see* Hernia, paraesophageal
perforation, 305–307
due to Sengstaken–Blakemore tube, 54
reflux, 4
resection
in reflux esophagitis with stricture, 4
in Zenker's diverticulum, 18
rupture, 307
sphincter
bethanechol for pressure of, 5
incompetence, test for, 5
metoclopramide for pressure, 5
stricture
after radiotherapy, 17
reflux esophagitis and, 2–5
tracheoesophageal fistual after radiotherapy, 17
varices, *see* Varices, esophageal
Estrogen receptors, 242
Extracorporeal circulation in pulmonary embolism with shock, 292
Extraperitoneal drainage of abscess with diverticulitis, 145
Extremity, *see* Limb

Fasciotomy in anterior compartment syndrome, 332, 333
Fasting in insulinoma, 217
Fecal peritonitis in Crohn's disease, 153
Feeding jejunostomy in acute pancreatitis, 94
Fever
in bowel obstruction, small, 124
in cholangitis, 77
in pancreatitis, 94
in septic shock, 276
in subphrenic abscess, 263
Fibrillation, atrial, and mesenteric artery embolism, superior, 112
Fibrinogen scan, ^{125}I, in deep venous thrombosis, 294, 295
Fibrinolytic drugs, 293
contraindications to, 293

Fibroadenoma of breast and cystosarcoma phyllodes, 254
Fibrosis, lung, after radiotherapy, 17
Fistula
anastomotic dehiscence and, postoperative, 264–265
arteriovenous, and gunshot wound, 331
colovesical, 143–144
in Crohn's disease, 153
enterovaginal, 265
mucous, in colonic obstruction, malignant, 111
pancreatic, after pancreatic pseudocyst treatment, 96
rectovaginal, radiation-induced, 163–169
excision of, 168
rectum, in Crohn's disease, 152
sigmoid mucous, in amebic colitis, 163
tracheoesophageal, after radiotherapy, 17
Flagyl, *see* Metronidazole
Fluid(s)
abnormalities in sigmoid volvulus, 118
intravenous
in cholangitis, 77
in cholecystitis, 72
resuscitation, *see* Resuscitation, fluid
retroperitoneal collections, ultrasound of, 95
Fluoroscopy for T tube insertion in retained common duct stone, 84
Fluorouracil in breast carcinoma, 241
Fogarty catheter in mesenteric artery embolus, 113
Fracture(s)
acetabulum, 325
pelvic, 324–236
Fulguration of rectal villous adenoma, 190
Fundic patch in esophageal perforation, 307
Fundoplication in achalasia, 14

Gallbaldder
calcified, and carcinoma, 178
carcinoma, 178–179
gangrene, and cholecystitis, 73
Gallstone(s)
asymptomatic, treatment, 78–79
in carcinoma
of gallbladder, 178
Gallstone(s) *(cont.)*
in carcinoma *(cont.)*
of hepatic duct bifurcation, 182
chenodeoxycholic acid for, 79, 80–81
cholecystectomy in, 78
cholecystitis and, 78
complications
cholangitis, 77
cholecystitis, 76
diabetes and, 78–79
after duodenal ulcer surgery, 33
ileus, 130–132
diagnosis, 131
pancreatitis, 92–93
ultrasound showing, abdominal, 72
Gangrene
in appendicitis, 148
bowel, small, in mesenteric vein thrombosis, 115
of gallbladder and cholecystitis, 73
of intestine, resection with revascularization, 113
in mesenteric artery embolism, 112
Gastrectomy
partial, tuberculosis after, 33–34
proximal, in adenocarcinoma of gastroesophageal junction, 176
subtotal
in duodenal ulcer, 26
in gastric ulcers, multiple, 44
total
in adenocarcinoma of gastroesophageal junction, 176
in endocrine neoplasia I syndrome, multiple, 213
in gastric ulcers, multiple, 44
Gastric, *see* Stomach
Gastrin
actions of, 38
decrease in, 4
elevated serum, 38–39
release, 38
Gastrinoma, diagnosis, 212
Gastritis
alkaline reflux, 35–37
pathophysiology, 35
atrophic, elevated gastrin in, 38
bile reflux and, 40
stress, 42
ulcer and, stress, 42–43

Gastroenterostomy in duodenal ulcer, 26
Gastroesophageal junction,
adenocarcinoma of, 176–177
Gastrointestinal
Gastrointestinal barium study in bowel obstruction, small, postoperative, 126
Gastrointestinal cancer, 173–199
Gastrointestinal hemorrhage, *see* Hemorrhage, gastrointestinal
Gastrointestinal inhibitory polypeptide and pancreatic diarrheagenic tumor, 216
Gastrointestinal obstruction after pancreatic pseudocyst, 95
Gastrointestinal perforation, and stress ulcer, 40
Gastrointestinal radiography, *see* Radiography, gastrointestinal
Gastropexy in paraesophageal hernia, 13
Gastroscopic electrocoagulation in gastrointestinal hemorrhage, 43
Gastroscopy
in adenocarcinoma of gastroesophageal junction, 176
in alkaline reflux gastritis, 35
Gastrostomy
in pancreatitis, acute, 94
tube, in paraesophageal hernia, 13
G cells, 38
hyperplasia, 39
Gentamicin in cholangitis, 77
GI, *see* entries under Gastrointestinal
GIP and pancreatic diarrheagenic tumor, 216
Globulin, tetanus human, 335
Glucagonoma, 214–215
Goiter
change in, and thyroid carcinoma, 228
diffuse toxic, 222–223
Granulomatous colitis, 160–162
toxic megacolon and, 158
Graves disease, 222–223
Growth in Crohn's disease, 152
G suit in hemorrhage with pelvic fracture, 326
Gunshot wound
arterial injury, 330–331
of colon, 312–313
exteriorization of injured segment, 312
Hartmann procedure
in colitis, ischemic, 165
in diverticulitis with abscess, 145
in sigmoid volvulus, 118
Heart
disease, and pulmonary embolism, 282, 288
failure, congestive, in ascites, intractable, 66
output decrease after vasopressin, 56
Heller cardiomyotomy in achalasia, achalasia, 14
Hemagglutination test, indirect, in amebiasis, 163
Hemotoma
duodenal, 308–311
pancreatitis and, 95
pelvic, 325
Hemicolectomy
in bowel obstruction, small, 111
in colitis, ischemic, 165
in colonic polyp, malignant, 188
in diverticulitis with abscess, 145
in volvulus, cecal, 123
Hemorrhage
complicating pancreatic abscess, 97
of duodenal ulcer, and pulmonary embolism, 290
gastrointestinal
control of, 43
in reflux esophagitis, 4
and stress ulcer, 40
pelvic, 324, 326
into pseudocyst, pancreatic, 95
respiratory distress syndrome after, adult, 270
of retroperitoneal vessels, embolization of, 324
of stomach mucosa, angiography of, 42
streptokinase and, 293
stress, cimetidine in, 43
urokinase and, 293
variceal
balloon tamponade for, 54–55
treatment, 52–53
vasopressin for, 56–57
Hemorrhagic diathesis after intractable ascites surgery, 67
Hemorrhagic pancreatitis, 94

Henle jejunal segment in alkaline reflux gastritis, 35
Heparin, 290
  common duct stone and, 84
  -induced thrombocytopenia, 294
  in pulmonary embolism, 284
  in thrombosis prevention, deep venous, 294
Hepatectomy, total, with transplant in carcinoma of hepatic duct bifurcation, 182
Hepatic, *see* Liver
Hepaticojejunostomy, Roux-en-Y, in carcinoma of hepatic duct bifurcation, 181
Hernia
  diaphragmatic, incarcerated
    prevention of, 6–7
    traumatic, 6–9
  diaphragmatic, symptoms of, 6
  hiatus
    reflux esophagitis and, 4
    with reflux, repair of, 5
  paraesophageal, 10–13
    closure of defect in, 10
    complications of, 10
    symptoms of, 10
5-HIAA in carcinoid, small bowel, 186
Hiatus hernia, *see* Hernia, hiatus
Hill repair for hiatus hernia with reflux, 5
Hormone, parathormone immunoassay, 220
Hospitalization, preoperative, length of, and wound infection, 258
HPP and pancreatic diarrheagenic tumor, 216
Hydration in renal trauma, 323
Hydrogen ion(s)
  back-diffusion of, and stress ulcer, 41
  duodenal ulcer and, 24
Hydrostatic barium enema in cecal volvulus, 121
17-Hydroxycorticosteroids in Cushing's disease, 202
Hyperalimentation, parenteral, in tetanus, 335
Hypercalcemia, differential diagnosis, 220
Hypercoagulable states and mesenteric vein thrombosis, 115
Hypergastrinemia, 213
Hyperinsulinemia, in children, 219
Hyperparathyroidism, primary, 220–221
Hyperplasia
  adrenal
    cortical, 206
    medullary, 230–231
  G cell, 39
Hypersplenism improvement after Warren shunt, 58
Hypertension
  in pheochromocytoma, 207
  portal, 51–69
    mesenteric vein thrombosis and, 115
  renovascular, 232–233
    diagnosis, 232
  after vasopressin, 56
Hypoalbuminemia and wound dehiscence, 260
Hypocalcemia and pancreatitis, 94
Hypochloremic alkalosis in chronic duodenal ulcer, 24
Hypoglycemia, in infant, 219
Hypokalemia
  in aldosteronoma, 206
  in chronic duodenal ulcer, 24
Hypophysectomy in Cushing's disease, 202
Hypotension in pancreatitis, 94
Hypovolemia and phlegmasia cerulea dolens, 297
Hypoxia
  atelectasis and, 268
  pulmonary embolism and, 282

Ileal carcinoid, 186
Ileo-ascending colostomy in Crohn's disease, 154
Ileocolectomy in Crohn's disease, 154
Ileocolic Crohn's disease, 154
Ileocolic resection in Crohn's disease, 154
Ileoproctostomy in colitis
  granulomatous, 160
  ischemic, 165
Ileostomy
  in colitis
    amebic, 163
    granulomatous, 160
  in colonic obstruction, malignant, 111
  in Crohn's disease, 162

Ileostomy *(cont.)*
in megacolon, toxic, 157
in proctitis, ulcerative, 156
in volvulus, cecal, 121
Ileus
adynamic, 127
gallstone, 130–132
diagnosis, 131
postoperative, 266
Iliofemoral thrombectomy in phlegmasia cerulea dolens, 296–297
Immunization of tetanus, 334
Immunoassay, parathormone, 220
Inderal
in Graves disease, 223
in pheochromocytoma, 207
Infant, hypoglycemia in, 219
Infarction, *see* Myocardial infarction
Inflammatory bowel disease, 141–172
Insulinoma, 217–218
diagnosis, 217
Intermittent positive pressure breathing and atelectasis, 268
Intestine, *see also* entries under Gastrointestinal
amebiasis, 163
cancer, 173–199
gangrene, resection with revascularization, 113
ischemia in mesentric artery embolism, 112
tube insertion, in bowel obstruction, small, 124
vasoactive polypeptide, and pancreatic diarrheagenic tumor, 216
Intussusception, 137–138
idiopathic, 137
Iodine-125 fibrinogen scanning of deep venous thrombosis, 294, 295
Iodine-131 therapy of Graves disease, 222
IPPB and atelectasis, 268
Iron
deficiency anemia after duodenal ulcer surgery, 33
therapy in carcinoma of colon, 191
Irradiation, *see* Radiation
Ischemia
intestinal, in mesenteric artery embolism, 112
of stomach and stress ulcer, 40
Ischemic colitis, *see* Colitis, ischemic
Isoperistaltic jejunal segment in alkaline reflux gastritis, 35
Isoproterenol with vasopressin, 57
IVP
drip infusion, in renal trauma, 323
in pneumaturia, 143
in renal trauma, 322, 323

Jaundice
in carcinoma of pancreas, 183
in cholangitis, 77
obstructive, of carcinoma of hepatic duct bifurcation, 182
after pancreatic pseudocyst, 95
postoperative, 275
Jejunostomy, feeding, in acute pancreatitis, 94
Jejunum, interposition in carcinoma of esophagus, 175

Kidney
aorto-renal bypass in renovascular hypertension, 232
artery stenosis, 233
failure
pancreatitis and, 94
postoperative, 274
treatment, 274
hypertension, renovascular, 232–233
diagnosis, 232
trauma, 322–323
complications of, 323

Laparoscopy in bowel obstruction, small, 124
Laparotomy in hernia, diaphragmatic, 6
Lavage, peritoneal
in abdominal trauma, blunt, 303, 312
postoperative, in perforated sigmoid diverticulitis, 142
Legs, *see also* Limb, lower
deep venous thrombosis of, prevention, 294–295
Leukocytosis and small bowel obstruction, 124
Levarterenol in gastrointestinal hemorrhage, 43
LeVeen shunt, *see* Shunt, LeVeen
Lidocaine in pheochromocytoma, 207

Limb, lower
orthopedic procedures, and pulmonary embolism, 282
thrombosis of, 290
Liver
abnormalities after chenodeoxycholic acid, 80
abscess, and cholecystitis, 73
arteriography in Budd–Chiari syndrome, 63
artery ligation after trauma, 317
carcinoid metastatic to, 186
carcinoma of hepatic duct bifurcation, 180–182
excision, wedge, in gallbladder carcinoma, 178
failure
in Budd–Chiari syndrome, 62
postoperative, 275
after Warren shunt, 59
lobectomy, *see* Lobectomy, hepatic
metastases, *see* Metastases, liver
scan, *see* Scanning, liver
–spleen scan in glucagonoma, 214
transplant in carcinoma of hepatic duct bifurcation, 181
trauma, 317–319
tumor in small bowel carcinoid, 186
vein thrombosis in Budd–Chiari syndrome, 62
Lobectomy, hepatic
in carcinoid, small bowel, 186
in carcinoma
of hepatic duct bifurcation, 181
of gallbladder, 178
Lobectomy, thyroid, for nodule, 224
L-Pam in breast carcinoma, 241
L-phenylalanine mustard in breast carcinoma, 241
Lung, *see also* entries under Pulmonary
failure, prolonged, and ARDS, 270
fibrosis after radiotherapy, 17
monitoring with Swan–Ganz catheter, 270
Lymph node(s)
in breast carcinoma, inflammatory, 248
metastases and carcinoma of anus, 195

Mammography, 224
Manometry of esophagus, 4
in Zenker's diverticulum, 18
Mastectomy
in breast carcinoma
intraductal noninvasive, 244
lobular, 249
in male, 252
in cystosarcoma phyllodes, 254
in Paget's disease of breast, 250
Meckel's diverticulum and intussusception, 137
Megacolon, toxic, 157–159
MEN, *see* Endocrine, neoplasia, multiple
Mental disturbance and insulinoma, 217
Mesenteric, superior
artery
embolism, 112–114
embolism, clinical picture in, 112
identification with Fogarty catheter, 113
thrombosis, 112
thrombosis, surgery of, 113–114
vein thrombosis, 115
Mesocaval shunt, *see* Shunt, mesocaval
Metanephrine and pheochromocytoma, 207
Metastases
in breast cancer, castration in, 252
of breast carcinoma, treatment, 242–243
of carcinoid of small bowel, to liver, 186
liver
CEA levels in, 192
excision of, 193
glucagonoma and, 214
treatment, 193–194
lymph node, and carcinoma of anus, 195
streptozotocin for, 215, 216
Methotrexate in breast carcinoma, 241
Metoclopramide
in bowel obstruction, small, postoperative, 127
effect on esophageal sphincter pressure, 5
Metronidazole in amebic colitis, 163
Monitoring of lung with Swan–Ganz catheter, 270
Morbidity of total thyroidectomy, 227
Mortality rate
in carcinoma of esophagus, 175
in cholangitis, 77
of cholecystectomy in gallstones, 78
in cholecystitis, 73
in hemorrhage into pancreatic pseudocyst, 95

Mortality rate *(cont.)*
in megacolon surgery, toxic, 158
in mesenteric artery embolism, superior, 112
operative, in carcinoma of colon, 191
in pancreatic abscess, 97
in pancreatitis
acute, 94
gallstone, 93
with Sengstaken–Blakemore tube, 54
in thyroid carcinoma, anaplastic, 228
Myeloproliferative disorders and splenectomy, 115
Myocardial infarction
cholecystitis and, 76
mesenteric artery embolism and, superior, 112
precipitated by vasopressin, 56
Myotomy, cricopharyngeal, in Zenker's diverticulum, 18

Nasogastric decompression and suction in pancreatitis, acute, 94
Nasogastric suction
in bowel obstruction, small, mechanical, partial, 133
in bowel obstruction, small, recurrent, 135
in cholecystitis, 74
in duodenal hematoma, 310
in mesenteric vein thrombosis, 115
Nasogastric tube
in bowel obstruction, small, 124
in bowel obstruction, small, postoperative, 127
in diverticulitis with abscess, 145
Necrosis, pancreatic, and pancreatitis, 94
Nelson's syndrome, 202
Neoplasia, *see* Tumors
Nesidioblastosis, 219
Nipple in Paget's disease, 250
Nisson repair for hiatus hernia with reflux, 5
Nobel plication in recurrent small bowel obstruction, 135
Norepinephrine and pheochromocytoma, 207
Normetanephrine and pheochromocytoma, 207

Nutrition, parenteral
in anastomotic dehiscence with fistula, 264
in pancreatic abscess, 97
in pancreatic ascites, 98

Oliguria and phlegmasia cerulea dolens, 297
Omental patch for perforated duodenal ulcer, 30
Omphalitis and portal vein thrombosis, 60
Oophorectomy in breast carcinoma
inflammatory, 246
metastatic, 242
o,p-DDD in Cushing's disease, 202
Orchiectomy in breast carcinoma in male, 252

Paget's disease of breast, 250–251
Pain
in cholangitis, 77
in duodenal hematoma, 309
in intussusception, 137
in mesenteric artery embolism, superior, 112
L-Pam in breast carcinoma, 241
Pancreas
abscess, 97
pancreatitis and, 95
recurrent, 97
signs and symptoms of, 97
ascites, 98–99
diagnosis, 98
pancreatitis and, 98
carcinoma, 183–185
cyst, in ascites, 98
fistula, after pseudocyst treatment, 96
necrosis, and pancreatitis, 94
polypeptide, human, and pancreatic diarrheagenic tumor, 216
problems, 71–106
pseudocyst, 95–96
complications of, 95
rupture of, 95
scan in Budd–Chiari syndrome, 62
trauma, 320–321
tumor, diarrheagenic, 216
Pancreatectomy
in carcinoma of pancreas, 183
subtotal
in ascites, pancreatic, 98

Pancreatectomy *(cont.)*
subtotal *(cont.)*
in nesidioblastosis, 219
in pancreatitis, chronic, 101
Pancreaticocystjejunostomy, Roux-en-Y
in ascites, pancreatic, 98
in pancreatic pseudocyst, 95
Pancreaticojejunostomy
distal, in pancreatitis, chronic, 101
longitudinal
in ascites, pancreatic, 98
in pancreatitis, calcific, 321
in pancreatitis, chronic, 101
Roux-en-Y, after pancreatic trauma, 320
Pancreaticolithiasis, 102
Pancreatitis
acute, prognostic factors, 94
alcoholic, 95, 98
ascites and, 98
calcific, Puestow procedure in, 321
chronic, 100–102
gallstone, 92–93
hemorrhagic, 94
"idiopathic," and cholecystopathy, acalculous, 91
mesenteric artery embolism confused with, 112
pancreatic abscess complicating, 97
splenic vein thrombosis after, 64
Pancreatoduodenentomy
in bile duct tumors, 182
in carcinoma of pancreas, 183
Pancreatography, endoscopic
in Budd–Chiari syndrome, 62
in pancreatitis, chronic, 100
Pancytopenia and portal vein thrombosis, 60
Papillotomy, endoscopic
in cholecystopathy, acalculous, 86
in common duct stone, 82
retained, 84
Paracentesis in pancreatic ascites, 98
Paraesophageal, *see* Hernia, paraesophageal
Parathormone immunoassay, 220
Parathyroid
adenoma, 220, 221
biopsy in hyperparathyroidism, 220
Parathyroidectomy
in multiple endocrine neoplasia I syndrome, 212
Parathyroidectomy *(cont.)*
subtotal, in hyperparathyroidism, 220
Parenteral hyperalimentation in tetanus, 335
Parenteral nutrition, *see* Nutrition, parenteral
Parietal cell, *see* Vagotomy, parietal cell
Patch, fundic, in esophageal perforation, 307
PEEP in respiratory distress syndrome, adult, 271, 272–273
Pelvic fracture, 324–326
Pelvic hematoma, 325
Pelvic hemorrhage, 324–326
Pelvic radiography in hemorrhage and fracture, 324
Penicillin in tetanus, 334
Penrose drainage
in pancreatic pseudocyst, 95
in pancreatitis, acute, 94
Peptic ulcer
disease, 23–49
recurrent, 33
Pericardiocentesis, 6
Peritoneal, *see* Lavage, peritoneal
Peritoneo-jugular shunt, *see* Shunt, peritoneo-jugular
Peritonitis
in diverticulitis, perforated sigmoid, 142
fecal, and Crohn's disease, 153
volvulus and, sigmoid, 118
Pernicious anemia, elevated gastrin in, 38
PGE and pancreatic diarrheagenic tumor, 216
Phenoxybenzamine in pheochromocytoma, 207
Phentolamine in pheochromocytoma, 207
L-Phenylalanine mustard in breast carcinoma, 241
Pheochromocytoma, 207–209, 231
Phlegmasia cerulea dolens, 296–297
Phlegmon
appendiceal, 150–151
pancreatitis and, 95
Phosphorus in hyperparathyroidism, 220
PIPIDA scan in cholecystitis, 72
Pitressin, *see* Vasopressin
Pituitary radiotherapy in Cushing's disease, 202
Plaques, atherosclerotic, and mesenteric artery embolism, superior, 112

Plastic ringed wound protectors and
wound infection, 258
Pleural effusion
in ascites, pancreatic, 98
esophageal perforation and, 307
Plication in recurrent small bowel
obstruction, 135
Pneumatic compression of calves in deep
venous thrombosis prevention, 295
Pneumatic dilatation in achalasia, 14
Pneumaturia
diagnosis, 143
evaluation of, 143
Pneumococcus in postsplenectomy sepsis,
314–315
Pneumomediastinum, 307
Pneumothorax, 273
PO_2 and pulmonary embolism, 282–283
Polyp, colon, malignant, 188–189
Polypectomy, colonoscopic, 188
Portacaval, *see* Shunt, portacaval
Portal blood flow, vasopressin reducing,
56
Portal hypertension, 51–69
mesenteric vein thrombosis and, 115
Portal node excision in carcinoma of
gallbladder, 178
Portal vein
pressure, vasopressin reducing, 56
thrombosis, 60–61
Porta-systemic shunt in variceal
hemorrhage, 54
Positive end expiratory pressure in
respiratory distress syndrome,
adult, 271, 272–273
Postoperative complications, 257–280
Postphlebitic syndrome, 297
Potassium and duodenal ulcer, 24
Prednisone in Crohn's disease, 154
Proctitis
radiation, 196
ulcerative, 156
complications, 156
Proctocolectomy
in colitis
amebic, 163
granulomatous, 160
ischemic, 165
in megacolon, toxic, 157
Proctoscopy in bowel obstruction, large,
108
Propranolol
in Graves disease, 223
in pheochromocytoma, 207
Propylthiouracil in Graves disease, 222
Prostaglandin E and pancreatic
diarrheagenic tumor, 216
Pseudocyst, *see* Pancreas, pseudocyst
Puestow procedure
in ascites, pancreatic, 98
in pancreatitis
calcific, 321
chronic, 101
Pulmonary angiography in suspected
embolis, 282, 287, 288
Pulmonary embolectomy in embolism with
shock, 292
Pulmonary embolism, *see* Embolism,
pulmonary
Pulmonary scan, in embolism, 283
suspected, 289
Pyelography, intravenous, *see* IVP
Pyloroplasty
in duodenal ulcer, 26
perforated, 30
in gastric ulcers, multiple, 44

Radiation, *see also* Radiography;
Radiotherapy
colitis, 169
enteritis, 133, 169
–induced
rectovaginal fistula, 168–169
rectovaginal fistula, excision of, 168
thyroid cancer, 226–227
proctitis, 169
Radiography
abdominal
in abscess, appendiceal, 147–148
in abscess, subphrenic, 261, 262
in bowel obstruction, large, 108
in bowel obstruction, small,
postoperative, 126
in duodenal hematoma, 309
in ileus, gallstone, 130
in megacolon, toxic, 157
in pancreatitis, chronic, 100
in volvulus, cecal, 120
in volvulus, sigmoid, 116
in abdominal trauma, blunt, 302
chest
in abscess, subphrenic, 261

Radiography *(cont.)*
chest *(cont.)*
in atelectasis, 267
in chest trauma, blunt, 327
in esophageal perforation, 305
in hernia, diaphragmatic, 6
in pulmonary embolism, 284
in pulmonary embolism, suspected, 287
in respiratory distress syndrome, adult, 272
gastrointestinal
in adenocarcinoma of gastroesophageal junction, 176
in cholecystopathy, acalculous, 86
of duodenal hematoma, 308
in esophageal reflux, 4
in paraesophageal hernia, 10
in reflux esophagitis with stricture, 4
pelvic, in hemorrhage and fracture, 324
Radioimmunoassay of CEA, 192
Radioiodine in Graves disease, 222
Radiotherapy
in adenocarcinoma of gastroesophageal junction, 176
Bowel problems after, small, 133
of cancer, thyroid, anaplastic, 228
in carcinoma
of breast, inflammatory, 246, 248
of breast, noninvasive intraductal, 244–245
of colon, 191
of esophagus, 16–17, 175
of gallbladder, 178
of hepatic duct bifurcation, 181
pituitary, in Cushing's disease, 202
Rectosigmoid carcinoma, 110
Rectovaginal fistula, radiation-induced, 168–169
excision of, 168
Rectum
abscess in Crohn's disease, 152
adenocarcinoma, differentiated from carcinoma of anus, 195
adenoma, *see* Adenoma, rectal
carcinoma, survival in, 193
extraperitoneal, injuries of, 312–313
fistula in Crohn's disease, 152
oversewing of, in diverticulitis with abscess, 145
Rectum *(cont.)*
oversewing of *(cont.)*
perforated sigmoid, 142
stump, oversewing
in colitis, granulomatous, 160
in toxic megacolon, 157
Reflex, bronchoconstriction, and pulmonary embolism, 286
Reflux
bile, and gastric ulcer and gastritis, 40
esophagitis with stricture, 2–5
esophagus, 4
gastritis, alkaline, 35–37
pathophysiology, 35
hernia and, hiatus, repair of, 5
Regitine in pheochromocytoma, 207
Renal, *see* Kidney
Renin, 232
in aldosteronoma, 206
Renovascular hypertension, 232–233
diagnosis, 232
Respiratory distress syndrome, adult (ARDS), 270–273
diagnosis, 270
evolution of, important factor in, 270
PEEP and, 272–273
treatment, 270–271
Respiratory failure and pancreatitis, 94
Resuscitation
in bowel obstruction, large, 110
in cholecystitis, 72
fluid
in esophageal injuries, 307
in gallstone pancreatitis, 92
mesenteric vein thrombosis, 115
in mesenteric artery embolism, superior, 112
in variceal hemorrhage, 52
volume
in bowel obstruction, small, 124
in ileus, gallstone, 131
in megacolon, toxic, 158
in volvulus, cecal, 123
Retroperitoneal
fluid collections, ultrasound of, 95
vessels, bleeding, embolization of, 324
Revascularization in gangrenous intestine resection, 113
Riopan in stress gastritis, 42

Roux-en-Y
choledochojejunostomy in common duct stone, 82
cystjejunostomy in pancreatic pseudocyst, 96
diversion in alkaline reflux gastritis,35
hepaticojejunostomy in carcinoma of hepatic duct bifurcation, 181
pancreaticocystjejunostomy, *see* Pancreaticocystjejunostomy, Roux-en-Y
pancreaticojejunostomy, after pancreatic trauma, 320
Rupture
aorta, 327, 329
duodenum, 308
esophagus, 307
of pancreatic cyst in pancreatic ascites, 98
of pancreatic pseudocyst, 95
spleen, 314–316
stomach, 310

Salt(s)
bile, and common duct stone, 84
restriction in Budd–Chiari syndrome, 62
Scanning
BIDA, in cholecystitis, 72
biliary exretion, in cholecystitis, 74, 75
bone, in breast carcinoma, 246, 247
in male, 252, 253
CAT, *see* CAT scan
fibrinogen, ^{125}I, in deep venous thrombosis, 294, 295
liver
in Budd–Chiari syndrome, 62
in carcinoid, small bowel, 186
liver–spleen, in glucagonoma, 214
pancreas, in Budd–Chiari syndrome, 62
PIPIDA, in cholecystitis, 72
pulmonary, in embolism, 283
suspected, 289
Sengstaken–Blakemore tube,54
complications of, 54–55
mortality rate with, 54
in variceal hemorrhage, 52
Sepsis
liver failure due to, 275
pancreatitis and, 94
Sepsis *(cont.)*
respiratory distress syndrome and, adult, 270
after splenectomy, 314
Septic shock, postoperative, 276–277
Septra in colovesical fistula, 143
Serotonin and carcinoids, 186
Sexual maturation, delayed onset in Crohn's disease, 152
Shock
pulmonary embolism and, 290
treatment, 292
septic, postoperative, 276–277
Shunt
LeVeen
in ascites, intractable, 66
in ascites, pancreatic, 98
in Budd–Chiari syndrome, 62
mesocaval
in splenic vein thrombosis with varices, 64
in variceal hemorrhage, 52
peritoneo-jugular, in ascites, intractable, 66
portacaval
end-to-side, in ascites, intractable, 66
end-to-side, in Budd–Chiari syndrome, 62
end-to-side, in variceal hemorrhage, 52
in portal vein thrombosis, 60
side-to-side, in ascites, intractable, 66
side-to-side, in Budd–Chiari syndrome, 62
side-to-side, in variceal hemorrhage, 52
in splenic vein thrombosis with varices, 64
porta-systemic, in variceal hemorrhage, 54
splenorenal
distal, *see below*
in portal vein thrombosis, 60
in splenic vein thrombosis with varices, 64
splenorenal, distal, 58–59
in ascites, intractable, 66
in splenic vein thrombosis with varices, 64
in variceal hemorrhage, 52

Shunt *(cont.)*
splenorenal *(cont.)*
varices disappearing after, 58
Warren, 58–59
in variceal hemorrhage, 53
varices disappearing after, 58
Sigmoid colopexy, 119
Sigmoid colostomy, *see* Colostomy, sigmoid
Sigmoid detorsion in volvulus, sigmoid, 118
Sigmoid diverticulitis, perforated, 142
Sigmoid fistula, mucous, in amebic colitis, 163
Sigmoid rectosigmoid carcinoma, 110
Sigmoid resection
in bowel obstruction, large, 109
in diverticulitis, perforated sigmoid, 142
in fistula, colovesical, 143
in volvulus, sigmoid, 118
Sigmoid volvulus, 116–119
recurrence, 118–119
Sigmoidoscopy
in colonic polyp, malignant, 188
in volvulus, sigmoid, 118
Sinography 264, 265
Sipple's syndrome, 230–231
Smoking and CEA levels, 192
Sphincter, *see* Esophagus, sphincter
Sphincteroplasty
in common duct stone, 82
in pancreatitis, chronic, 101
Sphincterotomy, in cholecystopathy, acalculous, 86
Splanchnic block in pancreatitis, chronic, 101
Spleen
–liver scan in glucagonoma, 214
rupture, 314–316
trauma, 314
vein thrombosis, varices secondary to, 64–65
Splenectomy
mesenteric occlusion after, 115
myeloproliferative disorders and, 115
in portal vein thrombosis, 60
sepsis after, 314
in splenic vein thrombosis with varices, 64
Splenomegaly and portal vein thrombosis, 60
Splenorenal, *see* Shunt, splenorenal
Splenosis, 316
Stab wound of abdomen, 304
Steatorrhea after pancreatectomy, subtotal, 102
Stenosis of renal artery, 233
Stent insertion in carcinoma of esophagus, 175
Stenting of small bowel, 135
Steroid enema
in colitis, ischemic, 165
in fistula, rectovaginal, radiation-induced, 168
Stomach, *see also* entries under Gastrointestinal
adenocarcinoma, 16
atony, postvagotomy, 127
cancer, 173–199
carcinoma, *see* Carcinoma, stomach
decompression in postoperative ileus, 266
interposition in carcinoma of esophagus, 175
ischemia, and stress ulcer, 40
mucosa, hemorrhage of, angiography of, 42
mucus, and stress ulcer, 40
outlet obstruction and duodenal ulcer, 24
resection, anemia after, 33
rupture, 310
ulcer(s)
bile reflux and, 40
multiple, 44–45
varices, endoscopy of, 64
Stone(s)
common duct, *see* Common duct, stone
gallstones, *see* Gallstones
Streptokinase, 293
in Budd–Chiari syndrome, 63
Streptozotocin for metastases, 215, 216
Stress
gastritis, 42
hemorrhage, cimetidine in, 43
ulcer, *see* Ulcer, stress
Subphrenic, *see* Abscess, subphrenic
Suit, G, in pelvic fracture with hemorrhage, 326

Sulfa
in proctitis, ulcerative, 156
–trimethoprim in colovesical fistula, 143
Sump drainage
in pancreatic pseudocyst, 95
in pancreatitis, acute, 94
Suture materials and wound dehiscence, 260
Swan–Ganz catheter for lung monitoring, 270

Tachycardia
bowel obstruction and, small, 124
pancreatitis and, 94
Tamponade, *see* Balloon tamponade
Temperature in mesenteric artery embolism, 112
Tetanospasmin, 334
Tetanus, 334–335
antitoxin, 334
diagnosis, 334
human globulin, 335
immunization for, 334
incubation period of, 334
prevention in, 334–335
Thoracolaparotomy
in carcinoma of stomach, 16
in diaphragmatic hernia, 6
Thoracostomy
in diaphragmatic hernia, 6
in respiratory distress syndrome, adult, 273
Thoracotomy
in adenocarcinoma of gastroesophageal junction, 176
in carcinoma of esophagus, 16
in chest trauma, blunt, 327
contrasted with celiotomy, 9
in esophageal perforation, 305, 307
in hernia
diaphragmatic, 6
paraseophageal, 10
Thorax, *see* Chest
Thrombectomy, iliofemoral, in phlegmasia cerulea dolens, 296–297
Thrombocytopenia, heparin-induced, 294
Thrombocytosis after splenectomy, 115
Thromboembolic disease, 281–299
Thrombolytic therapy, 293
Thrombosis
hepatic vein, in Budd–Chiari syndrome, 62
iliofemoral, venography of, 296
lower extremity, 290
mesenteric artery, superior, 112
surgery of, 113–114
mesenteric vein, superior, 115
portal vein, 60–61
splenic vein, varices secondary to, 64–65
venous, 282
deep, prevention, in leg, 294–295
deep, thrombolytic therapy of, 293
Thyroid
cancer, *see* Cancer, thyroid
carcinoma, 224
lobectomy for nodule, 224
nodule, 224–225
age and, 224
sex and, 224
Thyroidectomy
subtotal, in Graves disease, 222
total
in Graves disease, 222
morbidity of, 227
in thyroid cancer, radiation-induced, 226
Thyrotoxicosis, 223
Tolbutamide test in insulinoma, 217
Tomography, computed axial, *see* CAT scan
Toxic
goiter, diffuse, 222–223
megacolon, 157–159
Tracheoesophageal fistula after radiotherapy, 17
Tracheostomy in tetanus, 334
Transfusion
massive, respiratory distress syndrome after, adult, 270
in pelvic hemorrhage, 325
in toxic megacolon, 158
Transplantation of liver, in carcinoma of hepatic duct bifurcation, 181
Trauma, 301–340
abdomen, blunt, 302–303
kidney, 322–323
complications of, 323

Trauma *(cont.)*
liver, 317–319
pancreas, 320–321
complications of, 320–321
respiratory distress syndrome after, adult, 270
spleen, 314
thorax, blunt, 327–329
Traumatic diaphragmatic hernia, incarcerated, 6–9
Trimethoprim–sulfa in colovesical fistula, 143
T tube
in carcinoma of pancreas, 183
in common duct stone, 82
after liver trauma, 317
removal of retained common duct stone, 84
Tube
Baker, 135, 136
cholecystography after cholecystostomy, 76
duodenostomy, 310
intestinal, *see* Intestine, tube
nasogastric, *see* Nasogastric tube
Sengstaken–Blakemore, *see* Sengstaken–Blakemore tube
Tuberculosis after partial gastrectomy, 33–34
Tumors
bile duct, common, 182
colon, villous, 190
endocrine neoplasia, *see* Endocrine neoplasia
liver, in small bowel carcinoid, 186
pancreatic diarrheagenic, 216

Ulcer
in breast carcinoma, inflammatory, 248
duodenal
bleeding, and pulmonary embolism, 290
chronic, and cicatrix, 24
complications of 24–25
intractable, 27
intractable, parietal cell vagotomy in, 28
perforated, 30–32
perforated, antibiotics with fluids in, 24–25
Ulcer *(cont.)*
duodenal *(cont.)*
perforated, nasogastric suction in, 24–25
surgery, choice of, and lowest incidence of recurrence, 26–27
surgery, complications of, 33–34
gastric
bile reflux and, 40
multiple ulcers, 44–45
peptic
disease, 23–49
recurrent, 33
stress, 40–45
formation, factors contributing to, 40
gastritis and, 42–43
multiple gastric ulcers and, 44–45
pathogenesis, 40
pathophysiology of, 40
Ulcerative colitis, 156
megacolon and, toxic, 158
Ulcerative proctitis, 156
complications, 156
Ultrasound
abdominal
in cholecystitis, 74
in cholecystopathy, acalculous, 86
of common duct stone, 82
of gallstones, 72, 92
of pancreatic cyst, 98
of pancreatic pseudocyst, 95
of retroperitoneal fluid collections, 95
in carcinoma of pancreas, 183
Urecholine in bowel obstruction, small, postoperative, 127
Urokinase, 293

Vagina
enterovaginal fistula, 264
rectovaginal fistula, radiation–induced, 168–169
Vagotomy
in duodenal ulcer, 26
perforated, 30
gastric atony after, 127
in gastric ulcers, multiple, 44
in intussusception, 137
parietal cell, 28–29, 30
in duodenal ulcer, 26
in gastric ulcers, multiple, 44

Valium in tetanus, 335
Varices
disappearing after Warren shunt, 58
esophageal
in Budd–Chiari syndrome, 62
endoscopy of, 64
portal vein obstruction and, 60
gastric, endoscopy of, 64
hemorrhage, *see* Hemorrhage, variceal
ligation
in portal vein thrombosis, 60
transthoracic, 52
secondary to splenic vein thrombosis, 64–65
Vasocative intestinal polypeptide and pancreatic diarrheagenic tumor, 216
Vasopressin (Pitressin)
bolus administration, 56
in gastritis, stress, 42
as infusion, 56
in portal vein thrombosis, 60
for variceal hemorrhage, 52, 56–57
Vein
arteriovenous fistula and gunshot wound, 331
hepatic, thrombosis, in Budd–Chiari syndrome, 62
mesenteric, superior, thrombosis, 115
portal, *see* Portal vein
repair in gunshot wound, 330
splenic, thrombosis, varices secondary to, 64–65
thrombosis, *see* Thrombosis, venous
Vena cava
interruption, 290–291
ligation, 290–291
occlusion in Budd–Chiari syndrome, 62
Vena cavography in Budd–Chiari syndrome, 62
Venography of iliofemoral thrombosis, 296
Ventilatory support, continuous, in respiratory distress syndrome, adult, 273
Vessels
renal, hypertension, 232–233
diagnosis, 232
retroperitoneal, bleeding, embolization of, 324
Villous rectal adenoma, *see* Adenoma, rectal villous
Villous tumors of colon, 190
VIP and pancreatic diarrheagenic tumor, 216
Vitamin K supplements in toxic megacolon, 158
Volume, *see* Resuscitation, volume
Volvulus
cecal, 120–123
signs and symptoms, 123
sigmoid, 116–119
recurrence, 118–119
Vomiting
in duodenal hematoma, 309
in intussusception, 137
in mesenteric artery embolism, 112

Warfarin, 294–295
Warren shunt, 58–59
in variceal hemorrhage, 53
varices disappearing after, 58
Watery diarrhea syndrome, 216
Weight
in Crohn's disease, 152
loss in reflux esophagitis with stricture, 4
Whipple procedure
in bile duct tumors, 182
in carcinoma of pancreas, 183
Wound
debridement in tetanus, 334
gunshot, *see* Gunshot wound
postoperative
dehiscence, 260
infection, antibiotics for, prophylactic, 259
infection, etiology, 258
protectors, plastic ringed, and infection, 258
stab, of abdomen, 304

X ray, *see* Radiography
Xylocaine in pheochromocytoma, 207

Zenker's diverticulum, 18–19
pulsion, 18
Zollinger–Ellison syndrome, 212
gastrin in, 39

Batch number: 10620163

Printed by Printforce, the Netherlands